Surgery for
Cancer of the Larynx
and
Related Structures

Surgery for Cancer of the Larynx and Related Structures

Second Edition

Carl E. Silver, MD
Professor of Surgery
Professor of Otolaryngology
Albert Einstein College of Medicine
Chief, Head and Neck Surgery
Montefiore Medical Center
Bronx, New York

Alfio Ferlito, MD
Professor of Otolaryngology
University of Padua School of Medicine
Padua, Italy

Illustrator
Hugh Thomas

W.B. SAUNDERS COMPANY
A Division of Harcourt Brace & Company
Philadelphia   London   Toronto   Montreal   Sydney   Tokyo

W.B. SAUNDERS COMPANY
A Division of Harcourt Brace & Company

The Curtis Center
Independence Square West
Philadelphia, Pennsylvania 19106

Library of Congress Cataloging-in-Publication Data

Silver, Carl E.

Surgery for cancer of the larynx and related structures/
Carl E. Silver, Alfio Ferlito.—2nd ed.

p. cm.

ISBN 0–7216–5266–2

1. Larynx—Cancer—Surgery.   2. Hypopharynx—Cancer—Surgery.
3. Esophagus—Cancer—Surgery.   I. Ferlito, Alfio.   II. Title.
[DNLM: 1. Laryngeal Neoplasms—Surgery.   WV 520 S587s 1966]

RF516.S54 1996   616.99′422059—dc20

DNLM/DLC   95–17699

Surgery for Cancer of the Larynx and Related Structures   ISBN 0–7216–5266–2

Printed in the United States of America.

Last digit is the print number: 9   8   7   6   5   4   3   2   1

This book is dedicated to the memory of my parents,
Sylvia J. and Samuel A. Silver

CES

This book is dedicated to my wife,
Gianna, and our sons, Mario and Giuseppe

AF

Contributors

James Z. Cinberg, MD
Clinical Assistant Professor, Seton Hall University School of Graduate Medical Education, South Orange, New Jersey; Active Attending Otolaryngologist, Saint Barnabas Medical Center, Elizabeth General Medical Center, St. Elizabeth Hospital, Elizabeth, New Jersey
Laser Surgery for Cancer of the Larynx

Alfio Ferlito, MD
Professor of Otolaryngology, University of Padua School of Medicine, Padua, Italy
Squamous Cell Carcinoma and Its Precursors; Unusual Malignant Neoplasms; Total Laryngectomy; Neck Dissection; Prosthetic Voice Rehabilitation

Duncan R. Ingrams, MA, FRCS
Research Fellow, Department of Otolaryngology–Head and Neck Surgery, Tufts University School of Medicine and New England Medical Center, Boston, Massachusetts
Laser Surgery for Cancer of the Larynx

Roger J. Levin, MD
Assistant Professor of Surgery, Division of Otolaryngology–Head and Neck Surgery, Pennsylvania State University College of Medicine; Attending Otolaryngologist, The Milton S. Hershey Medical Center, Hershey, Pennsylvania
The Hypopharynx; Reconstruction of the Cervical Esophagus

Idel I. Moisa, MD
Assistant Clinical Professor, Department of Otolaryngology, Albert Einstein College of Medicine, Bronx, New York; Senior Assistant Attending, Department of Surgery, Section of Otolaryngology, North Shore Hospital, Manhasset, New York
Near-Total Laryngectomy

Gianfranco Recher, MD*
Formerly, Assistant-in-Chief, Division of Otolaryngology, San Bartolo Hospital, Vicenza, Italy
Prosthetic Voice Rehabilitation

---

*Deceased

Hector Rodriguez, MD

Assistant Professor of Otolaryngology, Columbia University College of Physicians and Surgeons; Attending Physician, Columbia-Presbyterian Medical Center, New York, New York
Tracheal Stomal Stenosis and Recurrence

Stanley M. Shapshay, MD

Professor and Chairman, Department of Otolaryngology–Head and Neck Surgery, Tufts University School of Medicine; Otolaryngologist-in-Chief, New England Medical Center, Boston, Massachusetts
Laser Surgery for Cancer of the Larynx

Carl E. Silver, MD

Professor of Surgery and Professor of Otolaryngology, Albert Einstein College of Medicine; Chief, Head and Neck Surgery, Montefiore Medical Center, Bronx, New York
Historical Aspects; Surgical Anatomy; Squamous Cell Carcinoma and Its Precursors; Conservation Surgery for Glottic Cancer; Conservation Surgery for Supraglottic Cancer; Total Laryngectomy; Near-Total Laryngectomy; The Hypopharynx; Reconstruction of the Cervical Esophagus; Neck Dissection; Tracheal Stomal Stenosis and Recurrence

Preface

The first edition of *Surgery for Cancer of the Larynx and Related Structures,* published in 1981, assembled for the first time in a single book the entire current surgical armamentarium for treatment of malignant disease of the larynx, hypopharynx, and cervical esophagus. The focus of the book was on detailed, step-by-step illustrations of operative procedures, some of which many surgeons may have had little opportunity to learn during residency training or in a subsequent practice. In particular, the various "conservation" operations were emerging from a period in which they could be performed by only a handful of pioneers into an era of widespread, although not universal, acceptance.

During the intervening 15 years, many of the most striking advances in the field of laryngeal oncology have been in the areas of cellular biology, multimodality therapy, and microvascular reconstruction. The functional extirpative techniques that represented the frontier of knowledge in 1981 are now commonplace. Nevertheless, the surgical armamentarium has been greatly expanded, and in this second edition we have attempted to depict the current status of oncologic surgery of the larynx and its adnexae. Procedures that have become obsolete have been deleted from the text, and many newer procedures are demonstrated. These include extended conservation operations for glottic and supraglottic carcinoma, the supracricoid laryngectomy (more popular in Europe than in the United States), subtotal laryngectomy with dynamic phonatory shunt, the use of revascularized "free" flaps for reconstruction, and various methods of primary and secondary prosthetic voice restoration. We have also included a discussion of recent concepts and procedures for management of metastatic disease in the cervical lymph nodes, as these concepts and procedures have changed considerably during the past decade and a half.

The distinctive illustrations of Hugh Thomas proved effective in demonstrating the surgical anatomy and methodology of the complex procedures described in the first edition as well as in other previous collaborations. We have been fortunate in retaining Mr. Thomas to illustrate the current edition. Residents and practicing surgeons found the presentation of the first edition to be useful and instructive. It is our hope that this revision will serve to update and replace its predecessor in an effective manner.

We would like to acknowledge the contributions of many individuals who assisted us with this project. We are grateful to our contributors for helping us to fill in the gaps in our knowledge and experience. The generous support of the Laryngeal Cancer Association has been very helpful in the production of this work.

CARL E. SILVER
ALFIO FERLITO

Contents

*Deceased

Chapter 1

Historical Aspects

Carl E. Silver

The history of laryngeal cancer has recently been reviewed by several authors[1, 2] and it is interesting to retrace developments in this field.

PATHOLOGY

The decade from 1850 to 1860 marked a turning point in the understanding of laryngeal pathology. The advent of laryngoscopy permitted examination of the larynx in the living subject, and the publication of Virchow's monumental work on histopathology[3] in 1858 enabled for the first time the accurate distinction of various laryngeal abnormalities and objective appraisal of the types of treatment. Before the mid-nineteenth century, there was much confusion concerning laryngeal disease, and knowledge was rudimentary. The earliest reference to laryngeal cancer is made by Aretaeus (circa A.D. 100).[4, 5] Galen (circa A.D. 200) described a malignant ulceration of the throat and apparently understood the nature and seriousness of laryngeal cancer. He also described the anatomy of the larynx in detail in a manuscript that was subsequently lost.[4, 5] There are no known references to laryngeal cancer in the Western literature of the Middle Ages, but during the Renaissance, Boerhaave (1688) described "cancerous angina," and in 1732 Morgagni clearly described autopsy findings in two cases of laryngeal carcinoma,[4, 5] though an understanding of the cellular nature of the disease had to wait for Virchow.

In the archaic terminology used before the eighteenth century, laryngeal diseases were classified as "cynanche trachealis." This was subsequently changed to "angina" and "phthisis," terms still used today, but with greatly altered meanings. The term "laryngeal phthisis" was originally applied to "any chronic alteration of the larynx which may bring on consumption or death in any way."[6] The term "sarcoma" was used to describe a lesion that was somewhere in between the benign and malignant categories, indicating the general lack of understanding of pathologic processes. By 1839, a number of authors had written on laryngeal phthisis. The most important work on this subject was by Trousseau and Belloc in 1837,[7] describing four types of phthisis; one of these was the cancerous type, termed "laryngophthisis carcinomatosa." Their paper indicates that granulomatous diseases, such as syphilis and tuberculosis, were not clearly distinguished from carcinoma. Indeed, these diseases often existed simultaneously, thus adding to the confusion of pathologists of the time. Trousseau is generally considered to have been the first to use tracheostomy for the treatment of laryngeal cancer.

After the introduction of laryngoscopy and histopathology in the mid-nineteenth century, understanding of laryngeal pathology improved considerably. In 1871, Luschka[8] published an accurate description of laryngeal anatomy. In 1876 Isambert[9] suggested the classification of intrinsic, extrinsic, and subglottic varieties of laryngeal carcinoma. Krishaber[10] modified Isambert's groupings in 1879, classifying laryngeal tumors as intrinsic or extrinsic. Krishaber recognized that intrinsic carcinoma, originating inside the larynx, tended to be slow growing and to remain localized within the larynx for months or years, spreading to the regional lymph nodes only at an advanced stage. Extrinsic cancer, however, because it originated around the laryngeal orifice or on its pharyngeal surface, followed a much more malignant course, with rapid progression and early lymphatic invasion. Krishaber's classification remained the basis for describing laryngeal tumors for the next 50 years, until it was replaced by the modern topographic classification and staging systems.

Krishaber's distinction between the differing behaviors of intrinsic and extrinsic carcinoma was a great contribution, enabling rational prognostication and therapy. Nevertheless, it took time before the actual frequency and proportional occurrence of these lesions was realized. As late as 1876, Cornil and Ranvier[11] described cancer of the larynx as an extremely rare disease, and in 1880 the great Professor Störk of Vienna wrote that "carcinoma is rarely found limited to the larynx and most frequently invades it from the mucous folds between the epiglottis and the tongue, or the epiglottis and the esophagus."[5] By 1883, however, Butlin had made an advance by noting that intrinsic carcinoma was much more frequent than extrinsic cancer and that the true vocal cords were the most common site of origin.[12] The frequency of intrinsic versus extrinsic carcinoma was confirmed by Semon (136 cases of intrinsic carcinoma out of a total of 212), Chevalier Jackson (98 out of 141 cases), Gabriel Tucker (144 out of 200 cases), and Schmiegelow (36 out of 48 cases).[5]

LARYNGOSCOPY

The Russian engineer Paul Jablochkov had illuminated the boulevards of Paris with arc lights in 1867, but it was not until 1879 that a practical incandescent electric light for use in homes and offices was invented by Thomas Edison. This underscores the difficulty involved in developing a method for viewing the larynx in the gaslit nineteenth century. Similarly, it was not until 1884 that Karl Koller introduced the use of cocaine as a local anesthetic. Observation of the larynx was generally considered impossible before 1854, and several attempts and claims of laryngeal observation were condemned because of this prevalent belief.

Alberti[6] credits Leverett with the first authenticated attempt to examine the throat with a bent mirror in 1743 and with the development of a snare for the removal of polyps. In 1807 Dr. Felipe Bozzini claimed to have observed the larynx with a double cannula, using an angled mirror, a wax candle, and a reflector.[13] In 1829 Dr. Benjamin Guy Babington presented the first effective laryngoscope to the Hunterian Society in London. This "glottiscope" consisted of a tongue depressor combined with a mirror that was held against the palate. Illumination was provided by reflected sunlight from a hand-held mirror. The instrument was used successfully by Babington for many years but was never accepted for general use, partly because it was bulky and cumbersome and partly because Babington never published his findings. The device thus remained unknown except within his immediate circle of colleagues and students.[6]

Further attempts to observe the glottis using mirrors, spatulas, and prisms were recorded by Sen, Liston, Baumes, Benati, and Warden.[6,13] The devices of these early laryngoscopists remained impractical because they were cumbersome, difficult to use, and poorly tolerated by patients. In London, Avery invented a similarly unwieldy laryngoscope that was noteworthy for its introduction of a headband and mirror reflector. The light source, a mineral oil lamp, was also attached to the headband, and according to Alberti,[6] "it required considerable skill, perseverance, perspicacity and a strong neck to use the instrument." Avery's laryngoscope was not publicly described until 1862, 18 years after its invention, although he had been successful in using it during that time.

A most unlikely individual developed the first simple, practical, and widely accepted method for laryngeal examination and was hailed as the "Father of Laryngology." Manuel Garcia, an expatriate singing teacher of Spanish descent, had fled to London from France during the revolution of 1848. Garcia's lifelong ambition had been to observe the phonating glottis. In a sudden flash of inspiration, while vacationing in Paris in 1854, he envisaged a method for laryngeal autoexamination with an angled mirror. After obtaining a small, long-handled dentist's mirror, he heated it in warm water, dried it, and succeeded in observing his own glottis by reflecting sunlight from a handheld mirror onto the dental mirror, which he had placed against his palate.[6] Although greeted with the usual skepticism accorded by the medical profession of the time to claims of laryngeal observation, Garcia had the foresight to present his findings to the Royal Society of London in 1855,[14] thus documenting and securing credit for inventing this technique.

Popular acceptance of mirror laryngoscopy still had to await the work of Ludwig van Türck of Vienna[15] and Johann Czermak of Budapest.[16] Although hampered by the lack of consistently available sunlight, van Türck successfully applied mirror laryngoscopy to the diagnosis of laryngeal disease in infants. Czermak, his former colleague, advanced the popularity of clinical laryngoscopy by using artificial light and a concave mirror held between the teeth, thereby keeping a hand free for instrumentation.[6] In a manner characteristic of the great European clinicians of the nineteenth century, van Türck and Czermak quarreled publicly and with increasing ill-feeling over claims for priority in the use of the laryngoscope. Czermak presented his findings to the Academy of Sciences of Vienna in 1858, giving full credit to Garcia, but van Türck claimed to have originated the laryngeal mirror with no knowledge of Garcia's work.[17] This claim was refuted by his own pamphlet, published in 1860,[18] which mentions his debt to Liston and Garcia.

In truth, although Garcia invented the technique of laryngoscopy, and van Türck was the first to apply it to medicine, it was Czermak who, by using lamplight and a collecting mirror, improving laryngeal mirrors, and publicizing the procedure, developed laryngoscopy into a practical and widely used diagnostic and surgical procedure.[17]

Laryngoscopy was introduced to North America in 1858 by Krackowizer.[6] The first recorded case of removal of a laryngeal tumor by indirect laryngoscopy was by Lewin in 1861.[13] As will be discussed below, Morell Mackenzie was instrumental in developing the art of surgical manipulation of the larynx using curved laryngeal forceps visually guided by mirror laryngoscopy.[19]

Direct laryngoscopy did not evolve until 1895, when Kirstein[20] used a procedure he called autoscopy. Using an instrument that resembled a tongue depressor, he was able to see a young man's vocal cords and tracheal bifurcation. Kirstein mentioned problems with the technique and with the electric lighting systems and mentioned the difficulty in observing the anterior commissure. Further modifications to the laryngoscope by Brunings,[21] Mosher,[22] Ingals,[23] and particularly Jackson[24–26] laid the foundations for the development of modern endoscopic techniques. Jackson created instruments that permitted relatively easy examination and biopsy of all regions of the larynx and brought together the endoscopic, diagnostic, and external surgical techniques in the management of laryngeal cancer.

LARYNGOFISSURE

Laryngofissure, or thyrotomy, is a surgical approach to the interior of the larynx that consists of splitting the thyroid cartilage at or near the midline. It represents the oldest form of surgical extirpation of laryngeal tumors. It is said that as early as 1778, Pelletan, a French surgeon, split the larynx to remove an impacted piece of meat.[27] In 1810, Desault of Paris reportedly incised the cricothyroid membrane, inserted a tracheostomy tube through the opening in a reversed upward direction, and performed a thyrotomy by transecting the midline of the larynx from within outward. Desault's operation was performed for removal of a foreign body.[5, 6] There is some question, however, whether Desault actually performed this procedure or merely suggested the technique.[28–30] In 1833, Brauers of Louvan entered the larynx of a 40-year-old man to "repeatedly cauterize" warty endolaryngeal growths "with various preparations and a hot iron."[5] The patient survived for 20 years. Brauers' case was reported in the literature by Albers of Bonn[31] in 1834. In 1844, Ehrman removed a laryngeal polyp from a 33-year-old woman by dividing the thyroid cartilage in the midline 2 days after preliminary tracheostomy, and then excising the lesion with a knife.[6, 29] The first laryngofissure for the treatment of intrinsic carcinoma of the larynx was performed on a 51-year-old woman in the United States in 1851 by Gurdon Buck.[32] The procedure was performed without anesthesia. Buck had believed the lesion to be a polyp, but a carcinoma too extensive for complete removal was found at surgery. It recurred, and the patient died 15 months after surgery while attempting to change her tracheostomy cannula.[5] In 1863, H.B. Sands of New York performed a laryngofissure for carcinoma of the larynx in a woman who died of unrelated causes 2 years later.[6] Duncan Gibb performed the first successful laryngofissure in Great Britain in 1867, with chloroform anesthesia. The patient died with recurrent tumor a year after surgery.[5] In 1867, the great American laryngologist Jacob da Silva Solis-Cohen of Philadelphia achieved the first documented permanent cure of carcinoma by laryngofissure.[33] His patient survived 20 years without recurrence.

Most of the early results of laryngofissure were not good, and the procedure was condemned by Mackenzie, Semon, and Butlin.[12, 17, 19] In the absence of a pathologic diagnosis, surgery was often done for benign lesions. Mackenzie noted that avulsion of benign lesions was better effected by laryngoscopy than by thyrotomy.[5] Removal of malignant tumors was usually piecemeal and was rightly condemned by Mackenzie, who noted that "radical removal of an ill-defined tumor cannot be efficiently accomplished by this method."[6] In 1878, Von Bruns collected statistics that served as a standard reference for many years.[34] He recorded the results of 19 thyrotomies performed in 15 patients: only two patients survived longer than 1 year, and only one patient, who died 22 months later of unrelated causes, remained free of recurrence. Similarly bad results were reported from Billroth's clinic between 1870 and 1884, and the procedure was condemned by Moure in 1891 and by Sendziak in 1897.[5]

With a better understanding of the limitations of laryngofissure and with improvements in the selection of patients, the results of this operation began to improve toward the end of the nineteenth century. In 1894, Semon published the results of eight thyrotomies with only two operative deaths, and in 1895 Butlin recorded 14 cases with one mortality.[5] Although there was little evidence of any improvement in cure rate, both Semon and Butlin became enthusiastic about the procedure. Improvements in anesthesia and aftercare were particularly helpful in reducing operative mortality. In 1919, St. Claire Thomson reported 38 cases with no operative mortality.[5] Thomson contributed greatly to reducing postoperative morbidity and mortality by abolishing the use of morphine and other sedatives, which were frequently used in conjunction with chloroform anesthesia, and by improving the management of bronchial toilet.

Cure rates began to improve after the beginning of the twentieth century. Semon, who had reported a 3-year-survival rate of 8.7% in 1897, achieved a 3-year-survival rate of 60% by 1907.[5] In 1912, Thomson reported on 10 patients operated on by himself or by his colleagues Semon and Butlin between 1900 and 1910:[35] "A lasting cure" was achieved in 8 of the 10 patients. Thomson comprehensively summarized the progress of laryngofissure as reported by various authors between 1878 and 1938. Among these were Chevalier Jackson's report of 3-year cures in 29 of 45 patients in 1927, Thomson's 1928 report of 3-year cures in 76% of the patients, and Gluck and Sorenson's 1930 report of "lasting" cures in 110 out of 125 patients, with 4 additional patients being salvaged by total laryngectomy.[5]

TOTAL LARYNGECTOMY

In 1829 Albers of Bonn experimented with total laryngectomy in dogs. These attempts were premature, and little more was undertaken for 25 years.[6] In 1870, Czerny reported the results of experimental laryngectomies on dogs at Billroth's clinic.[36] His initial work had been unsuccessful, temporarily discouraging further attempts in humans. Around the same time period, Langenbeck and his colleagues also experimented with dogs and were prepared to perform a human laryngectomy, but their patient refused the operation.[6]

Patrick Watson of Edinburgh has often been credited with performing the first human laryngectomy (for syphilis) in 1866. According to Stell,[37] however, Watson's own paper showed this to be untrue.[38] The patient had undergone only a tracheostomy during life. After his death, the larynx was demonstrated at a pathology meeting. The confusion resulted from a paper by Foulis[39] in 1881, which quoted a letter by Watson stating that he had removed some soft tissue from the larynx. It seems certain that a laryngectomy had not been performed.

The first laryngectomy was performed by Billroth. This famous case was reported to the Third Congress of the German Society of Surgeons by Billroth's assistant, Carl Gussenbauer, in 1874.[40] Philip Stell[37] and Adolf Schwartz[41] have provided fascinating reading with descriptions of this famous case. Billroth's patient was a 36-year-old instructor of religion who had been hoarse for 3 years. A subglottic tumor, mostly on the left side, had been treated by Professor Störk of Vienna by cauterization with silver nitrate and injections of liquor ferri. Pieces of tumor, removed to relieve stridor, were examined histologically, and the diagnosis of epidermoid carcinoma was made. The patient was admitted to Billroth's clinic in November 1873 for surgery. After a preliminary tracheostomy, a laryngofissure with division of the thyroid and cricoid cartilages was performed, and the tumor was removed with scissors and a sharp curette.

The lesion recurred, producing dyspnea. This was documented by reopening the wound under anesthesia on December 31, 1873. When cartilaginous invasion was detected, the anesthetic was discontinued, the patient was awakened, and consent was obtained for a total laryngectomy.

Billroth then proceeded to extirpate the larynx. The operation was periodically interrupted when the patient coughed large amounts of blood from the trachea. The larynx was excised, leaving the hyoid bone and part of the epiglottis in place. The edges of the tracheal and the pharyngeal mucosae were sutured to the skin. The procedure took 1 hour 45 minutes, after which the patient was revived by wine administered through a feeding tube. Hemorrhage occurred 4 hours after the operation and was treated by ligating the left superior laryngeal ar-

tery. The patient survived, and the remaining postoperative course was uneventful. A valved, air-diverting tracheostomy tube was designed for the patient by Gussenbauer, and this was successful in producing a voice.

Although the patient survived the surgery, he died within 7 months of recurrent tumor. Some authors have claimed that Billroth's patient had tuberculosis rather than cancer, but according to Alberti,[6] the diagnosis of carcinoma was well documented in this case.

The first completely successful laryngectomy was performed by Bottini of Turin in 1875 for mixed round and spindle cell sarcoma. The patient, a 24-year-old postman, survived 10 years after the operation.[5, 6] Other early laryngectomies were reported by Heine, Mores, Schmidt, Watson, and Schonlein.[42] Von Langenbeck combined a neck dissection with an extensive glossolaryngopharyngectomy; his patient survived the operation but died from the neoplasm.[42]

Despite the occasional spectacularly successful case, the results of early laryngectomies were generally disastrous because of hemorrhage, sepsis, mediastinitis, bronchopneumonia, shock, or heart failure.[5] Gluck reported an operative mortality of 54% between 1870 and 1880.[42] Mackenzie collected 19 cases from the literature in 1880 and noted operative and early postoperative deaths in nine, rapid recurrences in seven, and cure in only three patients[5]; one of these was a carcinoma, and the other two were sarcomas. These results led Mackenzie to recommend limiting treatment of carcinoma of the larynx to intralaryngeal removal, with tracheostomy when necessary. Similarly dismal statistics in larger series of cases were reported by Foulis 1881,[39] Hahn in 1885,[17] and Sendziak in 1888.[42] Although cure rates improved, the postoperative mortality remained approximately 50%, and widespread use of the procedure was discouraged by the extreme postoperative disability, caused not only by voice loss but also by the often persistent pharyngeal and pharyngotracheal fistulae (due to the then-customary procedure of leaving the wounds open to heal secondarily).

In 1892, Solis-Cohen[43, 44] devised the principle of diverting the tracheal stump to the skin. This technique was further developed by Gluck and his associates, particularly Sorenson, who systematically improved laryngectomy by separating the trachea to form a tracheostoma and also by accomplishing a permanent pharyngeal closure with a single-stage operation.[42]

Messerklinger added a neck dissection en bloc to the laryngectomy and also greatly reduced the incidence of postoperative fistulae.[42] A two-stage procedure, introduced by Gluck and Leller[29] in 1881, was revived by LeBec[45] in 1905, with improvements in survival. This procedure involved creating a tracheostoma as a preliminary procedure 2 weeks before the actual resection.

Themistokles Gluck and his colleague Sorenson dominated the progress of laryngectomy development for the first quarter of the twentieth century. By 1922, they had performed 160 total laryngectomies, the last 63 consecutive cases without a fatality.[4, 42, 46] This achievement contributed greatly to general acceptance of the operation. Cure rates also improved, although a review of a number of authors' series compiled by St. Claire Thomson between 1908 and 1938 revealed considerable variability in the results.[5] This was because of the failure to classify the cases according to site ("intrinsic" or "extrinsic") and extent (or stage) of the lesions. It was not until the widespread use of neck dissection, the development of the modern technique of "wide field" laryngectomy, and the proper classification of cases that the true value of total laryngectomy for curing laryngeal cancer became apparent.

VERTICAL HEMILARYNGECTOMY

At a meeting in 1903 of the Section of Laryngology and Otology of the British Medical Association, Semon[47] defined partial extirpation of the larynx as "an operation in which no less than an entire wing of the thyroid cartilage and possibly, additionally, an arytenoid and parts of the cricoid cartilage are removed." Procedures in which only small fragments of these cartilages were removed were considered to be laryngofissures. This distinction was helpful in evaluating claims and reports of "partial laryngectomies" performed in the past.

Billroth performed the first vertical hemilaryngectomy in July 1878,[29, 41] although it was Gluck who truly developed this procedure.[48, 49] Gluck's operation consisted of removing a complete anatomic half of the larynx, including the thyroid and the arytenoid cartilages and half of the cricoid cartilage. A large skin flap was rotated inward to resurface the defect, leaving a laryngostoma, which was subsequently closed. Although Kleinschmidt,[49] in describing Gluck's procedure, claimed that "with careful technique, complications are not usual," the operation was disabling and the temporary laryngostoma was objectionable. In addition, Gluck and other surgeons of his time performed hemilaryngectomy for tumors with fixed vocal cords and subglottic extension, resulting in high recurrence rates. Thus, during the early twentieth century, hemilaryngectomy fell into disuse until it was revived by

Hautant,[50] who attempted to avoid the laryngostoma by primary closure of the larynx over a tampon inserted to maintain the lumen. Hautant, however, still performed hemilaryngectomy for subglottic lesions.

It was not until a better appreciation of the limitations of vertical hemilaryngectomy prevailed that its true value for treatment of cancer was realized. Similarly, functional results were improved when the procedure was modified to avoid resection of the cricoid except under very particular and limited circumstances and when effective primary closure became possible. Thus, modifications of the operation by Clerf, Kemler, Leroux-Robert, and Norris[51–54] varied the amount of soft tissue and cartilage resection according to the site of the tumor. Improved methods for reconstruction evolved, including the use of an obturator by Goodyear,[55] intralaryngeal skin grafts by Figi,[56] skin flaps by Meurman,[57] and hypopharyngeal mucosa by Som.[58] The procedures developed by these authors, as well as a variety of partial laryngectomy techniques, will be described in detail in subsequent chapters.

PHARYNGOTOMY AND SUPRAGLOTTIC PARTIAL LARYNGECTOMY

The first, albeit rather primitive, supraglottic partial laryngectomy was apparently performed by Astley Cooper, who reportedly removed a large tumor of the epiglottis with his fingers early in the nineteenth century.[6] Alberti[6] cites Mackenzie's account of successful resection of an epiglottic tumor through a subhyoid pharyngotomy performed by Dr. Pratt, a French naval surgeon, at a naval base on a small Polynesian island. The suprahyoid, subhyoid, and transhyoid approaches to the hypopharynx were developed during the nineteenth century by von Langenbeck, Grünwald, Jermitsch, and Vallas,[49, 59] but these procedures were of little use because the limited exposures provided were inadequate for resecting most tumors. The same criticism of these procedures for the treatment of malignant disease holds true today.

Lateral subhyoid or suprahyoid pharyngotomy was developed by Kronlein to approach tumors of the lateral tongue base, pyriform sinus, and hypopharynx.[49] The lateral wall was entered deep to the transected hyoglossus muscle, and if a large tumor was resected, closure of the wound was "as a rule, impossible." Von Mikulicz described a similar procedure that included transection of the mandible for tumors simultaneously involving the epilarynx, faucial pillars, and tonsil[49]; the wound was left open to granulate. Obalinski modified this procedure by reuniting the divided mandible with silver wire.[49]

These procedures were of limited clinical use, and the procedure of lateral pharyngotomy received little attention until the work of Wilfred Trotter in 1913.[60, 61] Trotter described a practical, partial pharyngolaryngectomy suitable for resecting tumors of the epiglottis, aryepiglottic fold, and lateral pharyngeal wall. Colledge[62] and Orton[63] continued to develop these techniques. By 1938, Colledge reported a cure rate of 29% in 55 cases of lateral pharyngotomy and pharyngolaryngectomy.[64]

Despite the progress made by these surgeons, the resection of laryngeal and hypopharyngeal tumors by lateral pharyngotomy remained a surgical curiosity until after World War II, when Professor Justo M. Alonso of Montevideo, Uruguay, recognized the value of this technique for partial horizontal laryngectomy and "fought until the end of his long and brilliant career to spread his works not only to South American specialists, but also to those in North America and in Europe."[65] Alonso instituted various modifications, including a cutaneous flap and partial resection of the thyroid cartilage, and he increased the range of indications for the procedure from the treatment of benign laryngeal lesions to pharyngoepiglottic cancer.[66, 67] Barretto[65] has written an interesting dissertation on the many contributions of Alonso and several other South Americans to laryngeal cancer surgery.

The subsequent modifications and the development of supraglottic subtotal laryngectomy and partial pharyngolaryngectomy by Ogura and colleagues,[68–70] Som,[71] and Bocca et al.[72] represent the apex of progress in laryngeal surgery and have helped to realize the goal aspired to in all cancer operations: high cure rate with maximum preservation of function.

MORELL MACKENZIE AND THE CELEBRATED CASE OF EMPEROR FREDERICK III

The tragic story of Morell Mackenzie and his role in the treatment of the Prussian crown prince, later Emperor Frederick III of Germany, is inextricably woven into the history of laryngeal surgery. The story is worth telling in some detail, partly because it paints an excellent picture of the status of late-nineteenth-century laryngology and also because it is worthwhile to reiterate the enormous contributions made by Mackenzie to laryngology. The clouding of reputation from this case was undeserved. It has become a commonly held belief that Mackenzie failed to diagnose cancer of the larynx at an early

stage when called to examine the crown prince and, by preventing timely surgical intervention, was thus responsible for Frederick's death from this neoplasm. The liberal Frederick, who dreamed of establishing a representative democratic government in the German empire, was succeeded by his son, the famous Kaiser Wilhelm II. The strutting, pompous Wilhelm, insanely jealous of his uncle and of his cousin who ruled England and Russia, ultimately led Germany into World War I. Thus, Mackenzie has been blamed for practically causing this conflict and for the subsequent twentieth-century carnage that resulted from it. The story of Mackenzie and the crown prince has been told in considerable detail by Scott Stevenson[17] and was reported in an interesting article by McInnis et al.[73]

Morell Mackenzie

Early in his career, Mackenzie was awarded the Jacksonian Prize of the Royal College of Surgeons for his essay "On the Pathology and Treatment of Diseases of the Larynx: The diagnostic indications to include the appearance as seen in the living person." This volume was particularly notable for watercolor drawings by the author; these were some of the first representations of the larynx and laryngeal pathology as seen in the living subject. Mackenzie devoted himself intensively to the development of laryngoscopy and devised numerous instruments for removing polyps and other lesions from the larynx. The submission of pathologic material removed from the larynx for microscopic examination, together with the direct observation of laryngeal pathology for the first time, helped to put laryngology on a sound scientific basis.

In 1863 Mackenzie leased a house on Kings Street, London, which he turned into a dispensary for the treatment of diseases of the throat. This dispensary grew, became famous, and was eventually moved to larger quarters, becoming the Hospital for Diseases of the Throat. It was the first specialized facility for the diagnosis and treatment of laryngeal diseases. The large volume of clinical material concentrated there enabled Mackenzie to develop enormous experience and make great strides in the development of laryngology. In addition to his numerous publications, his *Diseases of the Throat and Nose*,[74] published in two volumes, was universally recognized throughout the world and became the standard textbook of laryngology, not only covering the whole field as it existed at the time but also anticipating many advances, which owed their inspiration to the author.

Political Background

The end of the Franco-Prussian War in 1871 saw the unification of the German states under the Prussian king, Wilhelm I, who was crowned emperor. Crown Prince Frederick, Wilhelm's son, had favored the unification, envisaging a government with an upper house of princes and a representative lower house elected by the people. The unification, however, had been engineered by the Prussian chancellor, Otto von Bismarck, who succeeded, instead, in accomplishing the absorption of Germany by autocratic Prussia under Wilhelm I. The conservative Junkers led by Bismarck firmly believed that representative democracy would lead inevitably to the downfall of the nation. At the time of unification in 1871, Wilhelm I was 73 years old. Frederick and his liberal supporters felt that they would soon have their chance to democratize the German autocracy. But the old Emperor Wilhelm lived another 17 years, and Frederick languished in ceremonial posts well into his middle age, while Bismarck's power grew.

Frederick had married Victoria, the daughter of Queen Victoria of England. The English crown princess, later the Empress Frederick, was a constant target of criticism from German conservative political figures and journalists. The fact that Mackenzie was British created a situation that was exploited by Frederick's and his wife's political enemies.

Frederick's Illness

In January 1887, the 55-year-old crown prince became hoarse. Examination by Professor Gerhardt of the University of Berlin revealed a pale red nodule about 4 mm in diameter, on the left vocal cord. Gerhardt attempted to remove the lesion with a snare, but he succeeded in obtaining only a fragment of material. He then attempted fulguration of the lesion by galvanocautery. After 13 such treatments, the nodule persisted, and cancer was suspected.

Gerhardt summoned von Bergmann, Professor of Surgery at the University of Berlin, for a consultation. Von Bergmann recommended immediate surgery. He apparently planned a laryngofissure but intended to proceed with a laryngectomy if required. There seems little question that von Bergmann minimized to Frederick the risk and extent of the procedure that was contemplated. This was not justifiable on the basis of his own or other contemporary results of laryngofissure or laryngectomy for treatment of cancer.

Additional laryngologic consultation was advised and the patient was examined by Professor Tobold, a senior Berlin laryngologist, who agreed that immediate surgical exploration was necessary.

At this point, Morell Mackenzie was called from London to give his opinion. There was doubt and endless controversy as to whether the request for Mackenzie's presence was initiated by Frederick's German physicians or through the influence of Frederick's wife and the British royal family. Being publicity shy was not one of Mackenzie's shortcomings. He was both friend and physician to a glittering array of theatrical and operatic celebrities of the day and enjoyed being interviewed and seeing his name in print, a tendency that was to exacerbate his later difficulties. Mackenzie was pleased and flattered to be summoned by a personal envoy of Queen Victoria to minister to as lofty a personage as the Crown Prince of Germany.

When he examined the prince, Mackenzie noted a pea-sized nodule on the posterior part of the left vocal cord, partly subglottic in position. There was slight limitation of motion of the vocal cord and slight congestion of the mucosa. Mackenzie recommended a biopsy, which he attempted with unfamiliar German forceps. He succeeded in removing only a small portion of the nodule, which was sent to the great pathologist, Virchow. Virchow could find no evidence of cancer in the small specimen and requested a second piece of the lesion. A second biopsy attempted a few days later was unsuccessful, partly because of congestion of the right vocal cord. In an action that was to set the stage for further animosity, Gerhardt examined Frederick immediately after the biopsy and accused Mackenzie of injuring the uninvolved right vocal cord with his forceps (an occurrence which was highly unlikely, since Mackenzie was renowned for his dexterity).

About 2½ weeks later, Mackenzie successfully removed about half of the tumor and again Virchow could find no evidence of cancer. Surgery was deferred indefinitely, and Mackenzie undertook responsibility for Frederick's further treatment. He eventually removed the remainder of the lesion from the left vocal cord, and again the specimen (examined by Virchow) was negative for cancer. After cauterization of a small recurrence on August 7, the left vocal cord healed completely and the growth did not recur. However, some transient posterior mucosal edema suggested to Mackenzie the possibility of perichondritis that could cause future difficulty.

The prince decided to winter in the mild climate of San Remo, in Italy. On November 5, immediately after Frederick's arrival there, Mackenzie's assistant, Mark Hovell, noted a sudden subglottic swelling. This time, when Mackenzie examined the prince, he suspected carcinoma. Almost immediately, recriminations began from all quarters. Mackenzie had detractors, such as Professor Störk of Vienna, and supporters, such as Schnitzler. The arguments were heightened by the intense personal hatreds that these Viennese teachers of the same subject held for each other. The most destructive aspect of the controversy was the daily appearance of the criticisms and of the most intimate details of Frederick's health in the public press. These reports were published with complete disregard for the feelings of the individuals involved, since "Royalties" were news and their most intimate affairs were of public interest. Newspaper reporters descended on San Remo, badgering Mackenzie and others and publishing daily reports.

Further consultations were obtained. Von Schnotter of Vienna recommended laryngectomy, while Mackenzie wanted to perform another biopsy. Kraus of Berlin suspected carcinoma but recommended treatment with potassium iodide to rule out syphilis. Moritz Schmidt of Frankfurt agreed with the trial of potassium iodide. Newspaper reports that Frederick was suspected of having syphilis caused him great personal embarrassment. The consultants, including Mackenzie, finally agreed that the prince had cancer and recommended a laryngectomy. The prince, however, refused to undergo a laryngectomy, but agreed to have a tracheostomy if it became necessary. Frederick's motives for declining laryngectomy were quite reasonable. Even if the operation were successful, the functional disability engendered by it would render him unsuitable to function as a ruler. He also felt that he had a better chance of surviving to become emperor by not undergoing surgery. Although he had publicly accepted news of his fate with great nobility and calmness, privately Frederick grieved over his illness. Of course, the confidential physician's report of Frederick's cancer was leaked to the press.

Again the controversy raged. Mackenzie was blamed for the delay in treatment. Virchow felt that Mackenzie was trying to blame him for missing the diagnosis. Mackenzie denied any such intention and tried to defend himself by noting that it was rare for carcinoma to remain undiagnosed after three separate biopsies. There were further recriminations in the newspapers and from political quarters against the Crown Princess, who shared the blame with Mackenzie for preventing the original surgery.

Meanwhile, the laryngeal edema fluctuated, creating optimism that the problem might be due to perichondritis. On January 17, 1888, Frederick expectorated a large necrotic slough, which by microscopic examination was found to be negative for cancer. On February 9, because of increasing stri-

dor, a tracheostomy was performed by Dr. Bramann, a young German surgeon.

Mackenzie remained at San Remo to attend the Prince and returned with him to Berlin on March 9, 1888, when Wilhelm I died and Frederick became emperor. While in San Remo, a sputum specimen had been examined by Waldeyer, and the findings were considered compatible with a diagnosis of cancer. This inconclusive report was nevertheless the most objective documentation of cancer ever obtained during Frederick's life.

The reign of Emperor Frederick III lasted 99 days, until his death from aspiration pneumonia on June 15, 1888. Mackenzie remained constantly in attendance during that time. An autopsy carried out by Professors Virchow and Waldeyer revealed that Frederick's larynx had been replaced by a large necrotic ulceration, containing a nodule of what was apparently carcinoma, according to the description from a microscopic examination. A large malignant lymph node was also present on the left side of the neck.

There was recently a suggestion from Pahor[75] that Frederick's illness should be considered a verrucous carcinoma of the larynx, the first such case known in history. This histologic diagnosis is excluded because a cervical lymph node metastasis was present; pure verrucous squamous cell carcinoma does not metastasize.

Repercussions After Frederick's Death

Following Frederick's death, Mackenzie returned to London a worn and haggard man. The £12,000 that he had been paid for 13 months of attendance to the Emperor did not begin to compensate him for the financial difficulties created by prolonged absence from his practice. He had lost many of his patients to several of the young laryngologists he had trained.

Calumny abounded. The German physicians, who wanted to fix the blame squarely on Mackenzie, published a vitriolic account of Frederick's case entitled *Die Krankheit Kaiser Frederick des Dritten*.[76] This report minimized the danger of laryngofissure and emphasized von Bergmann's reported seven successful cases (none of which were for cancer). Gerhardt's accusation that Mackenzie injured the vocal cords was reiterated, and the entire publication proceeded on the same rancorous note.

Angered by this attack, Mackenzie published *The Fatal Illness of Frederick the Noble*[77] in his own defense. Although his desire to attack his calumniators was understandable, the book was injudicious, to say the least. Mackenzie was advised to withhold publication, but he could not resist, and the book was sold widely in England. Among various points made was intense criticism of Gerhardt for his cauterization of the original lesion and of von Bergmann for causing an abscess by creating a false passage during a tracheostomy tube change. Both *Die Krankheit Kaiser Frederick des Dritten* and *The Fatal Illness of Frederick the Noble* were full of meaningless, petty criticisms that did nothing to enhance the stature of their authors. Although *Frederick the Noble* may have helped Mackenzie express his anger, it was looked on with considerable disfavor by the British medical establishment. He was criticized by the Royal College of Surgeons and the British Medical Association and found it necessary to resign from the Royal College of Physicians. Mackenzie retained some enthusiastic supporters, however, and before his death he founded the British Rhino-Laryngologic Association. He died of pneumonia on February 3, 1892, at the age of 54.

An Analysis

Stevenson,[17] after analyzing the details of the case, concluded that Frederick died of cancer of the larynx. The course of the disease, however, was far from typical. Most likely, the cancer supervened upon syphilis in this case. Waldeyer's examination of the sputum specimen was the best evidence for the cancer but was not conclusive. The postmortem examination was more conclusive for the ultimate diagnosis of cancer. The perichondritis and the autopsy finding of replacement of most of the larynx with a large necrotic ulceration was consistent with the diagnosis of syphilis, as was the temporarily favorable response to treatment.

The unfortunate result of this case was that laryngeal biopsy was discredited for decades. In modern times, of course, direct laryngoscopy would be performed. By his insistence on histologic confirmation of the diagnosis by biopsy, Mackenzie was well ahead of his time.

If Mackenzie had not interfered with the originally proposed surgery, the outcome would probably have been worse. The poor results of both laryngofissure and total laryngectomy before 1900 have already been discussed in some detail.

Perhaps the most dramatic scenario of what might have transpired had Frederick undergone surgery was described by Carl Ludwig Schleich, as quoted by Stevenson.[17] Schleich had gone to watch his old friend and colleague, von Bergmann, operate on the afternoon of the very day that *Die Krankheit Kaiser Frederick des Dritten* was published. Before commencing the operation, von Bergmann addressed his audience of students, explaining that the patient had exactly the same condition as Kaiser Frederick. The diagnosis of cancer had been confirmed by biopsy, and von Bergmann announced that he would demonstrate how he would have saved the Kaiser's life had he been allowed to operate. As the operation proceeded, however, von Bergmann discovered that the disease was not confined to one small area behind the vocal cord; it was a more extensive lesion, invading the "region above the larynx." After an interval of 1½ hours, von Bergmann announced, "Gentlemen, we have been mistaken. This is not carcinoma at all, it is diffuse tuberculosis of the larynx. I am discontinuing the operation." The patient died within the next 2 hours. As Schleich speculated, had a similar event occurred in the case of Frederick, the progress of surgery would have been impeded for a generation.

REFERENCES

1. Alberti PW. Historical aspects of laryngeal cancer. Invited lecture. Second World Congress on Laryngeal Cancer, Sydney, 1994.
2. Pratt LW. Historical perspective. *In* Ferlito A (ed): *Neoplasms of the Larynx,* pp 1–25. Edinburgh, Churchill Livingstone, 1993.
3. Virchow RLK. *Die Cellular Pathologie in ihren Begründung auf Physiologische und Pathologische Gewebelehre.* Berlin, A Hirschwald, 1858.
4. Myerson MC. *The Human Larynx.* Springfield, Charles C Thomas, 1964.
5. Thomson St C. The history of cancer of the larynx. *J Laryngol Otol* 1939; 54:61–87.
6. Alberti PW. The historical development of laryngectomy. II The evolution of laryngology and laryngectomy in the mid-19th century. *Laryngoscope* 1975; 85:288–298. Panel discussion.
7. Trousseau A, Belloc H. *Traité Pratique de la Phthisie laryngée.* Baillière, Paris, 1837.
8. Luschka H van. *Der Kehlkopf des Menschen.* Tubingen, Laupp'schen, 1871.
9. Isambert E. Contribution à l'étude du cancer laryngé. *Ann Mal Oreille Larynx* 1876; 2:1–23.
10. Krishaber M. Contribution à l'étude du cancer du larynx. *Gaz Bebd Med Chirug* 1879; 16:518–523.
11. Cornil AV, Ranvier L. *Manuel d'Histologie Pathologique.* Paris, 1876.
12. Butlin HT. *On Malignant Diseases of the Larynx.* London, J & A Churchill, 1883.
13. Goldman JL, Roffman JD. Indirect laryngoscopy. *Laryngoscope* 1975; 85:530–533.
14. Garcia M. Physiological observation on the human voice. *Proc R Soc Lond* 1855; 7:399–410.
15. van Türck L. *Klinik der Krankheiten des Kehlkopfes.* Vienna, 1866.
16. Czermak J. *Wien Med Wochenschr,* March 27, 1858.
17. Stevenson RS. *Morell Mackenzie, The Story of a Victorian Tragedy.* London, William Heinemann, 1946.
18. van Türck L. *Praktische Anletung zur Laryngoskopie.* Vienna, 1860.
19. MacKenzie M. *Essay on Growths in the Larynx.* London, J & A Churchill, 1871.
20. Kirstein A. Autoskopie der Larynx und der Trachea (Besichtigung ohne Spiegel). *Arch Laryngol Rhinol* 1895; 3:156–164.
21. Brunings W. *Die Direkte Laryngoskopie, Bronchoskopie und Oesophagoskopie.* Wiesbaden, Carl Ritter, 1909.
22. Mosher HP. Direct examination of the larynx and of the

upper end of the esophagus by the lateral route. *Boston Med Soc J* 1908; 48:189.

23. Ingals EF. Direct laryngoscopy. *Trans Am Laryngol Rhinol Otol Soc* 1911; 26–29.
24. Jackson C. *Tracheo-Bronchoscopy, Esophagoscopy and Gastroscopy.* St Louis, Laryngoscope Co, 1907.
25. Jackson C. *Peroral Endoscopy and Laryngeal Surgery.* St Louis, Laryngoscope Co, 1915.
26. Jackson C, Jackson CL. *Cancer of the Larynx.* Philadelphia, WB Saunders Co, 1939.
27. Thornwald J. *The Triumph of Surgery.* New York, Pantheon Books, 1957.
28. Durham AE. On the operation of opening the larynx by section of the cartilages etc, for the removal of morbid growths. *Med Chir Trans* (London) 1872; 37:17.
29. MacComb WS, Fletcher GH. *Cancer of the Head and Neck.* Baltimore, Williams & Wilkins Co, 1967.
30. MacKenzie M. *Diseases of the Pharynx, Larynx and Trachea.* New York, William Wood C, 1880.
31. Albers JFH. Über die Geschwülste im Kehlkopf. *J Chir Augen-Heilk* 1834; 21:517–536.
32. Buck G. On the surgical treatment of morbid growths within the larynx. *Trans Am Med Assoc* 1853; 6:509–535.
33. da Silva Solis-Cohen J. Modern procedures in excision of intrinsic malignant growths of the larynx. *Laryngoscope* 1907; 17:365–369.
34. Von Bruns P. *Die Laryngotomie zur Entfernung Intralaryngealer Neubildurgen.* Berlin, 1878.
35. Thomson St C. Intrinsic cancer of the larynx: Operation by laryngofissure: Lasting cure in 80% of cases. *Br Med J* 1912; 1:355–359.
36. Czerny V. Versuche über Kehlkopf-Extirpation. *Wien Med Wochenschr* 1870; 20:559–561.
37. Stell PM. The first laryngectomy. *J Laryngol Otol* 1975; 89:353–358.
38. Watson PH. Ulceration of the larynx, tracheotomy, haemoptysis. *Edinburgh Med J* 1866; 11:78.
39. Foulis D. Indications for the complete or partial extirpation of the larynx. Transactions of the Seventh International Congress in Otolaryngology, London, Kolcham, 1881; 57–64.
40. Gussenbauer C. Über die erste durch Th. Billroth am Menschen ausgeführte Kehlkopf-Extirpation und die Anwendung eines künstlichen Kehlkopfes. *Arch Klin Chir* 1874; 17:343–356.
41. Schwartz AW. Dr Theodore Billroth and the first laryngectomy. *Ann Plast Surg* 1978; 1:513.
42. Holinger PH. The historical development of laryngectomy. V A century of progress of laryngectomies in the northern hemisphere. *Laryngoscope* 1975; 85:322–332. Panel discussion.
43. da Silva Solis-Cohen J. Two cases of laryngectomy of adenocarcinoma of the larynx. *NY Med J* 1892; 56:533–535.
44. da Silva Solis-Cohen J. Two cases of laryngectomy for adenocarcinoma. *Trans Am Laryngol Assoc* 1893; 14:60–62.
45. LeBec. Laryngectomie totale en deux temps separés. *Ann Mal Oreille Larynx* 1905; 31:375.
46. Gluck T, Sorenson J. Die Resektion und Extirpation des Larynx, Pharynx und Esophagus. *In* Katz L, Presing H, Bumenfeld F (eds): *Handbuch des Spez Chir Ohres und der Obereu.* Leftwege, Vol IV. Wurzburg, C Kabitzch, 1931.
47. Semon F. A discussion on the operative treatment of malignant diseases of the larynx. *Br Med J* 1903; 2:1113–1118; 1125–1126.
48. Gluck T. A discussion on the operative treatment of malignant diseases of the larynx. *Br Med J* 1903; 2:1119–1124.
49. Kirschner M, Lautenschlager A, Kleinschmidt O. *Operative Surgery.* Philadelphia, JB Lippincott Co, 1937.
50. Hautant A. Hemilaryngectomie après mon procédé. *Ann Mal Oreille Larynx* 1929; May.
51. Clerf LH. Cancer of the larynx. An analysis of two hundred and fifty operative cases. *Arch Otolaryngol* 1940; 32:484–498.
52. Kemler JI. Bilateral thyrotomy for carcinoma of the larynx. *Laryngoscope* 1947; 57:704–718.
53. Leroux-Robert JL. Les possibilités therapeutiques du cancer du larynx par la chirurgie et les associations radiochirurgie à propos d'une statistique personelle de 1,000 cas operés depuis plus 5 ans. *Presse Med* 1965; 73:1031.
54. Norris CM. Technique of extended frontolateral partial laryngectomy. *Laryngoscope* 1958; 68:1240–1250.
55. Goodyear HM. Hemilaryngectomy: method of maintaining a satisfactory airway and voice. *Ann Otol Rhinol Laryngol* 1949; 58:581–585.
56. Figi FA. Removal of carcinoma of the larynx with immediate skin graft for repair. *Ann Otol Rhinol Laryngol* 1950; 59:474–486.
57. Meurman Y. Extended cordectomy for intrinsic laryngeal cancer: Application and results. Plastic covering of excision surface. Proceeding of the 5th International Congress of Otology, Rhinology and Laryngology, Amsterdam, 1953.
58. Som ML. Hemilaryngectomy—a modified technique for cordal carcinoma with extension posteriorly. *Arch Otolaryngol* 1951; 54:524–533.
59. Blassingame CD. The suprahyoid approach to surgical lesions at the base of the tongue. *Ann Otol Rhinol Laryngol* 1952; 61:483–489.
60. Trotter W. A method of lateral pharyngotomy for the exposure of large growths in the epilaryngeal region. *J Laryngol Otol* 1920; 35:289–295.
61. Trotter W. Operation for malignant disease of the pharynx. *Br J Surg* 1929; 16:485–495.
62. Colledge L. Repair of pharyngeal defects after operation for removal of malignant tumors. *Proc R Soc Med* 1931; 24:14.
63. Orton HB. Cancer of the laryngopharynx. *Arch Otolaryngol* 1938; 28:344–354.
64. Colledge L. Treatment of carcinoma in pharynx and larynx and its results. *Br Med J* 1938; 2:167–168.
65. Barretto PM. Panel discussion. The historical development of laryngectomy. IV The South American contribution to the surgery of laryngeal cancer. *Laryngoscope* 1975; 85:299–321.
66. Alonso JM. Conservative surgery of cancer of the larynx. *Trans Am Acad Ophthalmol Otolaryngol* 1947; 51:633–642.
67. Alonso JM, Jackson CL. Conservation of function in surgery for cancer of the larynx: Bases, techniques and results. *Trans Am Acad Ophthalmol Otolaryngol* 1952; 56:722–725.
68. Ogura JH. Supraglottic subtotal laryngectomy and radical neck dissection for carcinoma of the epiglottis. *Laryngoscope* 1958; 68:983–1003.
69. Ogura JH, Jurema AA, Watson RK. Partial laryngopharyngectomy and neck dissection for pyriform sinus cancer. *Laryngoscope* 1960; 70:1399–1417.
70. Ogura JH, Mallen RW. Partial laryngopharyngectomy for supraglottic and pharyngeal carcinoma. *Trans Am Acad Ophthalmol Otolaryngol* 1965; 69:832–845.
71. Som ML. Surgical treatment of carcinoma of the epiglottis by lateral pharyngotomy. *Trans Am Acad Ophthalmol Otolaryngol* 1959; 63:28–49.
72. Bocca E, Pignataro O, Mosciaro O. Supraglottic surgery of the larynx. *Ann Otol Rhinol Laryngol* 1968; 77:1005–1026.
73. McInnis WD, Egan W, Aust JB. The management of carcinoma of the larynx in a prominent patient, or did Morell MacKenzie really cause World War I? *Am J Surg* 1976; 132:512–522.
74. MacKenzie M. *Diseases of the Throat and Nose.* London, J & A Churchill, Vol I, 1880; Vol II, 1884.
75. Pahor AL. Tracheostomy. *J R Soc Med* 1993; 86:308. Letter to Editor.
76. Gerhardt E, von Bergmann E, Landgraf, et al. *Die Krankheit Kaiser Friedrich des Dritten.* Berlin, 1888.
77. MacKenzie M. *The Fatal Illness of Frederick the Noble.* London, Sampson Low, Marston Seale and Rivington Limited, 1888.

Chapter 2

Surgical Anatomy
Carl E. Silver

The following discussion makes no attempt at being a comprehensive treatise or even a beginner's textbook on the anatomy of the larynx. Such information is readily obtainable from the standard references on the subject.[1, 2, 3] Detailed discussions of laryngeal anatomy are also provided in Myerson's[4] and Tucker's[5] monographs on the human larynx. Descriptions of many fundamental anatomic features have therefore been omitted on the assumption that the reader has a basic medical school knowledge of laryngeal anatomy; detailed descriptions of features that are of interest only to anatomists have also been omitted.

The anatomic features that are presented are considered particularly important to the surgeon for performance of laryngeal surgery, for understanding the mechanism and routes of cancer spread in the larynx, and for being the basis for various forms of conservation surgery.

EXTERNAL FEATURES

The larynx is situated in the midline compartment of the neck, deep to the infrahyoid ("strap" or "ribbon") muscles (Fig. 2–1). The sternohyoids, or the more external of these muscles, insert on the body of the hyoid bone. The thinner and broader sternothyroid muscles are deep to the sternohyoids and insert on each side, on the oblique line of the thyroid ala. The thyrohyoid muscles arise from the oblique lines and insert into the lower border of the greater cornu of the hyoid bone, and the inferior constrictor muscles insert laterally into the oblique line and meet in a posterior midline raphe. The omohyoid muscles are in the same plane as the sternohyoids, inserting into the body of the hyoid bone lateral to the sternohyoids. The central tendon of the omohyoid crosses immediately superficial to the carotid sheath. During dissection this provides a useful landmark for safely dividing the supraclavicular soft tissue, including the sternomastoid muscles, because there are no important structures that cross superficial to the omohyoid muscles.

The mylohyoid and geniohyoid muscles arise from the superior border of the body of the hyoid bone, while the hyoglossus muscles arise from the greater cornua. The "slings" of the digastric muscles insert on the lesser cornua of the hyoid bone.

The hyoid bone, thyroid prominence, and cricoid

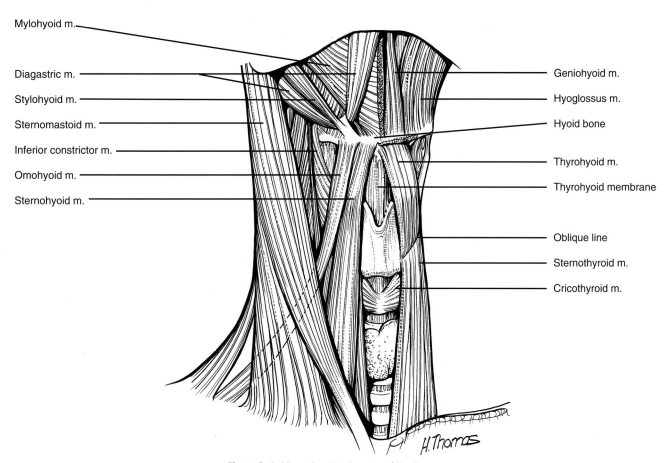

Figure 2–1. Muscular attachments of the larynx.

cartilage are generally palpable in the midline anteriorly (Fig. 2–2). Prior to commencing an operation on the larynx, the cervical trachea, or the thyroid gland, it is useful for the surgeon to palpate these landmarks, particularly the cricoid cartilage, which causes a prominent bulge. The thyroid isthmus crosses immediately below the cricoid cartilage, corresponding to the location of the upper tracheal rings. By carefully identifying the cricoid cartilage, the surgeon can avoid inadvertent placement of a tracheostomy either too high or too low. The level of the laryngotracheal structures can vary considerably. In a young patient with a long, thin neck the cricoid may be surprisingly high, whereas in an elderly "barrel chested" individual the laryngeal prominence may be barely palpable above the sternal notch. Proper orientation with regard to the level of the larynx, the hyoid bone, and the trachea greatly facilitates accurate placement of incisions, stomas, and planned fistulae.

MUCOSAL SURFACE FEATURES

The cavity of the larynx connects the laryngopharynx with the trachea. It is divided into glottic, supraglottic, and subglottic regions. The glottis consists of the true vocal cords, the anterior commissure, and the posterior commissure. The narrow, triangular space between the true vocal cords is called the rima glottis. The anterior two thirds of the vocal cords, called the membranous portions, insert into the midline of the thyroid cartilage at the anterior commissure. The level of the insertion at the anterior commissure is half the distance between the bottom of the thyroid notch and the bottom of the thyroid cartilage, at the midline. The membranous portions of the vocal cords are composed entirely of soft tissue, consisting of the vocal ligaments, covered by mucosa. The posterior third of the vocal cords consists of the vocal processes of the arytenoid cartilages covered by mucosa. The

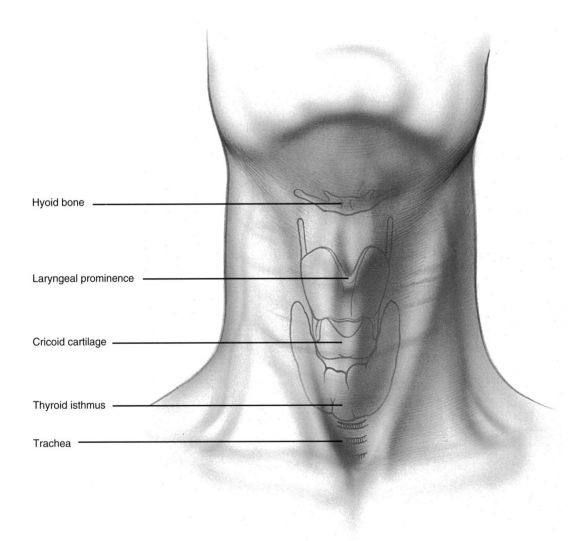

Hyoid bone

Laryngeal prominence

Cricoid cartilage

Thyroid isthmus

Trachea

Figure 2–2. Palpable landmarks of the larynx.

portion of the glottis containing the posterior thirds of both of the vocal cords and the posterior (interarytenoid) mucosa between them is called the posterior commissure (Fig. 2–3).

The supraglottic region contains the ventricles, the ventricular bands (false vocal cords), the epiglottis (both its lingual and laryngeal surfaces), and the aryepiglottic folds, as well as the expanse of supraglottic mucosa covering the arytenoids and extending from the false cords to the aryepiglottic folds. Most of the mucosal surface of the supraglottic region covers the epiglottis; thus, the majority of supraglottic tumors are epiglottic.

Unfortunately there are no precisely defined

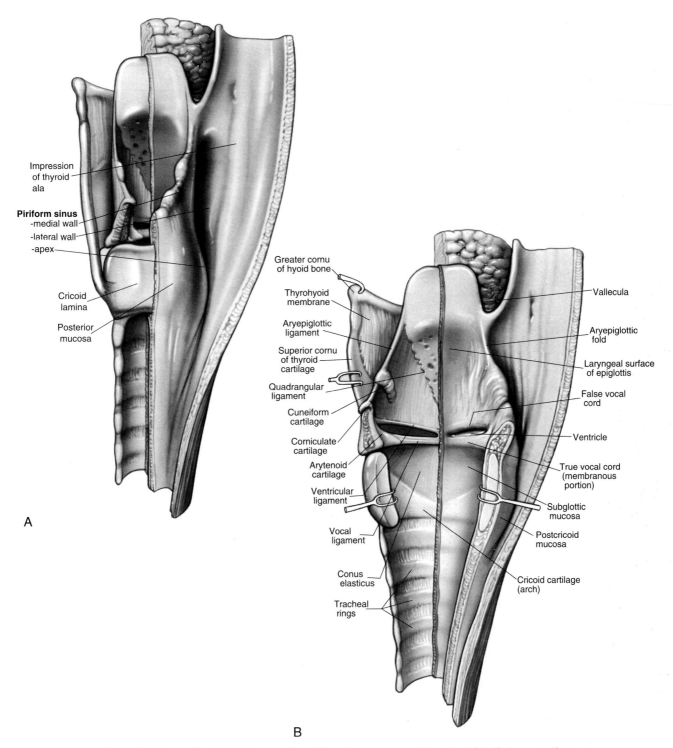

Figure 2–3. Larynx bisected in the posterior midline. Mucosa removed from the left half, demonstrating the relationship between mucosal features and underlying ligaments and cartilages.

boundaries within the larynx. The subglottic area, in particular, is not easy to define; it comprises the area at which the larynx merges with the trachea. The superior boundary of the subglottic region is arbitrary. Some suggest that the subglottic region is the area between the inferior border of the vocal folds and the inferior margin of the cricoid cartilage, including the areas caudal to the anterior and posterior commissures. Others consider it as beginning at the level of the conus elasticus (about 5 mm below the free margins of the vocal cords) and extending to the inferior border of the cricoid cartilage.

The subglottic region consists of a mobile upper half and a fixed lower half. The upper portion is formed by the mucosa over the conus elasticus, which covers the thyroarytenoid muscle. Mobility is caused by abduction or adduction of the vocal cords and the action of the muscles. During phonation,

the upper half of the subglottic region assumes the shape of a "Gothic arch"; this is nicely demonstrated by imaging in the coronal plane with techniques such as laryngography or polytomography, which were employed in the past, or by the current technique of magnetic resonance imaging. Subglottic extension of a glottic tumor disturbs the symmetry of this arch and is thus evident radiographically. The lower or fixed half of the subglottic space is lined by the mucosa on the inner aspect of the cricoid cartilage. The junction between the two parts is 1 cm below the vocal cord, coinciding with the cricothyroid membrane.

The mucosa of the glottis, the anterior surface of the epiglottis, and the upper half of the posterior surface of the epiglottis are covered with stratified squamous epithelium. The inferior half of the posterior surface of the epiglottis, the ventricles, and the subglottic region are lined with pseudostratified

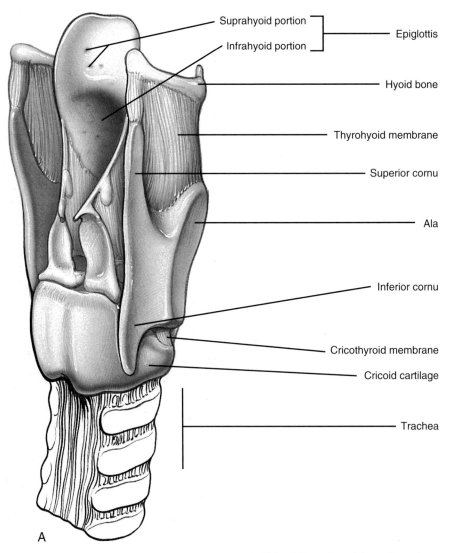

Figure 2–4. Laryngeal cartilages, ligaments, and spaces. *A.* Right oblique view with cartilages intact.

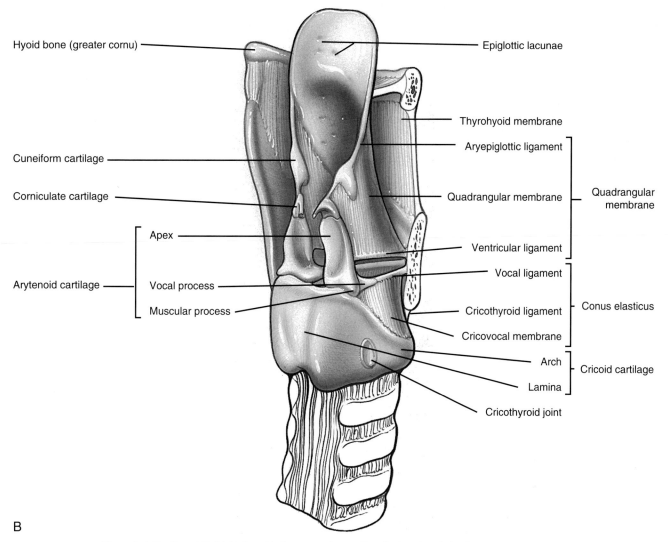

Hyoid bone (greater cornu)

Cuneiform cartilage

Corniculate cartilage

Apex

Arytenoid cartilage

Vocal process

Muscular process

Epiglottic lacunae

Thyrohyoid membrane

Aryepiglottic ligament

Quadrangular membrane

Quadrangular membrane

Ventricular ligament

Vocal ligament

Cricothyroid ligament

Cricovocal membrane

Conus elasticus

Arch

Cricoid cartilage

Lamina

Cricothyroid joint

B

Figure 2–4 *Continued B.* Right thyroid ala removed, revealing the interior of the right paraglottic space.

Illustration continued on following page

ciliated epithelium. Scattered islets of metaplastic squamous epithelium are often found in the larynx. The supraglottic and subglottic regions (particularly the ventricles and saccules) are rich in sero-mucous glands, which are scanty in the vocal cords and their immediate vicinity.

LARYNGEAL CARTILAGES

The framework of the larynx consists of nine cartilages—three single (the epiglottic, the thyroid, and the cricoid cartilages) and three paired (the arytenoid, the cuneiform, and the corniculate cartilages). Histologically, all the major cartilages (except for the epiglottic cartilage and the medial edge and tip of the arytenoid cartilage) are composed of hyaline cartilage.[6] The large single thyroid cartilage is shield shaped, open posteriorly, and angulated in

the front. The angulation is more acute and the protrusion of the thyroid prominence in the midline is greater in males than in females. The thyroid cartilage is aptly named. Its function is to shield the larynx from injury and also to provide an attachment for the vocal ligaments (Fig. 2–4).

The cricoid cartilage is a single signet ring–shaped cartilage that is thicker and stronger than the thyroid cartilage. The posterior portion, or lamina, measures 2 to 3 cm from the top down, being considerably broader and deeper than the anterior arch, which measures 5 to 7 mm vertically. The cricoid cartilage is the most important structure in the larynx from a functional and surgical point of view. It serves as a base or platform for the entire larynx. The arytenoid cartilages, which move the vocal cords, articulate with and are supported by the rostrum of the cricoid lamina. The intrinsic muscles of the larynx arise on the cricoid cartilage

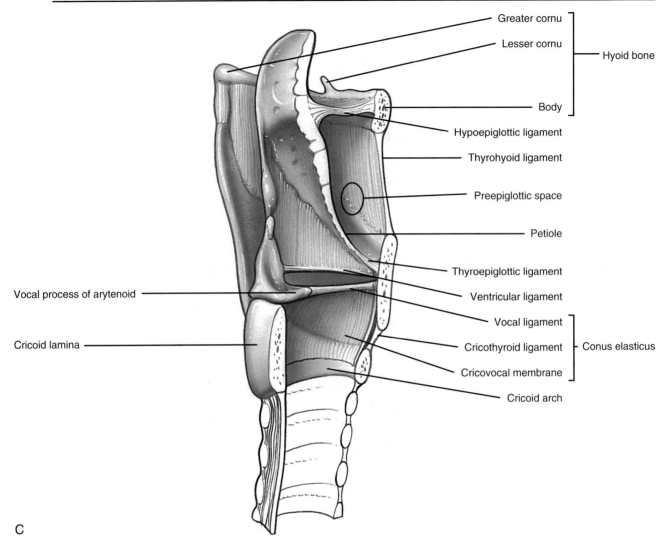

Figure 2–4 *Continued C.* Larynx bisected in the sagittal plane demonstrating the preepiglottic space.

and insert on the arytenoid cartilages, causing them to rotate, and the vocal cords thereby to adduct and abduct.

The cricoid cartilage is the only part of the cartilaginous framework of the respiratory tract that forms a continuous 360° ring of cartilage. This renders this cartilage and its underlying mucosa particularly susceptible to ischemic injury from a tightly fitting endotracheal tube. The rigid cartilaginous ring cannot expand to relieve pressure should mucosal edema occur. If the cricoid cartilage is injured or strictured, it is difficult to resect it and also preserve laryngeal function because it is critical in supporting the various laryngeal structures and also because of the proximity of the recurrent laryngeal nerves.

The paired arytenoid cartilages are pyramidal, each having three surfaces, a base, and an apex. The base of each arytenoid cartilage articulates with the cricoid cartilage in the manner already described. The important lateral and posterior cricoarytenoid muscles insert on the muscular process formed by the lateral angle of the arytenoid cartilage. The anterior angle is elongated into the vocal process, which receives the insertion of the vocal ligament and, as noted, comprises the posterior third of the vocal cord.

The epiglottis is a thin, leaf-shaped fibrocartilage situated in the anterior midline behind the angle of the thyroid cartilage and projecting upward behind the base of the tongue. The upper, free end is broad and rounded. The narrow base, called the petiole, is attached to the midline of the thyroid cartilage by the thyroepiglottic ligament. This attachment, which forms the lower limit to the preepiglottic space, is situated above the anterior commissure, a fact that has considerable surgical significance (see discussion of supraglottic tumors and supraglottic subtotal laryngectomy).

About half of the epiglottis projects above the

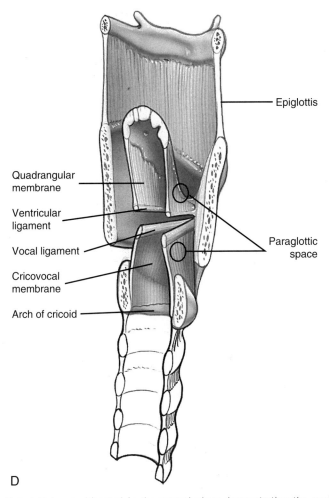

Epiglottis

Quadrangular
membrane

Ventricular
ligament

Vocal ligament

Cricovocal
membrane

Arch of cricoid

Paraglottic
space

D

Figure 2–4 *Continued D.* Larynx bisected in the coronal plane demonstrating the medial and lateral walls of the paraglottic spaces.

Illustration continued on following page

hyoid bone and is called the suprahyoid portion. This portion of cartilage is covered with mucosa on both sides and thus has a lingual surface and a laryngeal surface. The infrahyoid portion of the epiglottis has no free anterior surface. Instead, it forms the posterior wall of the preepiglottic space. The epiglottic cartilage contains many pits, or lacunae, which are filled with mucous glands, and thus provides little cartilaginous barrier between the infrahyoid portion of the laryngeal surface of the epiglottis and the preepiglottic space. The significance of this will be discussed in detail in subsequent chapters. It can also be seen that small tumors confined to the suprahyoid portion of the epiglottis do not have the same potential for preepiglottic spread as do tumors of the infrahyoid portion.

The paired corniculate and cuneiform cartilages are essentially vestigial structures situated within the aryepiglottic folds at the tips of the arytenoids. Their only surgical significance is that they tend to thicken the aryepiglottic folds, which are used for resurfacing the larynx after vertical hemilaryngectomy. Failure to thin the folds by excising the corniculate and cuneiform cartilages may result in some glottic obstruction from redundant mucosa.

NERVES AND VESSELS

The larynx has superior and inferior neurovascular pedicles. The superior pedicle consists of the superior laryngeal artery, which is a branch of the superior thyroid artery (a branch of the external carotid artery), the accompanying vein with the common facial artery, and the internal branch of the superior laryngeal nerve (Fig. 2–5). This pedicle enters the thyrohyoid membrane laterally and is best approached by mobilizing the superior cornu of the thyroid cartilage during dissection. The internal laryngeal nerves extend inferiorly anterior to the mucosa of the pyriform sinuses, where they can be topically anesthetized. These nerves are the sensory

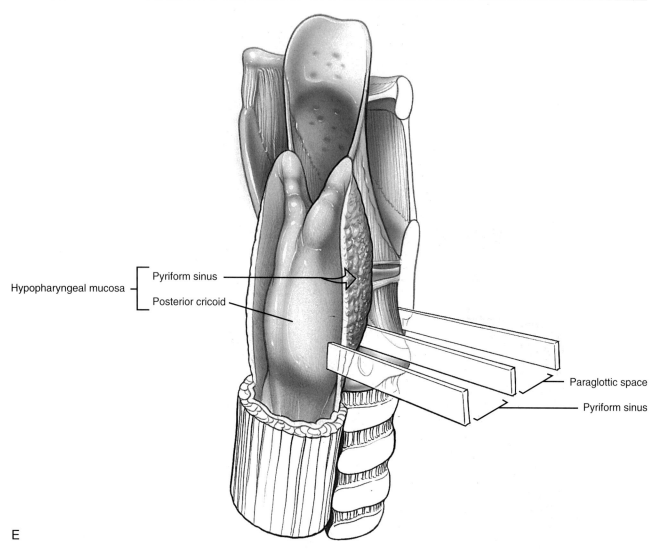

Hypopharyngeal mucosa — [Pyriform sinus

Posterior cricoid]

Paraglottic space

Pyriform sinus

E

Figure 2–4 *Continued E.* Hypopharyngeal mucosa shown in relation to the laryngeal framework. Note that the pyriform sinus forms the posterior wall of the paraglottic space.

nerves of the larynx. The cricothyroid muscles are innervated by the external branch of the superior laryngeal nerve and act to lengthen the glottis and therefore increase the tension of the vocal cords during phonation. Therefore, the consequence of injury to this nerve is a slight "bowing" of the vocal cords and hoarseness due to loss of tension of the cords.

The intrinsic muscles of the larynx are supplied by the recurrent or inferior laryngeal nerves. These mixed motor and sensory nerves also supply the esophagus, trachea, and inferior constrictor muscles. The nerves divide into anterior and posterior branches, which ascend at the lateral borders of the trachea, posterior to the thyroid gland, run deep to the cricothyroid muscles, and enter the larynx behind the cricothyroid joints. The inferior vascular supply is from branches of the inferior thyroid arteries, which closely parallel the nerves.

PYRIFORM SINUS MUCOSA

The mucosa of the pyriform sinus is reflected between the thyroid and cricoid cartilages posteriorly (see Fig. 2–4E). Removal of the posterior third of the thyroid ala will reveal the external aspect of the pyriform sinus, wider superiorly than inferiorly. The mucosa may be reflected posteriorly, revealing the cricoid lamina and the arytenoid. At surgery, incision of the inferior constrictor muscle over the posterior free border of the thyroid ala provides an approach to the pyriform sinus. Reflection of the mucosa from the cartilages permits preservation of

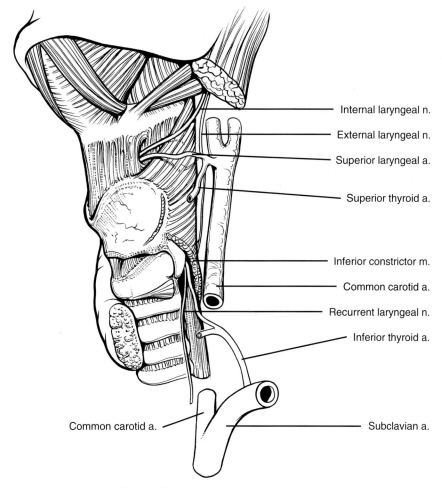

Figure 2–5. Vessels and nerves of the larynx.

- Internal laryngeal n.
- External laryngeal n.
- Superior laryngeal a.
- Superior thyroid a.
- Inferior constrictor m.
- Common carotid a.
- Recurrent laryngeal n.
- Inferior thyroid a.
- Subclavian a.
- Common carotid a.

uninvolved pyriform sinus mucosa during partial and total laryngectomy and an approach to the cricoarytenoid region for external arytenoidectomy. An oblique, vertical, posterior-third thyrotomy also provides access for partial pharyngolaryngectomy for tumors of the posterolateral or lateral walls of the hypopharynx.

LARYNGEAL CONNECTIVE TISSUE COMPARTMENTS

Beneath the laryngeal mucosa, the framework of the larynx consists of cartilages bound together by the intrinsic ligaments of the larynx (Fig. 2–6; see Fig. 2–4). These intrinsic ligaments are portions of a broad sheath of fibrous tissue containing many elastic fibers, which is well developed in some areas and rudimentary in others. The better-developed, lower portion (or conus elasticus) is separated from the less well developed upper portion (the quadran-

gular membrane) by the ventricles, where elastic tissue is almost absent.

The technique of whole organ serial section of the larynx developed by Tucker[7] has enabled accurate study of the relationship of the ligamentous, cartilaginous, and mucosal structures within the larynx. These connective tissue structures form barriers that divide the larynx into various compartments and serve to guide and limit the spread of cancer within the larynx. Tucker and Smith[8] have accurately delineated the various laryngeal connective tissue barriers and compartments by the study of whole organ sections at various stages of fetal development.

Intrinsic Ligaments

The conus elasticus, or cricovocal membrane, consists mainly of yellow elastic tissue. The anterior portion is fused with the median cricothyroid ligament in the midline of the thyroid cartilage and radiates to the vocal processes of the arytenoid car-

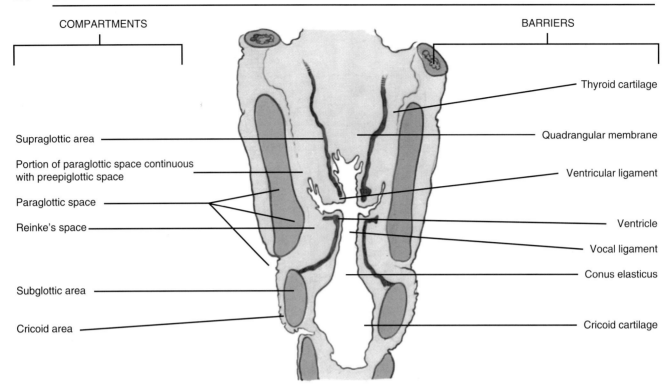

COMPARTMENTS

BARRIERS

Supraglottic area

Portion of paraglottic space continuous with preepiglottic space

Paraglottic space

Reinke's space

Subglottic area

Cricoid area

Thyroid cartilage

Quadrangular membrane

Ventricular ligament

Ventricle

Vocal ligament

Conus elasticus

Cricoid cartilage

Figure 2–6. Connective tissue compartments and barriers of the larynx.

tilages. The thickened upper borders of the conus extending from the anterior commissure to the vocal processes are the vocal ligaments. The thinner lateral portions of the conus extend from the superior border of the cricoid cartilage to the vocal ligaments with which they are continuous. The vocal ligaments are attached to the thyroid cartilage by the anterior commissure tendon, as described by Ridpath[9] and Broyles.[10] Broyles described the tendon as a band of fibrous tissue containing both lymph and blood vessels and thickened on both sides of the midline to receive the attachments of the various ligaments, membranes, and muscles of both sides of the larynx. The insertion directly into the thyroid cartilage is thought to account for the frequent involvement of the cartilage with tumor when the tendon is affected.

The elastic tissue is least evident in the region of the ventricle, except for a relatively heavy layer fanning out from the lateral margins of the vocal ligaments toward the internal perichondrium of the thyroid cartilage. This elastic layer beneath the floor of the ventricle corresponds roughly to the division between glottic and supraglottic portions of the larynx. The quadrangular ligaments are attached anteriorly to the lateral borders of the epiglottis and extend on both sides posteriorly to the medial surfaces of the arytenoid cartilages. The fibers are continuous with the aryepiglottic liga-

ments superiorly and the ventricular ligaments inferiorly.

Laryngeal Compartments

The ligaments, membranes, and skeletal structures present in the larynx delineate various spaces and compartments. These include Reinke's space, the supraglottic and subglottic spaces, the cricoid space, and the preepiglottic and paraglottic spaces.

Reinke's Space. The mucosa over the vocal ligaments is attached loosely to the ligaments themselves (see Figs. 2–4 and 2–6). There is, therefore, a submucosal space along almost the entire length of the free edge of the true vocal cord, extending slightly onto the superior surface. Pressman and associates[11] noted that injected dyes were confined to this space, which they called the laryngeal bursa.

Supraglottic Space. This is the area beneath the supraglottic mucosal surface of the lower edge of the vestibular ligaments and the petiole. This area is laterally limited in depth by the quadrangular membrane. The anatomic term "supraglottic space" must not be confused with the clinical term "supraglottic region."

Subglottic Space. This space extends from the vocal ligament and the elastic cone to the lower edge of the cricoid cartilage. It is a potential space, filled with fibroelastic submucosal tissue, between the mucosa and the conus elasticus. The subglottic space does not contain the vocal muscle, which is within the paraglottic space, deep to the conus elasticus.

Cricoid Space. This potential space contains the areolar tissue medial to the internal perichondrium of the cricoid cartilage. The compartment is situated between the subglottic area and the trachea.

Preepiglottic Space. This term is not synonymous with the "space of Boyer" (a term coined by Orton[5]), which is a bursa located anteriorly to the thyrohyoid membrane. The preepiglottic space lies anterior to the epiglottis and is bounded superiorly by the hyoepiglottic ligament, anteriorly by the thyrohyoid membrane and the thyroid cartilage, and posteriorly by the epiglottic cartilage and the thyroepiglottic ligament. The space is filled with fat and areolar tissue anterior and lateral to the epiglottis and it contains the saccule. This space is adjacent posteroinferiorly to the paraglottic space, from which it is separated by fibrous tissue (the so-called thyroglottic ligament), whereas posterosuperiorly the two spaces are not clearly distinguishable from each other.[12] Cancer on the laryngeal surface of the epiglottis spreads readily into the preepiglottic space.

Paraglottic Space. The submucosa of the ventricle is continuous with the paraglottic space, which is bounded by the conus elasticus below and the thyroid cartilage laterally. Above the ventricle, the paraglottic space is separated from the supraglottic space by the quadrangular membrane. The posterior limit of the paraglottic space is the mucosa of the pyriform sinus. Inferolaterally the paraglottic space is continuous with the cartilaginous defect between the thyroid and the cricoid cartilages (the cricothyroid space). The anatomic relationships of the paraglottic space are in keeping with the observation of Pressman et al.[13] that dyes injected into the ventricle spread extensively above and below the glottis deep to the mucosa. The paraglottic space has great significance in determining the spread of cancer within the larynx. Tumors involving the ventricle invade the paraglottic space and thus spread transglottically. Vocal cord tumors, which extend deep into the thyroarytenoid muscle, invade the paraglottic space with resultant potential subglottic and extralaryngeal spread. Lateral supraglottic tumors can travel laterally to the ventricle, along the inner surface of the thyroid ala, and thus spread subglottically. The proximity of pyriform sinus mucosa to the posterior paraglottic space makes this a potential route for spread of pyriform sinus carcinoma into the endolarynx, resulting often in fixation of the hemilarynx. Conversely, as noted by Tucker,[14] endolaryngeal carcinomas with paraglottic space involvement often resemble "icebergs" at the pyriform sinus mucosa. Thus, even in the absence of tumor of the pyriform mucosa, the preservation of this mucosa on the same side as an endolaryngeal lesion with fixed vocal cord during laryngectomy may place the plane of dissection too close to the paraglottic extent of the tumor.

LARYNGEAL INJECTION STUDIES

In the nineteenth century, Hajek[15] noted that laryngeal edema tended to remain localized in various portions of the larynx. Searching for the anatomic basis for this phenomenon, he demonstrated that a fluid injected into the human larynx was indeed confined to localized compartments beneath the mucosa. A sharp boundary could be demonstrated along the inferior edge of the false vocal cord; this prevented involvement of the vocal cords despite massive injections of fluid into the supraglottic region.

Pressman and his group[11, 13, 16] performed a sophisticated and comprehensive evaluation of the submucosal compartments and lymphatics of the larynx by injecting dyes and radioisotopes into living as well as cadaver human, canine, and porcine larynges. These studies were originally intended to serve as a guide for possible routes of therapeutic injection of radioisotopes into the larynx for the treatment of cancer. Pressman wished to establish that multiple injections would be required because of the anatomic compartmentalization. Although this modality of treatment never became clinically useful, the studies provided excellent documentation of the anatomic compartments and lymphatic flow within the larynx and afforded considerable insight into the nature of cancer spread within the larynx. The compartments demonstrated by Pressman and his colleagues in their injection studies of the 1950s correlated closely with the previously discussed connective tissue barriers and compartments demonstrated by Tucker's serial studies of the early 1960s.

Pressman and his colleagues demonstrated that the larynx is a highly compartmentalized organ with a physiologic and anatomic separation of the right and left halves, except on the mucous membrane surfaces. The compartments in which dye injections were confined were the following: the supraglottic compartment, including the aryepiglottic folds and ventricles; the ventricles; the margins of the true vocal cords; the subglottic area overlying the intrinsic muscles; and the cricoid area. The compartments on each side of the larynx were found to be totally independent of those on the opposite side, so that dyes injected on one side did not cross the midline.

Lymph flow was studied by in vivo injection of dyes and radioisotopes. The laryngeal lymphatics were found to consist of a superficial, intramucosal group and a deep, submucosal group. The superficial lymphatics formed an interlacing web spreading over the entire mucosal surface without compartmentalization. Conversely, the submucosal or deep lymphatics of each side were independent of each other, with practically no interconnection between the two sides. Radioisotope injected submucosally on one side of the larynx revealed no crossover beyond the midline for as long as 8 weeks after the injection, although the isotope entered the general lymphatic circulation rapidly and could be readily detected in the cervical nodes. Lymphatic drainage tended to be predominantly ipsilateral, except for that from the lowermost levels of the subglottic area. Lymphatic flow within the larynx was always cephalad, as opposed to tracheal lymphatic flow, which was always downward.

Lymphatic drainage from the lower levels of the larynx merged through the cricothyroid membrane into the cervical lymphatics, whereas lymphatic drainage from the higher levels was through the thyrohyoid membrane. When the lymphatic system of the homolateral side was surgically isolated from the larynx, injected dyes were recovered from the contralateral side.

Dyes injected into the free margin of the vocal cord remained confined to that space (Reinke's space), indicating the lack of communication of the lymphatics of this area with the general lymphatic circulation. Dyes injected into the ventricle did not appear on the surface of the larynx but spread deeply and widely between the soft tissue and the thyroid cartilage (paraglottic space) and then appeared in the tissues external to the larynx by direct extension through the cricothyroid membrane as well as the lymphatics. Pressman's group felt that studies on a large number of laryngeal cancers indicated that the disease was disseminated both within and beyond the larynx by direct extension as well as via lymphatic pathways and that the pattern of dissemination corresponded well to the observations emerging from the injection studies.

In 1989, Welsh and colleagues[17] used massive dye infusion techniques in 12 intact postmortem human larynges of young individuals and found that the supraglottic infusions paralleled the internal perichondrium and dissected inferiorly along the deep aspect of the vocal chord toward the supraglottic area. These authors postulated that large supraglottic cancers expand caudad. Essentially, the compartmentalization of the larynx tends to interfere with the spread of early carcinomas, but once these lesions enlarge, spread can readily occur beyond the site of origin.

REFERENCES

1. Berkovitz BKB, Hickey SA, Moxham BJ. Embryology and anatomy. *In* Ferlito A (ed): *Neoplasms of the Larynx,* pp 27–48. Edinburgh, Churchill Livingstone, 1993.
2. Grant JB. *An Atlas of Anatomy,* 3rd ed. Baltimore, Williams & Wilkins, 1951.
3. Gray H. *Anatomy of the Human Body,* 28th ed. Philadelphia, Lea & Febiger, 1966.
4. Myerson MC. *The Human Larynx.* Springfield, Charles C Thomas, 1964.
5. Tucker GF Jr. *Human Larynx Coronal Section Atlas.* Washington D.C., Armed Forces Institute of Pathology, 1971.
6. Cohen SR, Perelman N, Nimni ME, et al. Whole organs evaluation of collagen in the developing human larynx and adjoining anatomic structures (hyoid and trachea). *Ann Otol Rhinol Laryngol* 1993; 102:655–659.
7. Tucker GF Jr. A histological method for the study of the spread of carcinoma within the larynx. *Ann Otol Rhinol Laryngol* 1961; 70:910–921.
8. Tucker GF, Smith H. A histological demonstration of the development of laryngeal connective tissue compartments. *Trans Am Acad Ophthalmol Otolaryngol* 1962; 66:308–318.
9. Ridpath RF. Diseases of the larynx: Anatomy of the larynx. Part IV. *In* Jackson C, Coates GM (eds): *The Nose, Throat and Ear and Their Diseases.* Philadelphia, Saunders, 1929.
10. Broyles EN. The anterior commissure tendon. *Ann Otol Rhinol Laryngol* 1943; 52:342–345.
11. Pressman JJ, Dowdy A, Libby R. Further studies upon the submucosal compartments and lymphatics of the larynx by injection of dyes and radio-isotopes. *Ann Otol Rhinol Laryngol* 1956; 65:963–980.
12. Sato K, Kurita S, Hirano M. Location of the preepiglottic space and its relationship to the paraglottic space. *Ann Otol Rhinol Laryngol* 1993; 102:930–934.
13. Pressman JJ, Simon MD, Monell C. Anatomical studies related to the dissemination of cancer of the larynx. *Trans Am Acad Ophthalmol Otolaryngol* 1960; 64:628–638.
14. Tucker GF Jr. Some clinical inferences from the study of serial laryngeal sections. *Laryngoscope* 1963; 73:728–748.
15. Hajek M. Anatomische Untersuchungen über das Larynxödem. *Arch Klin Chir* 1891; 42:46–93.
16. Pressman JJ. Submucosal compartmentation of the larynx. *Ann Otol Rhinol Laryngol* 1956; 65:766–771.
17. Welsh LW, Welsh JJ, Rizzo TA. Internal anatomy of the larynx and the spread of cancer. *Ann Otol Rhinol Laryngol* 1989; 98:228–234.

Chapter 3

Squamous Cell Carcinoma and Its Precursors

Alfio Ferlito and Carl E. Silver

Approximately 85% to 90% of laryngeal malignancies are squamous cell carcinomas, ranging from the well differentiated through the poorly differentiated. Thus, study of the pathogenesis and natural history of this type of neoplasm is of fundamental importance in establishing treatment modalities and surgical procedures for management of laryngeal cancer.

ABERRATIONS OF SQUAMOUS EPITHELIUM

The stratified squamous epithelium of the upper aerodigestive tract is subject to a spectrum of abnormal epithelial proliferations, ranging from the various so-called premalignant lesions to frankly infiltrating squamous cell carcinoma. This field is complicated by considerable confusion in terminology, and it is therefore important to establish consistent definitions for the various epithelial lesions. The following terminology has evolved:

Leukoplakia. Leukoplakia means "white plaque" and is a clinical term describing any white lesion on a mucous membrane. The term cannot be considered a pathologic diagnosis and is not acceptable for biopsy reports by pathologists, although "premalignant leukoplakia" sometimes appears on reports.

Erythroplakia. Erythroplakia is a clinical term describing any reddish patch on the mucous membrane.

Erythroleukoplakia. Erythroleukoplakia is a clinical term for mixed forms of white and red mucosal changes. This term also is unsuitable as a diagnosis.[1]

Pachydermia. Pachydermia is a descriptive clinical term for large areas involved by leukoplakia. It should not be used in histologic diagnosis.

Hyperplasia. Hyperplasia refers to thickening of the epithelium caused by an increase in the prickle cell layer, basal cell layer, or both. This is a benign change that usually represents a response to injury and is reversible.

Squamous Metaplasia. Squamous metaplasia denotes the replacement of respiratory epithelium by stratified squamous epithelium. It is usually the result of persistent trauma or chronic irritation. There is no evidence that it is a potentially dangerous lesion.

Pseudoepitheliomatous Hyperplasia. Pseudoepitheliomatous hyperplasia is an exuberant and irregular overgrowth of squamous epithelium with epithelial extension in the stroma. This morphologic change may simulate well-differentiated squamous cell carcinoma. It is frequently associated with granular cell tumor but may also be associated with various specific chronic inflammatory conditions and mycotic diseases. There is no evidence that pseudoepitheliomatous hyperplasia is a potentially malignant lesion, and treatment depends on the nature of the subepithelial disease.

Keratosis. Keratosis is a pathologic feature resulting from the production of keratin on the surface of the epithelium. Squamous differentiation is well preserved, and a granular layer is often apparent. Keratinization may be without nuclei (orthokeratosis) or with nuclei (parakeratosis). Hyperplasia of the stratum spinosum (the prickle cell layer) (acanthosis) occurs with keratinization, and the proportions of acanthosis and keratinization can vary considerably. The basal membrane remains intact.[1, 2] There may be inflammatory cells in the lamina propria. Because the epithelium of the laryngeal mucosa is not normally keratinized, the term hyperkeratosis is redundant and should be avoided.[3] *Dyskeratosis* represents a faulty, premature keratinization of individual squamous cells.

Excisional biopsy or surgical stripping is generally a satisfactory form of treatment for keratosis. Although keratosis has been reported to have a potential for malignant transformation into cancer, it must not be regarded as a precancerous lesion from the histologic and photometric standpoints.[4] Keratosis may be associated with dysplasia (keratinizing dysplasia) or may occur on the surface of squamous cell carcinoma (keratinizing squamous cell carcinoma). Keratosis cannot be distinguished from carcinoma by clinical examination. Papillary keratosis may be confused with verrucous carcinoma.[5] In conclusion, simple keratosis is a lesion with no risk of progression.

Laryngeal Intraepithelial Neoplasia (LIN), Dysplasia, and Atypia. These are interchangeable terms describing the presence of atypical cytologic features in the laryngeal squamous epithelium. The lesion is characterized by a qualitative alteration toward malignancy in the appearance of the cells. The time-honored designation "dysplasia" has been largely replaced by the term "intraepithelial neoplasia" because the epithelial changes are considered a morphologic manifestation of a neoplastic process.[6]

Three grades of dysplasia are recognized, based on the degree of cellular atypia and structural alterations:

- mild or minimal dysplasia (LIN I)
- moderate dysplasia (LIN II)
- severe dysplasia and carcinoma in situ (LIN III)

Severe dysplasia and squamous cell carcinoma in situ are defined by Crissman et al.[7] as squamous intraepithelial neoplasia grade 3. Friedmann and Ferlito[1, 8] used the term "laryngeal intraepithelial neoplasia" to include both dysplasia and carcinoma in situ. Ferlito et al.[9] agreed with the notion that carcinoma in situ is a form of intraepithelial neoplasm and that the term "laryngeal intraepithelial neoplasia" (LIN) would encompass both carcinoma in situ and all grades of dysplasia. Other authors use the terms "high-grade dysplasia" and "carcinoma in situ" interchangeably in discussions of the esophagus and stomach.[10]

In carcinoma in situ, all layers of the epithelium are replaced by malignant cells. Stratification is lacking, and cellular polarity is often vertical.[11] The diagnosis of carcinoma in situ on the basis of a small biopsy specimen can be accepted only with reservation. Multiple sections should be processed in order to rule out an invasive lesion. Carcinoma in situ may occasionally occur as an isolated lesion, but it is more commonly associated with invasive cancer. Areas suggestive of carcinoma in situ have been found in spindle cell squamous carcinoma and in basaloid squamous cell carcinoma.

A fundamental distinction must be made among laryngeal epithelial abnormalities according to whether they show a significant risk of developing into an invasive neoplasm. Severe dysplasia and carcinoma in situ (LIN III) do carry this risk, whereas mucosal aberrations such as squamous metaplasia, squamous cell hyperplasia, and keratosis without atypia do not. These abnormalities of the surface epithelium have been erroneously considered to be premalignant, but prognosis is excellent. Hyperplastic, metaplastic, and dysplastic conditions are commonly found in the larynx in association with both in situ and invasive cancer. Unlike cancer of the uterine cervix, many carcinomas of the larynx do not go through the stage of carcinoma in situ and are invasive from the start.[1, 12]

LIN III lesions have an abnormal aneuploid DNA content indicating neoplastic transformation.[13] The changes occurring in laryngeal intraepithelial neoplasia are considered to be the morphologic manifestation of a neoplastic process and not those of a precancerous lesion.[14]

The diagnosis of LIN III on the basis of small biopsy specimens cannot be considered conclusive, and surgical specimens obtained by excisional biopsy should always be examined in order to establish a final diagnosis. Material obtained by stripping may not be adequate for a conclusive diagnosis. In a 1981 survey involving 52 otolaryngologists worldwide, Ferlito et al.[9] found a wide variation in treatment policy for laryngeal carcinoma in situ. Excisional biopsy with the carbon dioxide laser (that is, removal of the entire lesion together with a rim of healthy tissue) is ideal for the diagnosis and treatment of this lesion; if the margins are not free, reexcision or radiotherapy remain alternative options,[15] together with the elimination of all potential carcinogenic factors such as cigarette smoke, alcohol, and occupational factors. Radiotherapy has a definite but secondary role in the treatment of all cases of LIN. Close follow-up is required, especially during the first few years.[16, 17]

Microinvasive Carcinoma. Microinvasive carcinoma

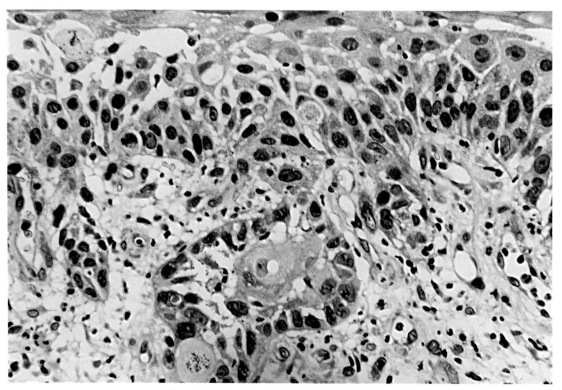

Figure 3–1. Microinvasive carcinoma of the larynx.

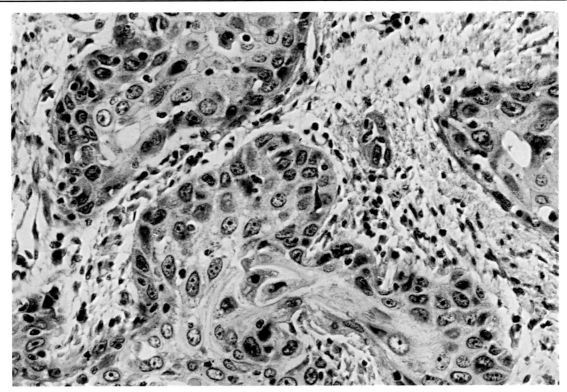

Figure 3–2. Moderately differentiated squamous cell carcinoma of the larynx.

is a term used to describe cases in which there is infiltration of the basement membrane with invasion into the underlying stroma (Fig. 3–1). Wenig[12] points out that this carcinoma is capable of metastasizing via either lymphatic or vascular channels.

Invasive Squamous Cell Carcinoma. Invasive squamous cell carcinoma is the most common malignancy arising in the larynx. This is a frankly malignant neoplasm that invades through the basement membrane and infiltrates the lamina propria and deeper tissues.

Well-differentiated squamous cell carcinoma is characterized by polygonal prickle cells, orderly stratification, clearly visible intercellular bridges, and keratinization with the formation of epithelial pearls. The nuclei are hyperchromatic and irregular in size and shape, and the nucleus/cytoplasm ratio is reduced. The connective tissue stroma is infiltrated with scattered nests or cords of malignant epithelial cells. There are few mitotic figures. The underlying stroma often contains a reactive inflammatory cellular infiltrate.

Moderately differentiated squamous cell carcinoma (Fig. 3–2) involves polygonal or prickle-type cells, stratification, and intercellular bridge formation. Epithelial pearls are scarce or absent. Mitoses are frequent and atypical.

Poorly differentiated squamous cell carcinoma (Fig. 3–3) consists of epithelial cells showing nuclear pleomorphism and hyperchromasia with

scanty but distinct intercellular bridge formation. Mitoses are atypical and abundant.

Squamous carcinoma usually arises from squamous epithelium or from respiratory epithelium (consisting of ciliated cells interspersed with goblet cells) that has undergone squamous metaplasia. Occasionally, it may arise directly from respiratory epithelium.

SPREAD OF LARYNGEAL CANCER

Laryngeal cancer may spread by direct infiltration or by the lymphatic (Fig. 3–4), hematogenous, and perineural routes. Tumor dissemination may be affected by various factors, such as the site of the primary neoplasm, the oncotype, the degree of cellular differentiation, and the presence or absence of any barriers to its spread (for example, perichondrium, ligaments, and fibroelastic membranes), as well as by certain biologic conditions (which are largely related to tumor-host relationships). All these factors may act independently or synergistically.[18, 19]

Spread of the Primary Laryngeal Cancer

Cancers of the larynx, in their early stages at least, are restrained by regional boundaries and partitions between compartments,[20] which were first studied by Pressman in 1956[21] using a dye injection technique. Whole-organ sections of laryngectomy specimens have led to a better understand-

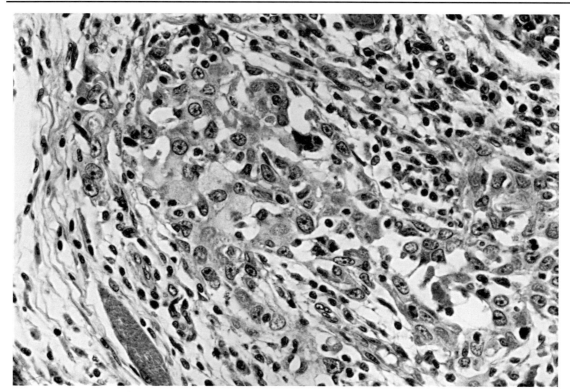

Figure 3–3. Poorly differentiated squamous cell carcinoma of the larynx.

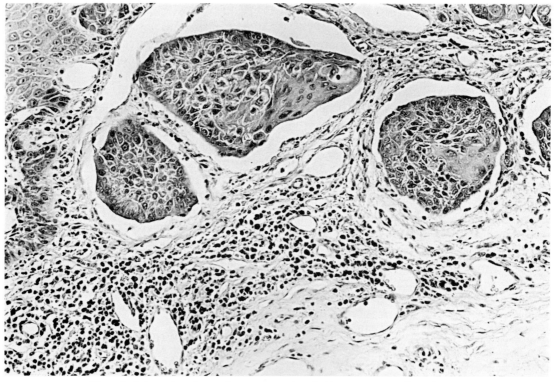

Figure 3–4. Some lymph vascular spaces are invaded by squamous cell carcinoma.

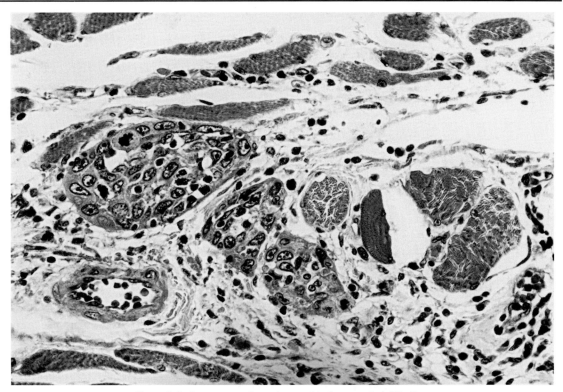

Figure 3–5. Squamous cell carcinoma showing muscle infiltration.

ing of tumor growth and spread,[22–43] but establishing the origin of the lesion is often arbitrary, especially for advanced lesions. Laryngeal cancer spreads in three dimensions, and the tumor may infiltrate the anatomic boundaries of the organ in various places.[38]

The principal structures forming a barrier to tumor spread are the hyoepiglottic ligament, the conus elasticus, and the nonossified cartilages with their perichondrium. The fibrous sheet, the so-called thyroepiglottic ligament, separating the paraglottic space and the preepiglottic space offers some resistance to tumor invasion in the early stages of laryngeal cancer[44] but is not a significant barrier.[45] Glandular structures may facilitate tumor spread. Muscle fibers are easily dissociated by neoplastic infiltration (Fig. 3–5). The tumor may extend directly into the adjacent normal structures, and it may infiltrate the valleculae, hypopharynx, thyroid, and trachea. Occasionally, the neoplasm may invade the prelaryngeal muscles, subcutaneous tissues, and overlying skin.

The growth and spread of laryngeal cancer is determined by its site of origin.

Glottic Tumors

Cancer of the vocal cords originating on the free margin of the anterior half spreads initially on the surface along the length of the cord. The progress of this tumor is usually slow and predictable. The anterior commissure and the contralateral cord may be invaded. Occasionally, the tumor may grow posteriorly, involving the vocal process or the anterior face of the arytenoid cartilage. In a few instances glottic cancer may involve the posterior commissure and the mucosa overlying the posterior plate of the cricoid cartilage.[46] The tumor may extend upward into the ventricle and vestibular fold and downward into the subglottic region, eventually escaping the confines of the larynx through the cricothyroid membrane.[41] Glottic cancer with more than 1 cm of subglottic extension tends to invade cartilage.[34]

Cancer of the anterior commissure spreads in all directions, involving both vocal cords, the ventricle, the ventricular fold, the base of the epiglottis, and the subglottis. Not uncommonly, cancer of the anterior commissure invades the lower margin of the thyroid ala and extends outside the laryngeal framework through the cricothyroid membrane. There may be infiltration of the Delphian lymph nodes.[42, 47] Squamous cell carcinoma of the vocal cord may be associated with areas of carcinoma in situ, dysplasia, and metaplasia.

Supraglottic Tumors

The behavior of supraglottic cancer is influenced by whether the tumors are exophytic or ulcerative, and by whether they primarily involve the epiglottis

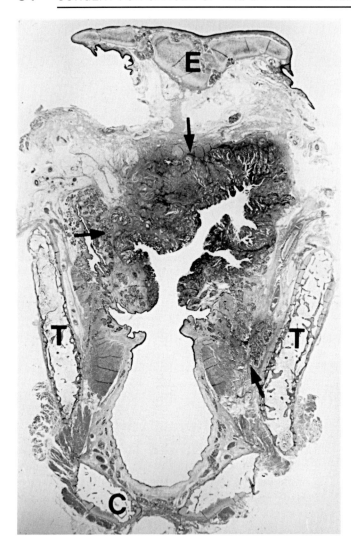

Figure 3–6. Supraglottic cancer with extension to the glottic region. This coronal section through the anterior part of the vocal cords shows a tumor that extends on the right side down into the vocal cord. C, cricoid cartilage; E, epiglottis; T, thyroid cartilage. Arrows indicate the extent of the tumor. (Courtesy of Prof. J. Olofsson.)

or the more posterior and lateral aspects of the supraglottic region (the false cords, arytenoid cartilages, and aryepiglottic folds). Thus, supraglottic cancers have been divided into suprahyoid laryngeal cancers (involving the suprahyoid epiglottis, aryepiglottic fold, and arytenoid cartilages) and infrahyoid laryngeal cancers (involving the infrahyoid epiglottis, ventricular fold, and ventricle). Infrahyoid cancers are more common and display a clear tendency to spread into the fatty areolar tissue of the preepiglottic space.[23, 28, 42] The tendency for invasion of the preepiglottic space has also been observed histologically in specimens of epiglottic cancer originally staged as T1 and T2.[48] Gregor[45] believes that tumor invasion of this space justifies a T4 classification, although both the International Union Against Cancer (IUAC) and the American Joint Committee for Cancer Staging and End Results Reporting (AJCC) imply a T3 grading for tumor invading this space.

The route of invasion of the preepiglottic space is through the lacunae or natural fenestrae in the epiglottic cartilage, which are normally filled with mucous glands. A less frequent route is laterally around the edge of the epiglottis. Kirchner[34] has emphasized that, anatomically, the entire preepiglottic space is confined to the supraglottic portion of the larynx, bounded posteriorly by the epiglottic cartilage and the thyroepiglottic ligament, anteriorly by the thyrohyoid membrane and the hyoid bone, and superiorly by the hyoepiglottic ligament. This space is thus totally extirpated by horizontal supraglottic laryngectomy. The hyoid bone may be preserved because only far-advanced lesions require its removal. Of 112 supraglottic lesions, the hyoid bone was removed in only 2 cases.[34] Kirchner[33] believes that carcinoma of the infrahyoid portion of the epiglottis with invasion of the preepiglottic space is relatively resistant to radiation therapy, possibly because of the poor blood supply that allows central necrosis of the tumor.

Suprahyoid epiglottic cancers tend to invade the tongue base and the pyriform sinus rather than the preepiglottic space. Lesions occurring more laterally and posteriorly in the supraglottic region also lack the tendency to spread to the preepiglottic space.

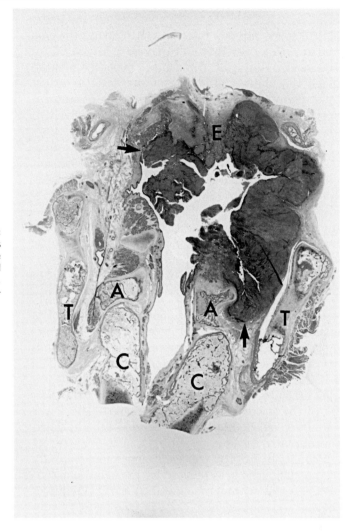

Figure 3–7. Another supraglottic cancer with extension to the glottic region. This coronal section through the arytenoid region shows how the tumor extends deep to the right arytenoid cartilage. Note also the partial destruction of the epiglottic cartilage. A, arytenoid cartilage; C, cricoid cartilage; E, epiglottis; T, thyroid cartilage. Arrows indicate the extent of the tumor. (Courtesy of Prof. J. Olofsson.)

They tend to be less invasive than similar growths in other parts of the larynx.[31] Occasionally, lateral supraglottic tumors penetrate the quadrangular membrane, where they can grow laterally to the ventricle through the paraglottic space, thus extending transglottically.[49] Lesions may invade laterally along the medial surface of the aryepiglottic fold as far as the arytenoid cartilage, usually without involving the cartilage itself. Cartilaginous involvement occurs only when there is extensive involvement of the mucosa overlying the arytenoid cartilage.[36]

When supraglottic tumors spread beyond the supraglottic region, they extend either superiorly to the valleculae and the pharyngeal wall or inferiorly to the glottis. Supraglottic cancers rarely extend in both directions.[42]

The supraglottic larynx arises embryologically from the buccopharyngeal anlage (branchial arches III and IV), while the glottis and subglottis arise from the tracheobronchial anlage (arches V and VI), but this does not justify the false assumption that supraglottic cancers (or so-called ascending cancers)

do not extend to the glottic region. Because of the ongoing nature of the process, a cancer may invade any neighboring tissue, regardless of whether it has the same embryologic origin; supraglottic cancers may infiltrate the glottic plane (Figs. 3–6 and 3–7) as well as the subglottic region.

Some authors have repeatedly postulated a barrier between the supraglottic and glottic regions,[50–53] but numerous pathologic studies, including those of whole-organ sections,[34] have shown that there is no such barrier.[54] Kirchner[34] believes that "whole-organ sections have failed to demonstrate an anatomic structure within the fundus of the ventricle that could qualify as a barrier to downward spread of cancer from the ventricular band." The existence of the so-called transglottic cancers, that is, of tumors with involvement of the glottis and supraglottis with fixation of the true vocal cord, is proof in itself. Nevertheless, supraglottic cancer often remains confined to the supraglottic area. However, if a supraglottic cancer invades the paraglottic space instead of the preepiglottic space, inferior invasion to the glottis can easily occur[20] and has often been reported.[35, 41, 42, 55–57] This is because the paraglottic space extends into the glottis along the medial surface of the thyroid cartilage.[20] In a series of 100 cases, Han and Yamashita[28] recently investigated the manner of spread of supraglottic cancer by studying whole-organ serial sections of surgical specimens, and they found the glottis involved in 48 cases and the anterior commissure in 12 cases.

Kirchner[34] demonstrated the rarity of involvement of the thyroid cartilage in supraglottic cancer, although this does occur in a small number of cases. Han and Yamashita[28] found it to be infiltrated in 9 of 100 cases of supraglottic cancer studied. Massive invasion of the upper aspect of the arytenoid cartilage causes fixation of the vocal cord in supraglottic carcinomas.

Subglottic Tumors

The rarity of primary tumors of the subglottis explains the limited experience that has been acquired, even in major institutions. The exact boundaries of the subglottis have been debated. The UICC[58] recently defined the subglottis as "the region extending from the lower boundary of the glottis to the lower margin of the cricoid." The lower boundary of the glottis was defined as "the horizontal plane, 1 cm below the apex of the ventricle."

Primary subglottic cancer arising independently in the subglottic area and not by infraglottic extension of a glottic tumor is extremely rare. Unequivocal and well-documented cases of true primary subglottic carcinoma are rarely found even in books devoted to laryngeal neoplasms, and the papers that discuss this tumor usually do not have macroscopic documentation. Subglottic extension of glottic carcinoma occurs much more frequently (about 20% of glottic cancers extended into the subglottic region). The primary tumors are insidious and often discovered at an advanced stage. They tend to spread circumferentially and invade intrinsic laryngeal muscles and cartilages and can spread anteriorly through the cricothyroid membrane and the thyroid gland, or caudally to invade the trachea. The presence of a neoplastic lesion in the subglottic region is linked with several conditions, which include the following:

1. Cancer involving the subglottic space by direct extension from glottic, transglottic, and pyriform sinus lesions
2. Cancer arising primarily in the subglottic space
3. Metastatic cancer from distant organs
4. Involvement of the subglottic space by systemic neoplastic disease (such as lymphoma, multiple myeloma, and leukemia)
5. Subglottic involvement by thyroid cancer
6. Subglottic involvement by esophageal cancer

Transglottic Cancer

None of the recently accepted clinical staging systems for laryngeal cancer include transglottic carcinoma as a separate category of tumor. Lesions that cross the ventricle and involve the glottic and supraglottic regions (with or without subglottic involvement) are variously classified as T2, T3, or T4 glottic or supraglottic tumors, depending on the clinician's opinion about the site of origin and the demonstrable presence of fixation or invasion of the laryngeal framework. The term "transglottic" is frequently used to describe such lesions and is indicative of a type of lesion that has certain clinical, pathologic, and prognostic characteristics. Usually transglottic cancers are associated with fixation of the true vocal cord.

Leroux-Robert[39] and Baclesse[59] described transglottic carcinoma in some detail, without calling it by that name. The term "transglottic" was first used by McGavran et al.[60] in their important study designed to correlate various characteristics of the primary tumor with the incidence of cervical lymph node metastases. These authors noted a greater than 2:1 prevalence of infiltrating to pushing margins at the periphery of transglottic tumors, a rate significantly higher than at any of the other sites. In addition, the rate of cervical lymph node metastases for transglottic carcinoma exceeded the rate for all other sites.

The pathology of transglottic cancer was studied in detail by Kirchner et al.[37] on whole-organ sections from 50 specimens. The study revealed that although all 50 specimens, on gross examination, appeared to be transglottic, the tumor actually crossed the ventricle or the anterior commissure in only 42 cases. All these lesions showed extensive invasion of the paraglottic space, and invasion of the laryngeal framework occurred in 32 out of 42 cases (76%). In the remaining 8 cases, the neoplasm crossed the arytenoid area downward from above or upward from below, without crossing the ventricle. The laryngeal framework was not invaded in any of these cases. The lesions that crossed the ventricle demonstrated a fairly typical pattern characterized by invasion of the paraglottic space.[31] Growth within this space was controlled inferomedially by the conus elasticus, laterally by the thyroid cartilage, and superomedially by the quadrangular membrane. The tumors were thus found to be directed downward and laterally, invading the lower region of the thyroid ala, and escaping from the larynx between the thyroid and cricoid cartilages. Despite extensive spread within the paraglottic space, there was often little involvement of the surface mucosa, sometimes making tissue diagnosis by biopsy difficult. Retraction of the false cord and biopsy directly into the ventricle were required in some cases.

Olofsson and van Nostrand[42] classified eight of their specimens as multiregional, that is, tumors so large that they could not be classified according to site of origin. All of these fit the criteria for transglottic cancer. All these tumors were bilateral, invaded laryngeal muscles and framework, and spread outside the larynx. The route of extralaryngeal spread was through the cricothyroid membrane in all eight cases and the cricotracheal space (laterally) in seven. The authors suspected that six of these tumors had initially arisen in the glottic region.

Kirchner et al.[37] believe that what is called transglottic cancer may follow more than one pattern of development. Such cancer includes true ventricular tumors that spread deeply upward and downward under relatively intact mucosa. In addition, both supraglottic and glottic carcinomas may cross the anterior commissure or ventricle with invasion of the paraglottic space. Tumors such as the eight specimens found by Kirchner et al. to cross the ventricle posteriorly, without involving it, do not exhibit the usual characteristics of transglottic tumors and, indeed, do not fit the definition, but they are clinically indistinguishable preoperatively.

Hypopharyngeal Tumors

Tumors of the pyriform sinus usually spread extensively beneath the mucosa because compartmentation is not present in the pyriform sinus or in other parts of the hypopharynx. Kirchner[34] found invasion of the posterior edge of the thyroid ala in 38% of 102 pyriform sinus specimens. Other studies confirm these observations.[20] Tumors involving the medial wall tend to invade laryngeal structures and produce vocal cord fixation.[42] The absence of anatomic barriers promotes infiltration of the laryngeal framework, the intrinsic muscles, and the paraglottic space.

Postcricoid neoplasms usually invade the cricoid cartilage and the posterior cricoarytenoid muscle and, when very extensive, may invade the trachea and the adjacent thyroid gland.[42, 47] Infiltration of the posterior cricoarytenoid muscles produces vocal cord fixation.[33] Carcinoma of the posterior wall of the hypopharynx usually shows extensive submucosal spread.

Spread to Cervical Lymph Nodes

It is generally acknowledged that cervical lymph node involvement is the most important factor for predicting the evolution of a laryngeal neoplasm, and it is taken into account in determining the clinical stage of the tumor. Spread to the lymphatic vessels is mainly by embolization, appearing first in the subcapsular sinus and subsequently spreading to the entire parenchyma of the node. Nodal deposits may be confined by an intact capsule, but the lesion can penetrate the capsule of the node and invade the surrounding fat and adjacent tissues. Transcapsular spread is common in laryngeal cancer. Metastases are usually ipsilateral, often bilateral, and exceptionally contralateral. The location of cervical lymph node metastases is closely linked to the site of the primary lesion.[19]

Primary Tumor Site

Glottic carcinomas have the lowest incidence of nodal metastases; subglottic, supraglottic, and transglottic lesions display a progressively increasing incidence of node involvement. There are inconsistencies among reported studies, and the overall results for the various sites do not always support generally accepted beliefs. There are many explanations for this, especially the inclusion of different types of cancers in the various reports. For example, McGavran et al.[60] found a 52% incidence of nodal metastases in patients with previously untreated transglottic carcinoma undergoing primary treatment by laryngectomy and radical neck dissection. Kirchner et al.[37] found only a 30% incidence of cervical lymph node metastases in 50 specimens studied, but their series included patients in whom radiation therapy had failed and whose originally positive nodes may have been sterilized by radiation. Olofsson and van Nostrand,[42] and Silver and Croft[61] noted a relatively low incidence of nodal metastases in specimens from patients who had received high-dose preoperative radiotherapy.

Skolnick et al.[62] reported the incidence of nodal metastases according to the T stage of the primary tumor in 264 cases of glottic carcinoma. Although the overall rate of node involvement was 20% (55 out of 264 patients), there was a marked increase in the frequency of involvement from T1- to T4-stage tumors. Many cases classified in this series as T3 and T4 glottic carcinoma would, in other reports, have been considered to be transglottic or subglottic (glottic with significant subglottic extension) tumors. This again emphasizes the difficulty in comparing various series in the literature with regard to the incidence of nodal involvement in relation to the primary tumor site.

In supraglottic carcinoma the incidence of positive nodes is usually reported to be around 30% to 35%.[60, 63] As previously noted, supraglottic tumors frequently invade the preepiglottic space, a factor that correlates strongly with positive cervical nodes.[52, 64] Shah and Tollefsen[65] noted a higher incidence of positive nodes (69%) in exolaryngeal supraglottic carcinoma (carcinoma that grows out of the laryngeal interior), as compared with endolaryngeal lesions (32%) (tumors confined within the larynx).

Tumors of the supraglottic region metastasize primarily to the subdigastric and upper jugular nodes, then to the midjugular nodes. The posterior triangle is seldom involved, and the nodes of the submandibular triangle and submental areas are rarely affected. Retrograde lymph flow may produce anomalous secondary deposits.[19]

Subglottic tumors metastasize to the lateral neck in about 20% to 25% of cases.[52, 60] However, the importance of paratracheal node involvement in subglottic carcinoma and its relation to stomal recurrence was first suggested by Norris[66] and subsequently emphasized in several papers by Harrison.[67–69] The latter author noted a 60% incidence of nodal metastases in subglottic carcinoma when paratracheal nodes were resected with the laryngeal tumor. Clearly these nodes may be undetectable by palpation.

In their study of transglottic carcinoma, Kirchner et al.[37] reported a higher incidence of positive nodes with primary tumors having a diameter of more than 4 cm (6 out of 11 cases) than with smaller-diameter tumors (10 out of 39 cases). Nodes were involved more often with poorly differentiated tumors (5 out of 8 cases) than with well-differentiated lesions (10 out of 42 cases). There was also a higher incidence of node metastases with tumors that involved the laryngeal framework.

Other Factors

Several authors have noted a lower incidence of metastases from well-differentiated tumors than from poorly differentiated or only moderately well differentiated lesions, a lower incidence from smaller than from larger tumors, and a lower incidence from lesions with pushing rather than with infiltrating margins.[37, 60, 64] McGavran et al.[60] noted an increased incidence of positive nodes in cases with nerve sheath invasion around the larynx. Recently, some authors noted that increased DNA content was associated with more aggressive laryngeal cancers that had a high rate of multiple lymph node metastases and a worse overall prognosis.[70]

Distant Metastasis

Although blood-borne metastases are uncommon in squamous cell carcinoma, widespread dissemination to various viscera may occur in advanced stages of laryngeal cancer. In a recent investigation, the

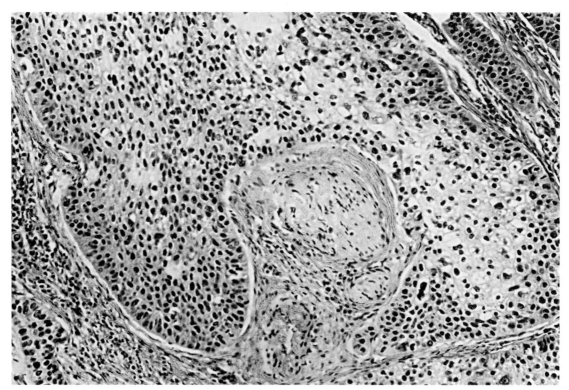

Figure 3–8. Squamous cell carcinoma of the larynx showing perineural invasion.

organs and structures most commonly involved at autopsy were (in decreasing order) mediastinal lymph nodes, lung, liver, pleura, skeletal system, kidney, heart, abdominal lymph nodes, spleen, pancreas, and adrenal glands.[71]

The distinction between lymphatic and hematogenous spread is artificial, because dissemination of most tumors occurs by both routes. Communications between the lymphatic and venous systems are present in the neck region. The collecting lymphatic trunks from the head and the neck terminate at the confluence of the subclavian and the internal jugular veins, on the right side in the lymphatic duct and on the left side in the thoracic duct.[72] Because the lymph nodes are well supplied with blood vessels and are usually situated in proximity to large veins, metastases in lymph nodes may infiltrate into veins and shed emboli into the venous stream. Lymph node involvement thus carries the threat of bloodstream dissemination.[73]

Perineural Spread

Perineural invasion (Fig. 3–8) is frequent and often occurs along the branches of the recurrent

---

Table 3–1. CLASSIFICATION OF THE PRIMARY TUMOR (T) FOR LARYNX (UICC and AJCC)*

Tx	Primary tumor cannot be assessed
T0	No evidence of primary tumor
Tis	Carcinoma in situ
Supraglottis	
T1	Tumor limited to one subsite of supraglottis or glottis with normal vocal cord mobility
T2	Tumor invades more than one subsite of supraglottis with normal vocal cord mobility
T3	Tumor limited to larynx with vocal cord fixation and/or invades postcricoid area, medial wall of pyriform sinus or preepiglottic tissues
T4	Tumor invades through thyroid cartilage and/or extends to other tissues beyond the larynx, e.g., to oropharynx, soft tissues of neck
Glottis	
T1	Tumor limited to vocal cord(s) (may involve anterior or posterior commissures) with normal mobility
	T1a Tumor limited to one vocal cord
	T1b Tumor involves both vocal cords
T2	Tumor extends to supraglottis and/or subglottis, and/or with impaired vocal cord mobility
T3	Tumor limited to the larynx with vocal cord fixation
T4	Tumor invades through thyroid cartilage and/or extends to other tissues beyond the larynx, e.g., to oropharynx, soft tissues of neck
Subglottis	
T1	Tumor limited to the subglottis
T2	Tumor extends to vocal cord(s) with normal or impaired mobility
T3	Tumor limited to the larynx with vocal cord fixation
T4	Tumor invades through cricoid or thyroid cartilage and/or extends to other tissues beyond the larynx, e.g., to the oropharynx or soft tissues of neck

*Data from International Union Against Cancer. *TNM Classification of Malignant Tumours.* 4th ed, 2nd rev. Berlin, Springer-Verlag, 1992; and American Joint Committee on Cancer (AJCC). *Manual for Staging of Cancer,* 4th ed. Philadelphia, JB Lippincott, 1992.

Table 3–2. CLASSIFICATION OF REGIONAL LYMPH NODES (N) (UICC and AJCC)*

Nx	Regional lymph nodes cannot be assessed
N0	No regional lymph node metastasis
N1	Metastasis in a single ipsilateral lymph node, 3 cm or less in greatest dimension
N2	Metastasis in a single ipsilateral lymph node, more than 3 cm but not more than 6 cm in greatest dimension; or in multiple ipsilateral lymph nodes, none more than 6 cm in greatest dimension; or in bilateral or contralateral lymph nodes, none more than 6 cm in greatest dimension
	N2a Metastasis in a single ipsilateral lymph node, more than 3 cm but not more than 6 cm in greatest dimension
	N2b Metastasis in multiple ipsilateral lymph nodes, none more than 6 cm in greatest dimension
	N2c Metastasis in bilateral or contralateral lymph nodes, none more than 6 cm in greatest dimension
N3	Metastasis in a lymph node more than 6 cm in greatest dimension

*Data from International Union Against Cancer. *TNM Classification of Malignant Tumours.* 4th ed, 2nd rev. Berlin, Springer-Verlag, 1992; and American Joint Committee on Cancer (AJCC). *Manual for Staging of Cancer,* 4th ed. Philadelphia, JB Lippincott, 1992.

Table 3–3. CLASSIFICATION OF DISTANT METASTASIS (M)*

Mx	Presence of distant metastasis cannot be assessed
M0	No distant metastasis
M1	Distant metastasis

*Data from International Union Against Cancer. *TNM Classification of Malignant Tumours.* 4th ed, 2nd rev. Berlin, Springer-Verlag, 1992; and American Joint Committee on Cancer (AJCC). *Manual for Staging of Cancer,* 4th ed. Philadelphia, JB Lippincott, 1992.

Table 3–4. STAGE GROUPING*

Stage 0	Tis	N0	M0
Stage I	T1	N0	M0
Stage II	T2	N0	M0
Stage III	T3	N0	M0
	T1	N1	M0
	T2	N2	M0
	T3	N3	M0
Stage IV	T4	N0,N1	M0
	Any T	N2,N3	M0
	Any T	Any N	M1

*Data from International Union Against Cancer. *TNM Classification of Malignant Tumours.* 4th ed, 2nd rev. Berlin, Springer-Verlag, 1992; and American Joint Committee on Cancer (AJCC). *Manual for Staging of Cancer,* 4th ed. Philadelphia, JB Lippincott, 1992.

laryngeal nerve into the thyroarytenoid muscle, near the lower end of the thyroid ala. The longitudinal arrangement of the nerve trunks and the tendency of cancer to invade nerve sheaths enable its spread from one region to another along the perineural spaces, centrally or peripherally, sometimes traversing long distances. The nerve axons can be affected secondarily by ischemia caused by the infiltrating neoplastic cells.[8, 19]

CLASSIFICATION BY STAGING

The precise location of a tumor and the existence of any metastases influence treatment and prognosis. Some classifications are essentially based on clinical findings.

From 1876 to the mid-twentieth century, laryngeal tumors were classified as "intrinsic" or "extrinsic" according to the proposals of Isambert[73] and Krishaber.[74] In 1953 the World Health Organization established a set of recommendations for the classification of clinical cancer cases by the characteristics of the primary lesions and of the metastases. The TNM system was devised with a view to representing the characteristics of the primary tumor (T), the regional nodes (N), and the distant metastases (M).[75] Efforts to establish a system of clinical classification and staging of laryngeal cancer were also made by the Latin American Committee for the

Study of Cancer of the Larynx and by the IUAC.[76] In 1956, the IUAC published a system classifying tumors with various TNM characteristics into larger groups with similar survival experience: stages I, II, III, and IV.[75] The first classification of cancer of the larynx was published in 1958. The second and third editions were published in 1974 and 1978, respectively, with several amendments.

A more universally accepted TNM staging system was developed in 1961 by the AJCC, based on the end results of 600 cases treated at seven representative institutions.[77] These criteria were revised in 1971. While the 1961 system classified primary tumors mainly on the basis of extent of mucosal surface involvement, the 1971 system was more three-dimensional in its approach, taking into account fixation of the larynx as an indication of in-depth tumor infiltration. Cases with fixation that were limited to the larynx were thus combined into a new T3 group, whereas cases with even fairly extensive mucosal involvement (confined to the larynx) without fixation were considered to be T2.

The AJCC staging system was further revised in 1976, and its comprehensive Manual for the Staging of Cancer was published in 1977, setting forth the current staging systems for cancers of various systems and organs. This manual has been revised and reprinted several times. A second edition was published in 1983, a third in 1988, and a fourth in 1992.[78] The most recent classifications[58, 78] (revised editions of the UICC and revised editions of the AJCC) have been unified (Tables 3–1, 3–2, 3–3, and 3–4). All classifications are compromises, however, and the unified TNM classification is still far from reliable. In applying them to matters concerning the diagnosis, prognosis, and treatment of laryngeal malignancies, therefore, it is worth bearing in mind that we must treat the lesion as it really exists, not as we think it exists.[79]

REFERENCES

1. Friedmann I, Ferlito A: Precursors of squamous cell carcinoma. *In* Ferlito A (ed): *Neoplasms of the Larynx.* Edinburgh, Churchill Livingstone, 1993.
2. Ferlito A: Precancerous lesions in the larynx: diagnostic and therapeutic problems. *In* Otorhinolaryngology, Head and Neck Surgery. Proceedings of the Fourteenth World Congress on Otorhinolaryngology and Head and Neck Surgery. Amsterdam, Kugler & Ghedini, 1990.
3. Barnes L, Gnepp DR. Diseases of the larynx, hypopharynx, and esophagus. *In* Barnes L (ed): *Surgical Pathology of the Head and Neck,* Vol 1, pp 141–226. New York, Dekker, 1985.
4. Hellquist H, Olofsson J, Gröntoft O. Carcinoma in situ and severe dysplasia of the vocal cords. A clinicopathological and photometric investigation. *Acta Otolaryngol* (Stockh) 1981; 92:543–555.
5. Barnes L, Peel RL. *Head and Neck Pathology: A Text/Atlas of Differential Diagnosis.* New York, Igaku-Shoin, 1990.

6. Crissman JD, Zarbo RJ. Quantitation of DNA ploidy in squamous intraepithelial neoplasia of the laryngeal glottis. *Arch Otolaryngol Head Neck Surg* 1991; 117:182–188.
7. Crissman JD, Zarbo RJ, Drozdowicz S, et al. Carcinoma in situ and microinvasive squamous carcinoma of the laryngeal glottis. *Arch Otolaryngol Head Neck Surg* 1988; 114:299–307.
8. Friedmann I, Ferlito A. *Granulomas and Neoplasms of the Larynx.* Edinburgh, Churchill Livingstone, 1988.
9. Ferlito A, Polidoro F, Rossi M. Pathological basis and clinical aspects of treatment policy in carcinoma in situ of the larynx. *J Laryngol Otol* 1981; 95:141–154.
10. Chejfec G. Atypias, dysplasias, and neoplasias of the esophagus and stomach. *Sem Diagn Pathol* 1985; 2:31–41.
11. Hellquist H, Lundgren J, Oloffson J. Hyperplasia, keratosis, dysplasia and carcinoma in situ of the vocal cords—a follow-up study. *Clin Otolaryngol* 1982; 7:11–27.
12. Wenig BM. *Atlas of Head and Neck Pathology.* Philadelphia, Saunders, 1993.
13. Crissman JD, Fu YS. Intraepithelial neoplasia of the larynx: a clinicopathologic study of six cases with DNA analysis. *Arch Otolaryngol Head Neck Surg* 1986; 112:522–528.
14. Friedmann I, Piris J. Nose, throat and ears. *In* Symmers W St C (ed): *Systemic Pathology,* 3rd ed, Vol 1. Edinburgh, Churchill Livingstone, 1986.
15. Gillis TM, Incze J, Strong SM, et al. Natural history and management of keratosis, atypia, carcinoma in situ, and microinvasive cancer of the larynx. *Am J Surg* 1983; 146:512–516.
16. Murty GE, Diver JP, Bradley PJ. Carcinoma in situ of the glottis: radiotherapy or excision biopsy? *Ann Otol Rhinol Laryngol* 1993; 102:592–595.
17. Rothfield RE, Myers EN, Johnson JT. Carcinoma in situ and microinvasive squamous cell carcinoma of the vocal cords. *Ann Otol Rhinol Laryngol* 1991; 100:793–796.
18. Ferlito A. Spread of cancer of the larynx. *In* Ferlito A (ed): *Cancer of the Larynx,* Vol II, pp 109–141. Boca Raton, CRC, 1985.
19. Ferlito A, Friedmann I. Squamous cell carcinoma. *In* Ferlito A (ed): *Neoplasms of the Larynx,* pp 113–133. Edinburgh, Churchill Livingstone, 1993.
20. Lam KH, Wong J. The preepiglottic and paraglottic spaces in relation to spread of carcinoma of the larynx. *Am J Otolaryngol* 1983; 4:81–91.
21. Pressman JJ. Submucosal compartmentation of the larynx. *Ann Otol Rhinol Laryngol* 1956; 65:766–771.
22. Bergman C, Gröntoft O, Olofsson J, et al. A technique for whole-organ sectioning and its applications. *Sci Tools* 1980; 27:46–50.
23. Bryce DP. The management of laryngeal cancer. *J Otolaryngol* 1979; 8:105–126.
24. Eckel HE, Sittel C, Sprinzl G, et al. Plastination: a new approach to morphological research and instruction with excised larynges. *Ann Otol Rhinol Laryngol* 1993; 102:660–665.
25. Ekem JK. Improved histological technique for the study of laryngeal carcinoma. *Can J Med Technol* 1972; 34:228–234.
26. Glanz H: Carcinoma of the larynx. *Adv Otorhinolaryngol* 1984; 32:1–123.
27. Goldman JL, Silverstone SM, Roffman JD, et al. High dosage preoperative radiation and surgery for carcinoma of the larynx and laryngopharynx: a 14-year program. *Laryngoscope* 1972; 82:1869–1882.
28. Han De-M, Yamashita K. The manner of spread of supraglottic carcinoma. *Larynx Jpn* 1991; 2:175–186.
29. Harrison DFN. Carcinoma of the larynx. *Br Med J* 1969; 2:615–618.
30. Kernan JD. The pathology of carcinoma of the larynx studied in serial sections. *Trans Am Acad Ophthalmol Otolaryngol* 1950; 55:10–21.
31. Kirchner JA. One hundred laryngeal cancers studied by serial sections. *Ann Otol Rhinol Laryngol* 1969; 78:689–709.
32. Kirchner JA. Pyriform sinus cancer: a clinical and laboratory study. *Ann Otol Rhinol Laryngol* 1975; 84:793–811.
33. Kirchner JA. What have whole organ sections contributed to the treatment of laryngeal cancer? *Ann Otol Rhinol Laryngol* 1989; 98:661–667.
34. Kirchner JA. Spread and barriers to spread of cancer within the larynx. *In* Silver CE (ed): *Laryngeal Cancer,* pp 6–13. New York, Thieme, 1991.
35. Kirchner JA, Som ML. Clinical and histological observations on supraglottic cancer. *Ann Otol Rhinol Laryngol* 1971; 80:638–645.
36. Kirchner JA, Som ML. The anterior commissure technique of partial laryngectomy: clinical and laboratory observations. *Laryngoscope* 1975; 85:1308–1317.
37. Kirchner JA, Cornog JL, Holmes RE. Transglottic cancer. *Arch Otolaryngol* 1974; 99:247–251.
38. Lam KH. Extralaryngeal spread of cancer of the larynx: a study with whole-organ sections. *Head Neck Surg* 1983; 5:410–424.
39. Leroux-Robert, J. *Les épitheliomas intra-laryngés. Formes anatomo-cliniques. Voies d'extension.* Thèse pour le doctorat en medecine. Paris, Gaston Doin & Cie, 1936.
40. MacComb WS, Fletcher GH. *Cancer of the Head and Neck.* Baltimore, Williams and Wilkins, 1967.
41. Olofsson J. Aspects on laryngeal cancer based on whole organ sections. *Auris Nasus Larynx* 1985; 12(suppl II):S166–171.
42. Olofsson J, van Nostrand AWP. Growth and spread of laryngeal and hypopharyngeal carcinoma with reflections on the effect of preoperative irradiation. 139 cases studied by whole organ serial sectioning. *Acta Otolaryngol* (Stockh) 1973; 308(suppl):1–84.
43. Tucker GF. A histological method for the study of the spread of carcinoma within the larynx. *Ann Otol Rhinol Laryngol* 1961; 70:910–921.
44. Sato K, Kurita S, Hirano M. Location of the preepiglottic space and its relationship to the paraglottic space. *Ann Otol Rhinol Laryngol* 1993; 102:930–934.
45. Gregor RT. The preepiglottic space revisited: is it significant? *Am J Otolaryngol* 1990; 11:161–164.
46. van Nostrand AWP, Brodarec I. Laryngeal carcinoma: modifications in surgical technique based on an understanding of tumor growth characteristics. *J Otolaryngol* 1982; 11:186–190.
47. Kleinsasser O. *Tumors of the Larynx and Hypopharynx.* Stuttgart, Thieme, 1988.
48. Zeitels SM, Vaughan CW. Preepiglottic space invasion in "early" epiglottic cancer. *Ann Otol Rhinol Laryngol* 1991; 100:789–792.
49. Tucker GF Jr: The anatomy of laryngeal cancer. *J Otolaryngol* 1974; 3:417–431.
50. Bocca E, Pignataro O, Mosciaro O. Supraglottic surgery of the larynx. *Ann Otol Rhinol Laryngol* 1968; 67:1005–1026.
51. Bocca E. Supraglottic cancer. *Laryngoscope* 1975; 85:1318–1326.
52. Ogura JH. Surgical pathology of cancer of the larynx. *Laryngoscope* 1955; 65:867–926.
53. Ogura JH. Supraglottic subtotal laryngectomy and radical neck dissection for carcinoma of the epiglottis. *Laryngoscope* 1958; 68:983–1003.
54. Million RR, Cassisi NJ, Mancuso AA. Larynx. *In* Million RR, Cassisi NJ (eds): *Management of Head and Neck Cancer: A Multidisciplinary Approach,* 2nd ed. Philadelphia, Lippincott, 1994.
55. Ferlito A. Histological classification of larynx and hypopharynx cancers and their clinical implications. Pathologic aspects of 2052 malignant neoplasms diagnosed at the ORL Department of Padua University from 1966 to 1976. *Acta Otolaryngol* (Stockh) 1976; 342(suppl):1–88.
56. McDonald TJ, DeSanto LW, Weiland LH. Supraglottic larynx and its pathology as studied by whole laryngeal sections. *Laryngoscope* 1976; 86:635–648.
57. Szlezak L. Histological serial block examination of 57 cases of laryngeal cancer. *Oncologia* 1966; 20:178–194.
58. International Union Against Cancer. *TNM Classification of Malignant Tumours.* 4th ed, 2nd rev. Berlin, Springer-Verlag, 1992.

59. Baclesse F. Carcinoma of the larynx. Radiotherapy of laryngeal cancer. Clinical, radiological and therapeutic study. Follow-up of 341 cases treated at the Foundation Curie from 1919 to 1940. *Br J Radiol* 1949; 3(suppl):1–62.

60. McGavran MH, Bauer WC, Ogura JH. The incidence of cervical lymph node metastases from epidermoid carcinoma of the larynx and their relationship to certain characteristics of the primary tumor: a study based on the clinical and pathological findings in 96 patients treated by primary en bloc laryngectomy and radical neck dissection. *Cancer* 1961; 14:55–66.

61. Silver CE, Croft CB. Elective dissection of the neck. *Surg Gynecol Obstet* 1979; 149:65–68.

62. Skolnick EM, Yee KF, Wheatley MA, et al. Carcinoma of the laryngeal glottis: therapy and results. *Laryngoscope* 1975; 85:1453–1466.

63. Som ML. Conservation surgery for carcinoma of the supraglottis. *J Laryngol Otol* 1970; 84:655–678.

64. Kashima HK. The characteristics of laryngeal cancer correlating with cervical lymph node metastasis (analysis based on 40 total organ sections). *J Otolaryngol* 1975; 4:893–902.

65. Shah JP, Tollefsen HR. Epidermoid carcinoma of the supraglottic larynx: role of neck dissection in initial surgical treatment. *Am J Surg* 1974; 128:494–499.

66. Norris CM: Causes of failure in surgical treatment of malignant tumors of the larynx. *Ann Otol Rhinol Laryngol* 1959; 68:487–508.

67. Harrison DFN. Pathology of hypopharyngeal cancer in relation to surgical management. *J Laryngol Otol* 1970; 84:349–367.

68. Harrison DFN. The pathology and management of subglottic cancer. *Ann Otol Rhinol Laryngol* 1971; 80:6–12.

69. Harrison DFN. Laryngectomy for subglottic lesions. *Laryngoscope* 1975; 85:1208–1210.

70. Wolf GT, Fisher SG, Truelson JM, et al. DNA content and regional metastases in patients with advanced laryngeal squamous carcinoma. *Laryngoscope* 1994; 104:479–483.

71. Silvestri F, Bussani R, Stanta F, et al. Supraglottic versus glottic laryngeal cancer: epidemiological and pathological aspects. *ORL J Otorhinolaryngol Relat Spec* 1992; 54:43–48.

72. Haagensen CD. The spread of cancer in the lymphatic system. *In* Haagensen CD, Feind CR, Herter FP, Slanetz CA Jr, Weinberg JA (eds): *The Lymphatics in Cancer.* Saunders, Philadelphia, 1972.

73. Isambert E. Contribution à l'étude du cancer laryngé. *Ann Mal Oreille Larynx* 1876; 2:1–23.

74. Krishaber M. Contribution à l'étude du cancer du larynx. *Gaz Hebd Med Chir* 1879; 16:518–523.

75. Barretto PM. Nomenclature and staging of malignant tumors of the larynx and of the hypopharynx. *Arch Otolaryngol* 1958; 68:160–164.

76. Jackson CL, Norris CM. *Cancer of the Larynx.* New York, American Cancer Society, 1963.

77. Smith RR, Caulk, RM. Russell WO, et al. End-results in 600 laryngeal cancers using the American Joint Committee's proposed method of stage classification and end-results reporting. *Surg Gynecol Obstet* 1961; 113:435–444.

78. American Joint Committee on Cancer (AJCC). *Manual for Staging of Cancer,* 4th ed. Philadelphia, JB Lippincott, 1992.

79. Ferlito A, Harrison DFN, Bailey BJ, et al. Are clinical classifications for laryngeal cancer satisfactory? *Ann Otol Rhinol Laryngol* 1995; 104:741–747.

Chapter 4

Unusual Malignant Neoplasms
Alfio Ferlito

The morphologic spectrum of laryngeal neoplasms has expanded considerably in recent years as new variants have been identified. The specific morphologies revealed are frequently associated with differing biologic behavior. Thus, the relevant classification and terminology have continued to evolve. This variety is illustrated by the recently published second edition of the World Health Organization's *Histological Typing of Tumours of the Upper Respiratory Tract and Ear*,[1] which also considers the larynx (Table 4–1).

This chapter deals with a selection of the less common malignant tumors arising in the larynx, chosen for their particular clinical interest, because their incidence is not so sporadic, because of their particular biologic behavior, or because they have only recently been identified. Though it is not usually malignant in the larynx, paraganglioma also is discussed here because, until recently, the literature has given the impression that it is malignant in 25%

of cases. The terminology used in this chapter is as recommended by the World Health Organization.

VERRUCOUS SQUAMOUS CELL CARCINOMA

Clinical Features

Verrucous squamous cell carcinoma is a distinct pathologic and clinical variant of highly differentiated squamous cell carcinoma and may present diagnostic problems.[2] The lesion is not rare in the larynx; more than 500 cases have been reported.[3] The tumor shows certain unique features of clinical significance. It does not manifest a capacity for cervical and distant metastases, but it is locally invasive and destructive. An untreated tumor may destroy adjoining tissues, including muscle, cartilage, and thyroid gland. The tumor has a propensity for local recurrence after radiation, and anaplastic transformation is an occasional finding after such treatment.

Table 4–1. HISTOLOGIC TYPING OF LARYNGEAL TUMORS*

Epithelial Tumors and Precancerous Lesions	Leiomyoma
Benign	Rhabdomyoma
Papilloma	Hemangioma
Papillomatosis	Hemangiopericytoma
Pleomorphic adenoma	Lymphangioma
Basal cell (basaloid) adenoma	Neurilemmoma
Dysplasia and carcinoma in situ	Neurofibroma
Squamous cell dysplasia	Granular cell tumor
Mild dysplasia	Paraganglioma
Moderate dysplasia	***Malignant***
Severe dysplasia	Fibrosarcoma
Carcinoma in situ	Malignant fibrous histiocytoma
Malignant	Liposarcoma
Squamous cell carcinoma	Leiomyosarcoma
Verrucous squamous cell carcinoma	Rhabdomyosarcoma
Spindle cell carcinoma	Angiosarcoma
Adenoid squamous cell carcinoma	Kaposi's sarcoma
Basaloid squamous cell carcinoma	Malignant hemangiopericytoma
Adenocarcinoma	Malignant nerve sheath tumor
Acinic cell carcinoma	Alveolar soft part sarcoma
Mucoepidermoid carcinoma	Synovial sarcoma
Adenoid cystic carcinoma	Ewing's sarcoma
Carcinoma in pleomorphic adenoma	***Tumors of Bone and Cartilage***
Epithelial-myoepithelial carcinoma	***Benign***
Clear cell carcinoma	Chondroma
Adenosquamous carcinoma	***Malignant***
Giant cell carcinoma	Chondrosarcoma
Salivary duct carcinoma	Osteosarcoma
Carcinoid tumor	***Malignant Lymphoma***
Atypical carcinoid tumor	***Miscellaneous Tumors***
Small cell carcinoma	***Benign***
Lymphoepithelial carcinoma	Mature teratoma
Soft Tissue Tumors	***Malignant***
Benign	Malignant melanoma
Aggressive fibromatosis	Malignant germ cell tumors
Myxoma	***Secondary Tumors***
Fibrous histiocytoma	***Unclassified Tumors***
Lipoma	

*Adapted from Shanmugaratnam K. Histological typing of tumours of the upper respiratory tract and ear. *In* World Health Organization: International Histological Classification of Tumours, 2nd ed. Berlin, Springer-Verlag, 1991, with permission.

Verrucous carcinoma constitutes 1% to 4% of laryngeal malignancies. The larynx is the most common site for this tumor within the respiratory tract and the second most common location in the body, after the oral cavity. The most frequent location within the larynx is the glottis.[4] The tumor occurs in both sexes but predominantly in elderly males, and most patients have a history of smoking. The presenting symptoms may be insignificant in the early stages of this slowly developing tumor. Long-standing hoarseness and dyspnea develop owing to obstruction of the laryngeal lumen by the fungating neoplasm.[5] Occasionally dysphagia or hemoptysis may be the symptoms. Emergency tracheostomy may be necessary for the obstruction before a definitive diagnosis is made.[6]

Different biotypes of human papillomavirus DNA have been identified by polymerase chain reaction in laryngeal verrucous carcinoma, and an etiologic relationship has been proposed.[7–9] Several authors have suggested that the cells are genetically abnormal.[6, 10]

Pathology

Macroscopically the tumor appears to be a broadly implanted, nonulcerated, exophytic, gray-white fungating mass with papillary fronds and a locally invasive nature. The gross appearance of the tumor is characteristic and virtually pathognomonic. Histologically it is composed of islands and solid cords of highly differentiated squamous epithelial cells. Cytologic criteria of malignancy are lacking (Fig. 4–1) or minimal. Anaplasia is absent, and this may lead to an incorrect diagnosis. The tumor surface is covered by a thick layer of keratinized cells (Fig. 4–2) arranged in invaginating bulbous acanthotic folds. Typically there is considerable inflammation in the stroma, consisting of lymphocytes and plasma cells that tend to surround the tumor mass, the margins of which appear to be pushing and blunt rather than infiltrating. Epithelial pearls, keratinous cysts, microabscesses, and macroabscesses may be seen. The neoplasm stains positively for epithelial membrane antigen (EMA) and cytokeratin (CK).

Microspectrophotometric studies may be helpful in establishing the diagnosis.[2] Image analysis of cells may assist in the initial histologic diagnosis of verrucous carcinoma, particularly in distinguishing the tumor from squamous papilloma. Mean cell areas and nuclear areas are significantly larger in verrucous carcinoma than in squamous papilloma. A mean cell area greater than 300 μm^2 supports a

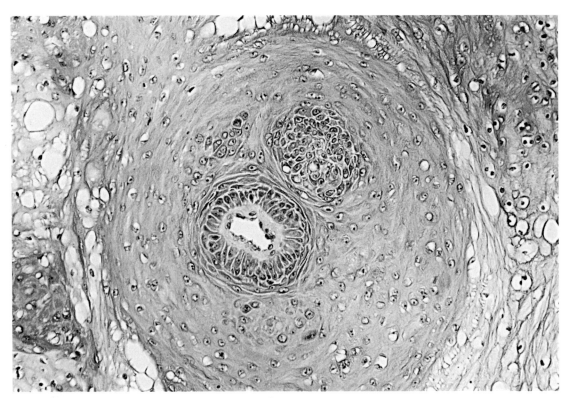

Figure 4–1. Microscopic appearance of verrucous carcinoma.

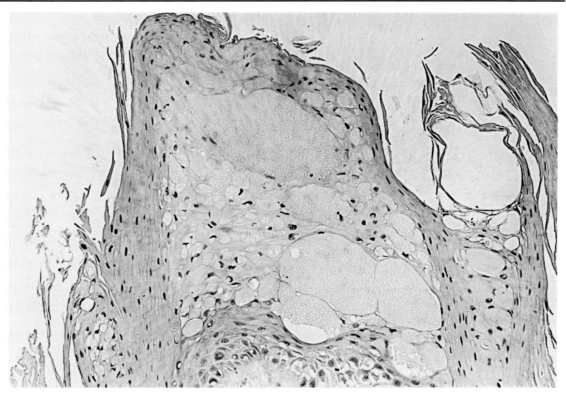

Figure 4–2. Verrucous squamous cell carcinoma of the larynx. The tumor surface is covered with a thick layer of keratinized cells.

diagnosis of verrucous carcinoma, whereas an area less than 250 μm^2 is suggestive of squamous papilloma.[11]

Although pathologists have little difficulty in diagnosing verrucous carcinoma when an entire surgical specimen is studied, it is often hard to diagnose this neoplasm accurately from a biopsy specimen.[12] The tumors lack the usual histologic features of malignancy and are often misdiagnosed as benign keratoses. On the other hand, the exophytic nature of the lesions is suggestive of malignancy. Fisher's claim that "the grading of malignancy of verrucous carcinoma is often overestimated by the clinician examining the endolarynx, and the biopsy section is often underdiagnosed by the surgical pathologist"[12a] accurately reflects our experience. Diagnosis stems from a combined clinical and histologic decision, and both aspects must be properly considered.[13]

A correct diagnosis therefore depends largely on close cooperation between clinician and pathologist, particularly when repeated biopsy examinations show a morphologic pattern of diffuse hyperkeratosis while the clinical appearance suggests a neoplastic lesion.[14, 15] Criteria for diagnosing verrucous squamous cell carcinoma are as follows:

1. The patients are usually elderly men
2. The glottis is the most common site
3. Tumor formation is warty, fungating, and exophytic with multiple filiform projections
4. The margins are advancing, pushing, and well demarcated
5. Deeply projecting, cleftlike spaces are present, with degenerating keratin, and there is subsequent cystic degeneration of the central portion of the filiform projection
6. Cellular differentiation is of a high degree
7. Cytologic features of malignancy are absent (small focal areas of cellular atypia may occasionally be present in large lesions)
8. A chronic inflammatory reaction is prominent in the stroma (the presence, especially, of lymphocytes and plasma cells)
9. Foreign body granulomas are evident near epithelial pearls or keratinized matter
10. The tumor shows nonmetastatic behavior

The tumor should be distinguished from keratosis, keratotic squamous papilloma, verruca vulgaris, conventional well-differentiated squamous cell carcinoma, and papillary squamous cell carcinoma.

Treatment

There is a consensus that surgery is the treatment of choice for verrucous carcinoma. Cure rates are excellent. Surgery should preserve as much laryngeal structure and function as possible, although total laryngectomy should be performed if necessary. Because cervical metastases have not been reported in nonirradiated true verrucous carcinoma, neck dissection is not indicated, even though enlarged and tender lymph nodes may be palpated. In documented cases of verrucous carcinoma, histologic examination of these nodes has revealed only an inflammatory reaction.[16] Excisional biopsy is ideal for diagnosis and treatment of glottic verrucous carcinoma.[17] Carbon-dioxide laser excision is the recommended treatment for stage T1.[6]

The tumor is highly curable when adequate surgical treatment is performed without delay. Hagen et al.[6] recently presented a report on 12 new cases of this lesion and reviewed the literature for the outcomes of radiation therapy versus surgery. Primary radiotherapy in 37 patients resulted in a 49% cure rate and a 51% failure rate (84% of these treatment failures showed no response); 11% of the patients died from anaplastic transformation. Primary surgery in 144 patients resulted in a 92.4% cure rate with an initial failure rate of 7.6%; the mortality attributed to the neoplasm was 3.5%.

The major contraindication for radiation appears to be the high recurrence rate of the neoplasm, coupled with the risk of postirradiation anaplastic or sarcomatoid changes observed in the larynx and at other sites. Primary radiotherapy is ineffective in half of the cases; it is also associated with an increased mortality and yields poor surgical salvage results.[6]

The prognosis for verrucous carcinoma is excellent when adequate treatment is adopted from the beginning, even when the tumor is extensive.

SPINDLE CELL CARCINOMA

Clinical Features

Spindle cell carcinoma is a rare, bimorphic carcinoma with a component identifiable as squamous cell carcinoma, together with an underlying or adjacent spindle cell or pleomorphic cell component.[1] Most of the neoplasms classified in the past as laryngeal sarcomas were actually cases of spindle cell squamous carcinoma. Squamous cell carcinoma with an extensive spindle cell component is the most common spindle cell tumor of the larynx.

It comprises about 1% of all laryngeal malignant neoplasms. Men in the fifth to seventh decades of life are more frequently affected than women.

The lesion arises mainly in the glottic region, particularly in the anterior commissure. Symptoms are similar to those of a squamous cell carcinoma affecting the same regions of the larynx.

Pathology

The histogenesis of spindle cell carcinoma is controversial, which explains the variety of terms used to designate this neoplasm, such as pseudosarcoma, pleomorphic carcinoma, carcinosarcoma, Lane tumor, biphasic spindle cell carcinoma, and collision tumor. It has been suggested that this tumor is not a homogeneous entity but consists of (1) spindle cell squamous carcinoma, (2) squamous cell carcinoma with pseudosarcomatous stroma, and (3) rare examples of true carcinosarcoma.[18] Brodsky[19] devised six hypothetical histogenetic schemes for this tumor.

Two thirds of spindle cell carcinomas occur as a polypoid, pedunculated mass attached to the mucosa by a stalk; the remainder are infiltrative or sessile. The tumor surface is frequently ulcerated. Microscopically there is usually a squamous cell carcinoma (often inconspicuous or in situ) together with a sarcoma-like component. The squamous component is sometimes difficult to find, especially when the lesion is ulcerated. Multinucleated tumor giant cells may occur (Fig. 4–3), and there may be some osteoid, chondroid, or osseous metaplasia. A storiform pattern may be detected. Lymph node and distant metastases usually contain either squamous epithelial elements alone, or both a squamous and a spindle cell element; they occasionally have only a spindle cell component. This tumor may stain positively for CK, EMA, and vimentin; it may also be positive for alpha$_1$-antitrypsin, alpha$_1$-antichymotrypsin, and albumin.

The tumor may be confused with reactive fibroblastic proliferation, fibromatosis, fibrosarcoma, malignant fibrous histiocytoma, and spindle cell malignant melanoma. Electron microscopy or immunocytochemical investigations should be used to make a correct diagnosis.[20, 21]

Treatment

Surgery is the preferred treatment. Neck dissection is often indicated. Radiotherapy has also been successfully employed for limited lesions but is not the treatment of choice. The prognosis of spindle cell squamous carcinoma, especially the nonpolypoid variant, is generally unfavorable. Metastases

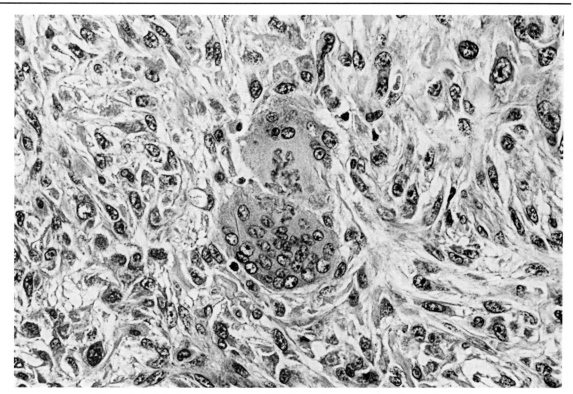

Figure 4–3. Spindle cell carcinoma of the larynx showing multinucleated giant cells.

to lymph nodes are frequent, and distant metastases have also occurred.

BASALOID SQUAMOUS CELL CARCINOMA

Clinical and Pathologic Features

Basaloid squamous cell carcinoma is a rare, separate histopathologic entity, first described by Wain et al. in 1986[22] and recently accepted by the World Health Organization.[1] In recent years, however, it has been reported with increasing frequency.[23–29] It manifests a predilection for the supraglottis and the pyriform sinus.[22, 26, 29] Macroscopically the tumor may appear either as an exophytic polypoid mass or as an infiltrative lesion. It is considered a distinct variant of squamous cell carcinoma and is composed of a carcinoma with a basaloid pattern associated with in situ or invasive squamous cell carcinoma, which is usually well or moderately differentiated. The basaloid component consists of small, crowded cells with hyperchromatic nuclei, scant cytoplasm, and small cystic spaces (Fig. 4–4) containing material resembling mucin that stains with periodic acid–Schiff (PAS) or alcian blue stains. There are foci of coagulative necrosis within the central areas

of the tumor lobules together with hyalinosis. Sometimes an abrupt transition between the basaloid cells and keratin pearls can be demonstrated (Fig. 4–5). Immunohistochemically the tumor shows reactivity for CK, EMA, carcinoembryonic antigen (CEA), neuron-specific enolase (NSE), S-100 protein, and vimentin.[23–26, 28–29a]

Ultrastructural studies show that the basaloid epithelial cells possess rare tonofilaments and varying amounts of desmosomes. The tumor displays highly aggressive behavior[25] and has to be distinguished from adenoid cystic carcinoma, mucoepidermoid carcinoma, adenosquamous carcinoma, and combined small cell neuroendocrine carcinoma.

Treatment and Prognosis

Surgery followed by radiation appears to be the treatment of choice. The high incidence of distant metastases (most commonly to the lung) indicates that adjuvant chemotherapy deserves investigation.[30]

Biologically this tumor is considered to be a high-grade malignancy, and therefore it has a distinct prognostic significance, usually worse than that of the common type of squamous cell carcinoma.[30a]

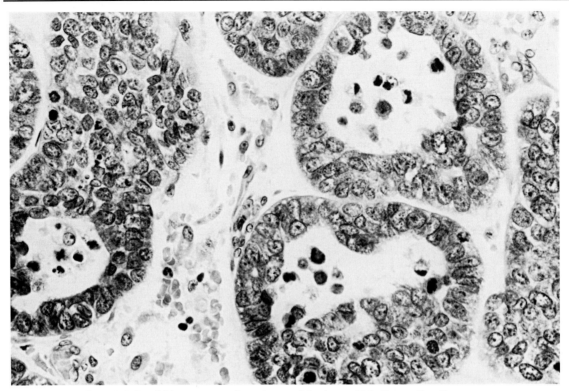

Figure 4–4. Basaloid squamous cell carcinoma of the larynx. Note the small cystic spaces.

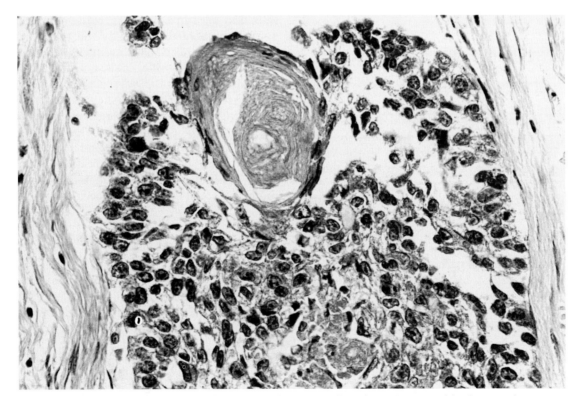

Figure 4–5. Basaloid squamous cell carcinoma of the larynx. There is an abrupt transition between the basaloid cells and the keratin pearl.

LYMPHOEPITHELIAL CARCINOMA

A rare but well-documented tumor,[31] lymphoepithelial carcinoma occurs most frequently in male patients from 50 to 70 years of age. The lesion is composed of large, poorly differentiated, nonkeratinized cells intermingled with lymphocytes (Fig. 4–6). The tumor cells have oval or round vesicular nuclei and prominent nucleoli. Cell margins are indistinct, and the tumor often has a syncytial appearance. The lymphocytes are not a neoplastic component of the tumor. Electron microscopy shows that the malignant epithelial cells form tonofilaments, desmosomes, and keratin fibrils.

The neoplasm must be distinguished from lymphoma. Immunocytochemical staining for EMA and CK gives positive results, and negative staining for leukocyte common antigen provides further documentation of epithelial differentiation. The rare possibility of metastatic spread from a nasopharyngeal primary carcinoma should be excluded before a tumor is classified as being of laryngeal origin.[18]

This neoplasm metastasizes to the cervical lymph nodes and occasionally to the lungs, bones, and other organs. The paucity of cases reported in the literature precludes any conclusions as to treatment and prognosis.

MUCOEPIDERMOID CARCINOMA

Clinical Features

Mucoepidermoid carcinoma is a malignant epithelial tumor consisting of a mixture of keratin-forming cells, mucin-secreting cells, and cells of intermediate type in varying proportions (Fig. 4–7). There is a male preponderance, with the mean age of occurrence in the seventh decade, while the mean age of female patients is in the sixth decade.[32] It has also been reported in a child.[33]

Approximately 100 cases of this tumor arising in the larynx have been described, but the true incidence is certainly higher because some cases probably escape detection, particularly at initial laryngeal biopsy. The epiglottis is the most commonly affected site, but the lesion may also involve other laryngeal regions.

Pathology

Macroscopically, the lesion has no characteristic feature to distinguish it from the much more common squamous carcinoma. Mucoepidermoid carcinomas have been divided into two categories: low-grade and high-grade carcinomas. Epidermoid cells and frequent mitoses are predominantly found in

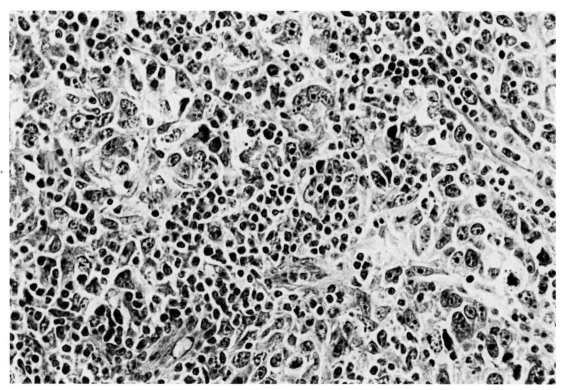

Figure 4–6. Typical appearance of a lymphoepithelial carcinoma of the larynx.

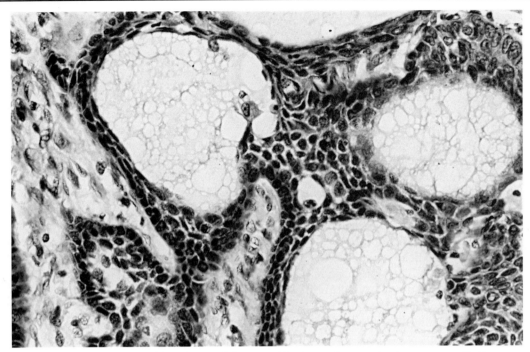

Figure 4–7. Mucoepidermoid carcinoma of the larynx. The tumor shows nests of squamous epithelium and glandular structures containing mucous secretions.

high-grade lesions, but mucus-secreting cells are scarce. Clear cells may be present. Low-grade tumors contain a higher proportion of mucus-secreting cells.

The tumor may stain positively for EMA, CEA, CK, vimentin, glial fibrillary acidic protein (GFAP), S-100 protein, smooth muscle actin, and myosin. Ultrastructural studies confirm the presence of mucous, epidermoid, and intermediate cell types, as well as of some amorphous mucin material. Mucoepidermoid carcinoma, unlike adenoid cystic carcinoma, rarely contains myoepithelial cells.

Mucoepidermoid carcinoma may be mistaken for squamous carcinoma, especially in small biopsy fragments in which the glandular component may be absent or may be neglected because of its paucity. Ho et al.[34] recommended that a mucicarmine stain be used to distinguish all cases of laryngeal carcinoma except for unmistakable squamous cell carcinoma.

Treatment

Mucoepidermoid carcinoma responds poorly to radiotherapy; partial regression is the most that may be expected from this treatment. The treatment of choice is complete surgical removal. Neck dissection for low-grade tumors is justified only in cases with clinical or radiographic evidence of cervical node metastases. However, elective neck dissection has been advocated for high-grade tumors.[34a]

The biologic behavior of this tumor is less aggressive than that of squamous cell carcinoma. It may, however, recur or metastasize to the cervical lymph nodes and lungs. Prognosis depends on the histologic grading and the stage.[35] The 5-year survival rate is 91% to 100% for low-grade neoplasms and 50% for high-grade neoplasms,[34, 36] with overall survival of 80%.[34]

ADENOID CYSTIC CARCINOMA

Clinical Features

Adenoid cystic carcinoma is the most common of the laryngeal minor salivary gland carcinomas; about 130 cases have been reported.[37–39] There is no significant gender difference, which is unusual for laryngeal neoplasms. It occurs more frequently between 50 and 70 years of age. About two thirds of these neoplasms are found in the subglottic region, the remainder being supraglottic.[40]

Patients with subglottic tumors may complain of shortness of breath, exertional dyspnea, and coughing, which is occasionally accompanied by hemoptysis. Supraglottic tumors produce dysphagia, sore throat, and hoarseness. Pain may be a prominent symptom in some adenoid cystic carcinomas of the larynx regardless of site, probably because of the propensity of the tumor to invade nerves. Paralysis of the recurrent laryngeal nerve is a frequent finding.

Distant metastasis occurs frequently in adenoid cystic carcinoma of the larynx. The tumor metastasizes to the lungs and, less frequently, to the liver, bones, and other organs. It does not usually metastasize to the cervical lymph nodes, and therefore the absence of metastases in the cervical area cannot be considered a favorable prognostic sign (as in squamous cell carcinoma) because multiple visceral metastases may nevertheless be present.

Pathology

The lesion appears grossly as large nonulcerated and well-defined polypoid exophytic masses that are sharply circumscribed but not encapsulated. They are covered by a generally intact, nonulcerated mucosa. Cyst formation and hemorrhage are unusual. The thyroid gland is often invaded.

Microscopically the lesion is composed mainly of small basaloid cells forming tubules, cords, or compact masses surrounded and intersected by cylinders of hyaline or mucoid material, typically giving a cribriform (Fig. 4–8) or lacelike pattern.[1] Three subtypes of this tumor are recognized, based on their pattern of growth: cribriform or cylindromatous type (grade I); tubular or trabecular type (grade II); and solid or basaloid type (grade III). The tubular spaces may contain material that stains positively with PAS, PAS with diastase predigestion (DPAS), mucicarmine, alcian blue, and alcian blue/ PAS stains. Immunocytochemical staining for S-100 protein has shown positivity in the myoepithelial cells of the tumor. Ultrastructural studies may also prove useful to confirm the presence of myoepithelial and intercalated duct cells.

The differential diagnosis includes small cell neuroendocrine carcinoma, mucoepidermoid carcinoma, basaloid squamous cell carcinoma, and salivary duct carcinoma, the last of which may produce a pseudocribriform pattern.

Treatment

The propensity of this tumor to metastasize widely without lymph node involvement makes evaluation for distant metastases essential for determination of appropriate therapy. The tests should include panendoscopy, chest x-ray examination, computed tomography (CT) of the lung and brain, liver echotomography, bone scintigraphy, and appropriate blood tests.

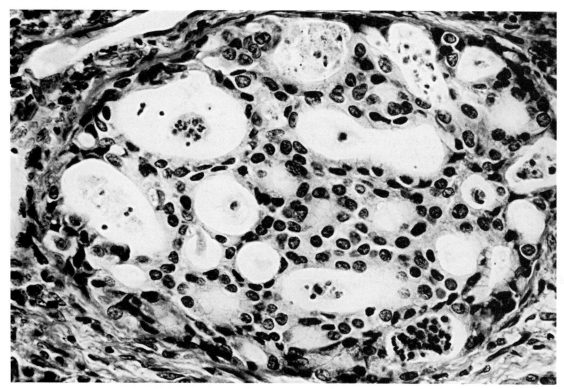

Figure 4–8. Typical appearance of an adenoid cystic carcinoma of the larynx.

The treatment of choice is surgical removal, by partial or total laryngectomy according to the size and site of the neoplasm.[41] Total laryngectomy should always be combined with subtotal thyroidectomy. Large subglottic tumors may necessitate resection of the pharynx and cervical esophagus. Pulmonary metastases, which are often symptom free, should not discourage surgical eradication of the primary tumor because single or multiple metastases may remain dormant for a decade or more.[37] Neck dissection is not indicated unless the patient has clinically enlarged or histologically confirmed nodal metastases.[41] A cervical mass is not always caused by a metastatic lymph node; it may be a recurrence or persistence of the primary tumor or a metastasis from a basaloid squamous cell carcinoma that is sometimes misdiagnosed as adenoid cystic carcinoma.

The role of chemotherapy in the management of this lesion is still undefined.

The tumor is slow growing but is markedly infiltrative and has a unique tendency to grow along nerves. The success of treatment and ultimate prognosis is best assessed in terms of a 15- to 20-year survival rate. Cohen et al.,[42] in 1985, reported survival rates of 87.5% at 2 years and 44.4% at 10 years at the M.D. Anderson Cancer Center in Houston, Texas. More recently, Irish et al.[38] reported survival rates of 89% at 2 years, 50% at 4 years, and 20% at 10 years, suggesting a more dismal long-term outlook than was previously believed.

NEUROENDOCRINE NEOPLASMS

Neuroendocrine neoplasms of the larynx are uncommon lesions of considerable scientific interest and clinical importance. Recent advances in immunohistochemistry and ultrastructural analysis have permitted clarification of previously confusing nomenclature as well as recognition of a greater number of these lesions. The designation "neuroendocrine" is unrelated to the embryologic derivation of the cells and is used in a morphologic sense. The term "neuroendocrine neoplasms" is employed as a convenience to encompass different neoplastic morphologies that possess certain features in common.

Neuroendocrine neoplasms have recently been reported with increasing frequency in the larynx and form the largest group of nonsquamous carcinomas. Approximately 500 cases have been reported in the world literature to date.[43] The actual incidence of these tumors is difficult to determine because many cases encountered clinically have been diagnosed simply as "undifferentiated carcinomas" or confused

with other oncotypes. It is also difficult to determine the exact number of each type of neuroendocrine neoplasm reported in the literature because of the disparity in the diagnostic criteria used.[44]

Neuroendocrine neoplasms can be conveniently divided into two main groups: those of "epithelial type" and those of "neural type." The epithelial neuroendocrine carcinomas include the typical carcinoid tumor, the atypical carcinoid tumor, and the small cell neuroendocrine carcinoma. The last of these may be further divided into small cell or oat cell carcinoma, intermediate cell type, combined cell carcinoma, and hybrid cell type[45]; these are malignant lesions with divergent differentiation patterns along both epithelial and neuroendocrine cell lines. Paraganglioma, which represents the neural type of neuroendocrine tumor, is unquestionably a neuroendocrine neoplasm but should not be classified with the laryngeal neuroendocrine carcinomas because of its different biologic behavior.[46]

Another method of classifying neuroendocrine carcinomas considers carcinoid tumor as well-differentiated neuroendocrine carcinoma, atypical carcinoid tumor as moderately differentiated neuroendocrine carcinoma, and small cell neuroendocrine carcinoma as poorly differentiated neuroendocrine carcinoma.

The neuroendocrine features shared by these tumors include the presence of neurosecretory cytoplasmic granules and the immunohistochemical identification of a variety of immunoreactive peptides within the tumor cells.[47, 47a] Electron microscopy has contributed greatly to the diagnosis of these tumors by demonstrating membrane-bound neurosecretory granules in their cells,[45] but it fails to discriminate between different neuroendocrine neoplasms. The secretory granules may also be demonstrated by special histochemical stains. The diverse group of neuroendocrine tumors can express a great variety of immunoreactive peptides identifiable by means of the immunoperoxidase technique. Comprehensive immunocytochemical analysis of laryngeal neuroendocrine tumors demonstrates that these lesions represent specific entities but have immunostaining patterns similar to those of neuroendocrine tumors at other sites.[48]

There is controversy among investigators as to the histogenesis of neuroendocrine carcinomas. They are believed to originate from endocrine cells or from uncommitted epithelial stem cells that are normally capable of differentiating into several cell types. The latter hypothesis appears more likely and would explain the occurrence of neoplasms exhibiting simultaneous squamous, glandular, exocrine, and neuroendocrine differentiation. Indeed, laryngeal carcinomas have been reported as featuring multidirectional epithelial, neuroendocrine, and even sarcomatous differentiation.[44] Paraganglioma clearly arises from paraganglia normally present in the larynx.

Neuroendocrine neoplasms of the larynx exhibit very different clinical behavior, ranging from the benign course of paraganglioma to the extreme virulence of small cell neuroendocrine carcinoma. The treatment of paraganglioma and of neuroendocrine carcinomas is therefore also different.[49]

Carcinoid Tumor

Carcinoid tumor is the rarest neuroendocrine carcinoma of the larynx; only 17 cases have been reported. The tumor mainly affects men, 60 to 70 years of age, who have been heavy cigarette smokers. The supraglottic region, particularly the arytenoid and the aryepiglottic fold, is the most commonly affected site. The lesion presents as a submucosal nodular or polypoid mass, usually without surface ulceration. Carcinoid tumor of the larynx is usually nonfunctional, although one patient developed carcinoid syndrome following liver metastasis.[50]

Microscopically this carcinoma is composed of nests and sheets of large and uniformly bland cells with abundant granular, eosinophilic cytoplasm and centrally placed, small, round-to-oval nuclei arranged in an organoid or trabecular growth pattern, with fibrovascular or hyalinized stroma. The tumor may occasionally produce amyloid. Mitoses and pleomorphism are scant, and necrosis is absent. Glandular or squamous differentiation may be seen. The overlying epithelium is usually intact. There is no vascular, lymphatic, or perineural invasion.

Argyrophilic staining is usually positive, whereas argentaffin staining is often negative. Epithelial mucin (diastase resistant, PAS positive) is a common finding. The tumor cells may express reactivity for CK, chromogranin, serotonin, NSE, and somatostatin. By electron microscopy, the neoplastic cells always exhibit numerous round and oval neurosecretory granules in the cytoplasm with a mean size of about 110 to 140 nm, preferentially located in the periphery of the cytoplasm. Cellular junctional complexes and intercellular and intracellular lumina are also present. The tumor must be distinguished from the atypical carcinoid tumor and from paraganglioma.

The treatment of choice is surgical excision. Conservative laryngeal surgery is often indicated because the supraglottis is the area involved. Neck dissection should not be performed because this tumor does not usually metastasize. The prognosis is usually favorable, and the biologic behavior of the typical carcinoid tumor is less aggressive than that of the more frequent atypical carcinoid tumor. Carcinoid tumor of the larynx is an indolent lesion that is capable of metastasizing but is rarely lethal.

Atypical Carcinoid Tumor

Atypical carcinoid tumor, although rare, is nevertheless the most frequent neuroendocrine tumor of the larynx. Approximately 250 cases have been reported in the literature, including cases described as atypical carcinoid tumor, together with those originally given other diagnoses and then reclassified as atypical carcinoids. The tumor is more common in men, with a peak incidence in the sixth and seventh decades. Atypical carcinoid of the larynx occurring in a patient with laryngotracheal papillomatosis has been reported.[51] More than 90% of the reported tumors occurred in the supraglottic region.

The tumor appears as a subepithelial lesion (Fig. 4–9), and surface ulceration is often present. The tumor displays a variable pattern showing a trabecular or mosaic arrangement of pleomorphic cells of atypical size and shape. There is enhanced mitotic activity, nuclear irregularity, pleomorphism, and focal necrosis. Amyloid may be found, and mucin production has been reported. Oncocytic or oncocytoid changes may occur, and there may be vascular, lymphatic, and perineural invasion. Argyrophil staining is usually positive, but argentaffin staining is often negative. The glandular lumen may contain diastase-resistant, PAS-positive, and alcian blue–positive material.

Immunohistochemically the tumor may be positive for CK, chromogranin, NSE, synaptophysin, neurofilaments, protein gene product 9.5 (PGP 9.5), Leu 7, calcitonin, serotonin, endocrine granule constituent, S-100 protein, EMA, CEA, bombesin, substance P, calcitonin gene–related peptide (CGRP), neuropeptide Y, and somatostatin. Electron microscopy reveals many round and oval neurosecretory granules in the cytoplasm but in smaller numbers than in the typical carcinoid tumor. The membrane-bound granules have an electron-dense core separated from the membrane by a clear space. Cellular junctional complexes and intercellular and intracellular lumina are present.[52]

Morphologic diagnosis is based primarily on conventional light microscopy and is confirmed by histochemical, immunohistochemical, and ultrastructural investigations. The differential diagnosis includes poorly differentiated squamous cell carcinoma, adenocarcinoma, small cell neuroendocrine carcinoma, acinic cell carcinoma, paraganglioma, and medullary carcinoma of the thyroid gland; atypical carcinoid tumor may be distinguished from carcinoma of the thyroid gland by the lack of elevated

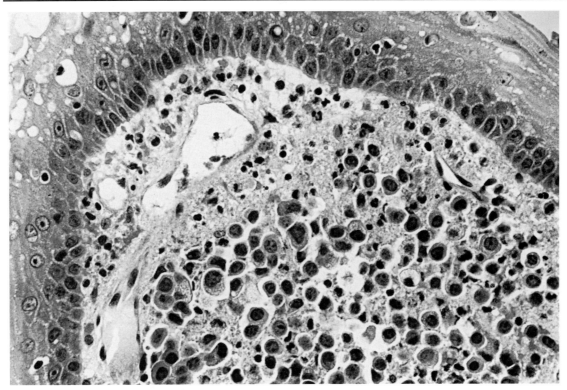

Figure 4–9. Atypical carcinoid tumor of the larynx.

serum calcitonin level. A marked elevation of 5-hydroxy-indoleacetic acid, caused by impaired tryptophan metabolism, is considered pathognomonic for carcinoid tumor.

The clinical behavior of this tumor is aggressive. Cervical lymph node metastases are common; other sites of metastases include the skin, subcutaneous tissues, bones, lung, liver, heart, and mediastinum. Carcinoid syndrome has been an exceptional finding in atypical carcinoid tumor.[53] Because regional and distant metastases often occur with this neoplasm, a careful routine workup is recommended before any treatment is undertaken. Pretreatment staging includes endoscopic examination of the upper aerodigestive tract, chest radiography, CT of the lung and brain, bone scintigraphy, liver echotomography, iliac crest bone marrow aspiration and biopsy, and laboratory investigations.

Surgical resection is the treatment of choice, and conservative laryngeal surgery should be employed if the tumor can be adequately removed. Large lesions may require total laryngectomy. Neck dissection should be performed because of the high likelihood of cervical lymph node metastases.

The survival rate is 48% at 5 years and 30% at 10 years and is uninfluenced by adjuvant irradiation.[54]

Small Cell Neuroendocrine Carcinoma

The larynx is one of the most common sites of extrapulmonary small cell neuroendocrine carcinoma. The first case in the larynx was reported by Olofsson and van Nostrand in 1972.[55] The total number of cases described in the literature is approximately 130.[45] The neoplasm mainly affects men 50 to 70 years of age who have been heavy cigarette smokers. The supraglottis is the most commonly affected site.

Symptoms and signs are similar to those of other laryngeal tumors and depend on the region involved, although in some cases a neck mass may be the first presenting sign.

Grossly the tumor presents as a submucosal lesion, and surface ulceration is often present. Microscopically (Figs. 4–10 and 4–11) the tumor is composed of small cells of various shapes with scanty cytoplasm and relatively large, hyperchromatic, oval, round, or spindle-shaped nuclei with delicate chromatin and inconspicuous nucleoli. Necrosis is prominent. Typical crush artefact may be present. Mitoses are numerous and vascular, and perineural and lymphatic invasion is commonly seen. The stroma is scanty and rarely mucoid. Scattered neo-

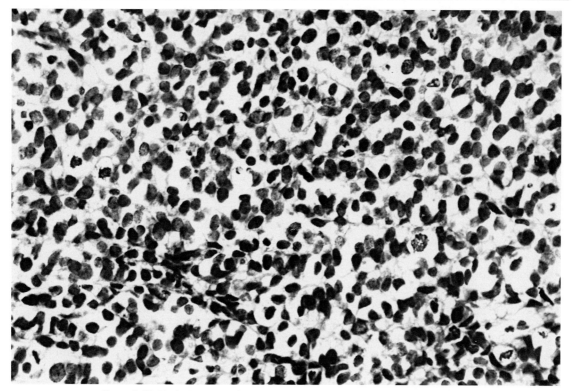

Figure 4–10. Typical pattern of small cell neuroendocrine carcinoma of the larynx.

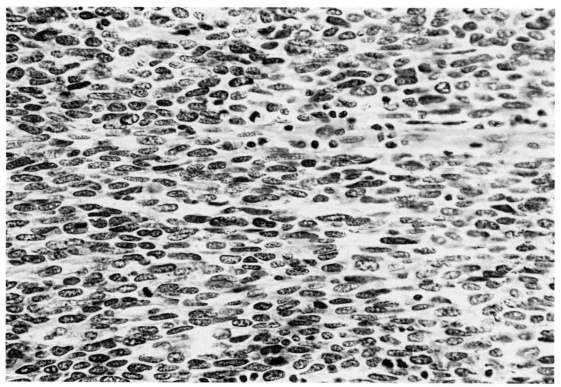

Figure 4–11. Small cell neuroendocrine carcinoma of the larynx containing fusiform and spindle-shaped cells.

plastic multinucleated giant cells may be present. The cells sometimes appear to cluster around alveolar-like spaces containing DPAS-positive material. Rarely, glandular structures may be seen. Reticulin staining is negative. Staining for argyrophilic and argentaffin cells with the Grimelius method and Fontana-Masson stain, respectively, is frequently negative.

The neoplasm may show positivity for chromogranin, NSE, PGP 9.5, synaptophysin, neurofilaments, bombesin, calcitonin, CK, CGRP, CEA, and somatostatin. Ultrastructurally there are scanty dense-core neurosecretory granules preferentially located in the periphery of the cytoplasm. Cellular junctional complexes and intercellular and intracellular lumina are usually absent.[52]

The differential diagnosis includes poorly differentiated squamous cell carcinoma, basaloid squamous cell carcinoma, typical and atypical carcinoid tumors, lymphoma, paraganglioma, melanoma, and medullary carcinoma of the thyroid. It is also important to ascertain whether the small cell carcinoma is a primary tumor or results secondarily from a bronchogenic, tracheal, or prostatic neoplasm.[45]

Tumor staging is mandatory for therapeutic and prognostic reasons, and examination should include panendoscopy, chest x-ray examination, CT of the lung and brain, bone scintigraphy, liver echotomography, iliac crest bone marrow aspiration biopsy, and laboratory tests. Systemic polychemotherapy and irradiation, with or without surgical resection, is the treatment of choice. Commonly used cytotoxic agents include cisplatin, vincristine, methotrexate, doxorubicin (Adriamycin), cyclophosphamide, and etoposide.[56, 57] Irradiation alone has been used successfully to control neoplasms with limited growth. Radical procedures have failed in the majority of cases reported.[47]

Cerebral metastases are rare and usually occur as a terminal event. In small cell lung cancer, prophylactic cranial irradiation may reduce the incidence of brain metastases but does not enhance survival.

The prognosis for this carcinoma is usually poor and the clinical course is rapidly fatal. The most common sites of metastatic spread from this very aggressive neoplasm are the cervical lymph nodes, liver, lungs, bones, and bone marrow. A few paraneoplastic syndromes, such as Schwartz-Battner syndrome, Eaton-Lambert syndrome, or ectopic ACTH syndrome, have occasionally been reported in association with laryngeal small cell neuroendocrine carcinoma. The 2- and 5-year survival rates are 16% and 5%, respectively.[58]

Paraganglioma

The most common sites of occurrence of paraganglioma in the head and neck region are the carotid body (carotid body tumor) and the temporal bone (glomus jugulare and glomus tympanicum).[59] The larynx represents a rare site of occurrence of this tumor. Laryngeal paragangliomas arise from superior and inferior paraganglia or aberrant paraganglionic tissue.

This neoplasm has been confused with a variety of other primary and secondary laryngeal neoplasms, especially with typical carcinoid and atypical carcinoid tumors. After critical review of the world literature, Ferlito et al[60] accepted as true paraganglioma only 62 cases out of 116 reported paragangliomas. Of these 62 cases, only 1 possible case of malignant paraganglioma of the larynx was identified. This occurred in a 36-year-old woman who developed a metastasis to the lumbar spine 16 years after diagnosis.[61]

This neoplasm is three times more common in women than in men and occurs most often after middle age. The lesion is frequently located in the supraglottic region, in particular in the right aryepiglottic fold. Some tumors described as "thyroid paraganglioma" are actually laryngeal paraganglioma deriving from the inferior laryngeal paraganglia.[45]

Macroscopically the lesion almost always appears to be encapsulated and intramucosal. Microscopically (Fig. 4–12) it is composed of chief cells arranged in clusters and round cell nests ("Zellballen" pattern), surrounded by a delicate stroma containing numerous vascular channels. The cell number varies from a few to more than 10 cells. The cells have abundant granular eosinophilic cytoplasm and large vesicular nuclei. Mitoses, necrosis, and vascular invasion are infrequent and do not necessarily indicate aggressive or malignant behavior. Dendritic spindle cells or sustentacular cells are found interspersed among the clusters of polygonal cells. Reticulin staining accentuates the organoid pattern. The tumor contains no mucin, and a fibrous capsule may be present.

Cytoplasmic argyrophilic granules may be demonstrated by the Grimelius method. With the Fontana-Masson stain the cells are negative for argentaffin granules. The lesion may express reactivity for chromogranin, synaptophysin, NSE, PGP 9.5, somatostatin, substance P, CGRP, neuropeptide Y, met-enkephalin, serotonin, and vasoactive intestinal polypeptide. S-100 protein and GFAP are not identified in the tumor cells but may be present in the sustentacular cells. Nuclear ploidy, whether

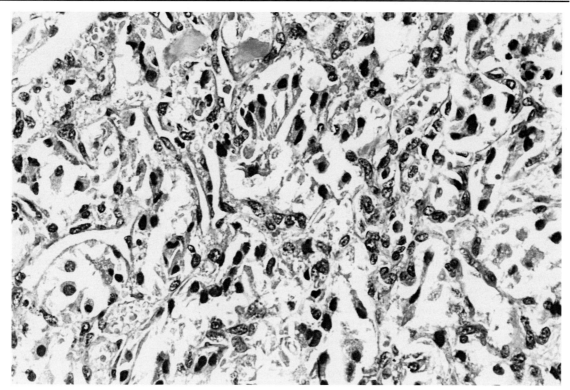

Figure 4–12. Typical pattern of a paraganglioma of the larynx.

diploidy or aneuploidy, cannot be correlated with prognosis. Electron microscopy reveals large, oval or polygonal cells with round-to-oval nuclei. Large numbers of dense-core neurosecretory granules are visible in the chief cells. The sustentacular cells have occasionally been described as containing lysosomes.

Differential diagnosis from atypical carcinoid, malignant melanoma (primary or secondary), metastatic renal cell carcinoma, and medullary carcinoma of the thyroid has to be considered and is not always easy. The most useful diagnostic method for differentiating paraganglioma from atypical carcinoid is immunohistochemistry.[49, 62, 62a] Paraganglioma is distinguished from atypical carcinoid by failing to stain for CK, CEA, and calcitonin.[63] The immunocytochemical profile of paraganglioma is typical of a neuroendocrine neoplasm of neural type and is therefore negative for CK.[64]

Surgery represents the treatment of choice. The majority of laryngeal paragangliomas are supraglottic submucosal masses, and these neoplasms are amenable to surgical resection by modified lateral pharyngotomy. The superior thyroid artery should be ligated as an initial step.[65, 66] Endoscopic excision should be avoided because bleeding, which may be profuse even from biopsy, may be difficult to

control.[63, 65] Local recurrence after endoscopic excision is common.

The rare cases of subglottic paraganglioma should be treated without complete removal of the larynx, although a total laryngectomy may sometimes be necessary. Neck dissection is not indicated because this neoplasm does not metastasize to cervical lymph nodes. The presence of a neck mass may be indicative of a metachronous carotid body paraganglioma.

Paraganglioma has often been overtreated.[49] The biologic behavior of "true" paraganglioma of the larynx is benign.[60, 63] Almost all the cases in the literature reported as malignant paraganglioma, especially those associated with chronic pain, were atypical carcinoids.

CHONDROSARCOMA

Clinical Features

Laryngeal sarcoma accounts for less than 1% of all malignancies of the larynx; of these unusual tumors, chondrosarcoma is the most common. Approximately 260 cases have been reported in the literature.[67–70] The number is probably higher, however, if we consider that many cases reported as chondroma were actually well-differentiated chondrosarcomas.

Traves[71] is credited with the first description of this lesion in the larynx, in 1816, at the Medico-Surgical Society of London; New[71a] first used the term "chondrosarcoma of the larynx" in 1935. This lesion is now being diagnosed more frequently than in the past, probably because of more accurate diagnoses by pathologists.[72]

The neoplasm is most frequent in patients between the ages of 40 and 70, but it may also occur in young people. The male/female ratio is 3:1. The most common site of origin is the cricoid cartilage (75% of cases), especially the anterior surface of the lamina. However, there are also reports of its onset in the thyroid cartilage, arytenoid cartilages, and accessory cartilages. The finding of some chondrosarcoma cases originating from the epiglottis[73] disproves the commonly held belief that this tumor occurs only in hyaline and not in elastic cartilage. Chondrosarcoma may occasionally involve the hyoid bone,[74, 75] but anatomically this is not a part of the larynx.

Symptoms consist of progressive hoarseness, dyspnea, and dysphagia, depending on the tumor location. Dyspnea will predominate if the neoplasm extends anteriorly into the lumen of the airway; if it develops posteriorly into the pharynx, dysphagia will result. As the neoplasm is usually slow growing, the patient may adapt to progressive narrowing of the airway until an episode of acute inspiratory dyspnea leads to emergency tracheostomy.[76] When the neoplasm originates from the thyroid cartilage, the major complaint may be the presence of a hard lump in the neck produced by the tumor mass. As in some cases reported in the literature, the first clinical sign may be vocal cord paralysis, apparently unassociated with other laryngeal or nonlaryngeal lesions, and therefore labeled as being idiopathic. Vocal cord paralysis is almost exclusively an early sign of cricoid chondrosarcoma and may be related to involvement of the recurrent nerve or fixation of the cricoarytenoid joint. On routine radiographs of the neck, the neoplasm usually appears as a mass with variable patterns of calcification.[77]

CT with contrast medium is very useful for demonstrating both the size and the extent of the lesion and for leading up to the diagnosis of a cartilaginous tumor. A lesion with calcified areas, extensively involving one or more cartilages and being moderately enhanced after injection of intravenous contrast medium, is a typical CT finding for laryngeal cartilaginous tumor.[78] However, there are no reliable radiographic criteria to enable differentiation between chondrosarcoma and chondroma. Magnetic resonance imaging (MRI) can also demonstrate the lesion within the larynx and has the additional advantage of better contrast resolution between the neoplasm and the paralaryngeal tissues.

Pathology

Macroscopically the tumor presents as a lobulated submucosal, rounded or oval, firm mass covered by intact mucosa. The neoplasm may be uniformly hard or may have soft and cystic areas of degeneration. Even in the more advanced stages the tumor tends to develop within the cartilage; only rarely, or in the event of a recurrence, does it extend beyond the external perichondrium and invade the surrounding tissues.

Microscopically chondrosarcomas must be distinguished as low-grade (grade I) (Fig. 4–13), medium-grade (grade II), or high-grade (grade III) tumors according to degree of differentiation and mitotic activity. A particular variant, called dedifferentiated chondrosarcoma, has also been reported in the larynx.[79, 80] This term indicates a neoplasm in which a spindle cell component is associated with cartilaginous proliferation (Fig. 4–14). Another morphologic variant of chondrosarcoma occasionally found in the larynx is myxoid chondrosarcoma. This tumor is composed of rounded or elongated cells arranged in nests or ribbons embedded in basophilic, homogeneous myxoid material. No laryngeal mesenchymal chondrosarcoma has been reported to date.[81]

On immunostaining, the cells express positivity for S-100 protein and vimentin. Electron microscopic examination shows malignant chondrocytes that are mostly round with short processes and scalloping of the membrane. Nuclei are indented or very irregular and have dispersed chromatin, occasionally with large nucleoli. Cytoplasm is abundant and contains numerous short, branching segments of rough endoplasmic, often distended, reticulum with variable amounts of flocculent material. The Golgi apparatus is prominent, and small clusters of glycogen and a few lipid droplets are also visible. The matrix is composed of fine elements and small proteoglycan granules. Binuclear cells are often present.

Biopsy may be difficult and is often unsuccessful because of the hardness and submucosal depth of the mass. It is advisable to take the biopsy sample under general anesthesia, and it often proves necessary to perform a preliminary tracheostomy for easier access to the lesion. Laryngeal chondrosarcomas often contain areas with different degrees of differentiation, so only a generous biopsy sample provides a reliable definition of the nature and micro-

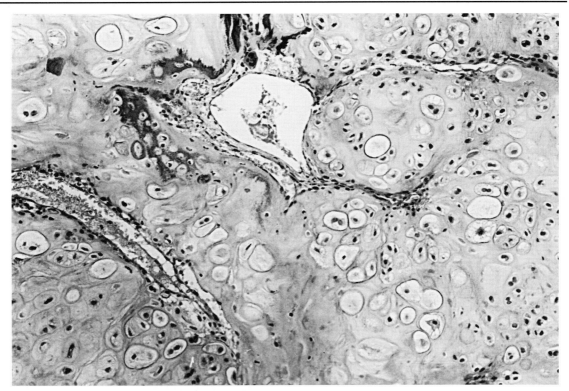

Figure 4–13. Well-differentiated chondrosarcoma of the larynx.

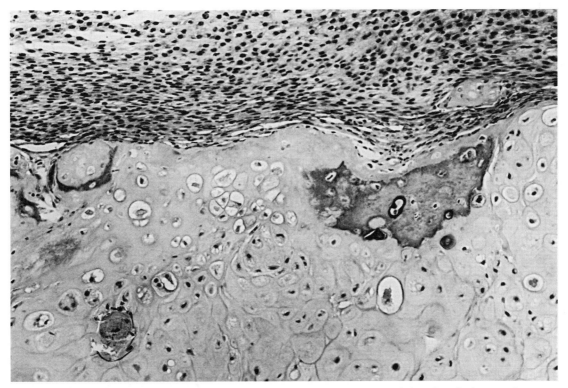

Figure 4–14. Dedifferentiated chondrosarcoma of the larynx. Note the association of cartilaginous and spindle cell components.

scopic features of the tumor. A correct diagnosis has also been obtained by needle biopsy with guidance from a CT scan. It is often difficult to distinguish between benign and malignant varieties of cartilaginous neoplasms of the larynx. It is not uncommon to find cases reported in the literature as benign chondromas that were actually chondrosarcomas, the correct diagnosis not being established until recurrence or development of metastases. In many instances, however, the so-called recurrence represents persistence, because resections are not always adequate.[82]

Differential diagnosis from chondroma, myxoid liposarcoma, embryonic rhabdomyosarcoma, spindle cell squamous carcinoma with cartilaginous metaplasia, and chondrometaplasia must be made. Chondrosarcoma of the larynx is primarily locally invasive, but lymphogenous and hematogenous metastases have been observed in 22 cases, which corresponds to 8.5% of reported cases.[83] When metastasis occurs, the secondary deposits are usually in the lungs and cervical lymph nodes. Tumor-related deaths are generally from uncontrolled local disease.[84]

Complete excision of the tumor, together with its perichondrial capsule and a reasonably generous margin of normal tissue, is generally regarded as the treatment of choice.[83] Recurrences, which developed in about 25% of reported cases, are probably related to piecemeal excision that spared the external perichondrium. Recurrences are most often seen in patients with high-grade chondrosarcoma. They tend not to be catastrophic because they can be treated surgically, and they also usually occur after relatively long intervals (from 2 to 20 years).

Supraglottic laryngectomy is indicated when the lesion is restricted to the supraglottic region. The problem becomes more complex when dealing with cricoid lesions because this cartilage is considered essential to the maintenance of an adequate laryngeal airway. When the lesion is limited in size and involves less than half of the cricoid, conservative removal through a laryngofissure may be adequate. Different techniques have been described for reconstructing the laryngeal lumen and preventing stenosis. Neis et al.[85] have reported using a rib graft after removing more than half the cricoid for a grade I chondrosarcoma. Though the results of these reconstruction techniques seem encouraging, the number of cases treated by this technique is so limited that no conclusions can be drawn as yet.[69] Extensive involvement of the cricoid cartilage may necessitate total laryngectomy.[83]

Because cervical lymph node metastases are rare, neck dissection must be reserved for cases in which the clinical picture or the imaging techniques suggest lymph node involvement. Radiotherapy and chemotherapy have not proved to be effective therapeutic modalities for laryngeal chondrosarcoma.

This tumor is considered to be a slow-growing malignant lesion, but it actually ranges from a locally aggressive, nonmetastasizing lesion, with occasional invasion of the thyroid gland, to a high-grade malignancy with metastatic spread via the bloodstream to the lungs. Laryngeal chondrosarcomas are much less aggressive than chondrosarcomas originating in other anatomic areas.

The clinical course of this neoplasm depends on the degree of differentiation and extent of the tumor, as well as on the adequacy of primary treatment. Grade I chondrosarcomas usually show a local malignancy with a minimal propensity for metastatic spread. Metastases increase in frequency with grades II and III tumors. Chondrosarcoma with a myxoid appearance seems to be associated with a worse prognosis than is conventional chondrosarcoma.[68] Dedifferentiated chondrosarcoma also shows an aggressive behavior pattern.[80, 86, 87] Careful follow-up is mandatory; 5-year follow-up is inadequate for these patients, who should be monitored for the rest of their lives.

REFERENCES

1. Shanmugaratnam K. Histological typing of tumours of the upper respiratory tract and ear. *In* World Health Organization: *International Histological Classification of Tumours*, 2nd ed. Berlin, Springer-Verlag, 1991.
2. Ferlito A, Antonutto G, Silvestri F. Histological appearances and nuclear DNA content of verrucous squamous cell carcinoma of the larynx. *ORL* 1976; 38:65–85.
3. Ferlito A. Verrucous squamous cell carcinoma. Second World Congress on Laryngeal Cancer, Sydney, 1994. Abstract.
4. Olsen KD. Verrucous carcinoma of the larynx. Second World Congress on Laryngeal Cancer, Sydney, 1994. Abstract.
5. Friedmann I, Ferlito A. *Granulomas and Neoplasms of the Larynx*. Edinburgh, Churchill Livingstone, 1988.
6. Hagen P, Lyons GD, Haindel C. Verrucous carcinoma of the larynx: role of human papillomavirus, radiation, and surgery. *Laryngoscope* 1993; 103:253–257.
7. Brandsma JL, Steinberg BM, Abramson AL, et al. Presence of human papillomavirus type 16 related sequences in verrucous carcinoma of the larynx. *Cancer Res* 1986; 46:2185–2188.
8. Fliss DM, Noble-Topham SE, McLachlin CM, et al. Laryngeal verrucous carcinoma: a clinicopathologic study and detection of human papillomavirus using polymerase chain reaction. *Laryngoscope* 1994; 104:146–152.
9. Kasperbauer JL, O'Halloran GL, Espy MJ, et al. Polymerase chain reaction (PCR) identification of human papillomavirus (HPV) DNA in verrucous carcinoma of the larynx. *Laryngoscope* 1993; 103:416–420.
10. Sllamniku B, Bauer W, Painter C, et al. Clinical and histopathological considerations for the diagnosis and treatment of verrucous carcinoma of the larynx. *Arch Otorhinolaryngol* 1989; 246:126–132.
11. Cooper JR, Hellquist HB, Michaels L. Image analysis in the discrimination of verrucous carcinoma and squamous papilloma. *J Pathol* 1992; 166:383–387.

12. Silver CE. *Surgery for Cancer of the Larynx and Related Structures*. New York, Churchill Livingstone, 1981.
12a. Fisher HR. Verrucous carcinoma of the larynx. A study of its pathologic anatomy. *Can J Otolaryngol* 1975; 4:270–277.
13. Strong MS. Diagnosis and treatment of verrucous squamous cell carcinoma of the larynx: a critical review. *Trans Am Laryngol Assoc* 1985; 106:163–164. Discussion.
14. Ferlito A. Diagnosis and treatment of verrucous squamous cell carcinoma of the larynx: a critical review. *Ann Otol Rhinol Laryngol* 1985; 94:575–579.
15. Ferlito A, Recher G. Ackerman's tumor (verrucous carcinoma) of the larynx: a clinicopathologic study of 77 cases. *Cancer* 1980; 46:1617–1630.
16. Ferlito A. Atypical forms of squamous cell carcinoma. *In* Ferlito A (ed): *Neoplasms of the Larynx*, pp 135–167. Edinburgh, Churchill Livingstone, 1993.
17. Blakeslee D, Vaughan CW, Shapshay SM, et al. Excisional biopsy in the selective management of T1 glottic cancer: a three-year follow-up study. *Laryngoscope* 1984; 94:488–494.
18. Shanmugaratnam K, Sobin LH. The World Health Organization histological classification of tumours of the upper respiratory tract and ear: a commentary on the second edition. *Cancer* 1993; 71:2689–2697.
19. Brodsky G. Carcino(pseudo)sarcoma of the larynx: the controversy continues. *Otolaryngol Clin North Am* 1984; 17:185–197.
20. Ellis GL, Langloss JM, Heffner DK, et al. Spindle-cell carcinoma of the aerodigestive tract: an immunohistochemical analysis of 21 cases. *Am J Surg Pathol* 1987; 11:335–342.
21. Zarbo RJ, Crissman JD, Venkat H, et al. Spindle-cell carcinoma of the upper aerodigestive tract mucosa: an immunohistologic and ultrastructural study of 18 biphasic tumors and comparison with seven monophasic spindle-cell tumors. *Am J Surg Pathol* 1986; 101:741–753.
22. Wain SL, Kier R, Vollmer RT, et al. Basaloid-squamous carcinoma of the tongue, hypopharynx, and larynx: report of 10 cases. *Hum Pathol* 1986; 17:1158–1166.
23. Banks ER, Frierson HF Jr, Mills SE, et al. Basaloid squamous cell carcinoma of the head and neck: a clinicopathologic and immunohistochemical study of 40 cases. *Am J Surg Pathol* 1992; 16:939–946.
24. Ferlito A. Basaloid squamous cell carcinoma. Second World Congress on Laryngeal Cancer, Sydney, 1994. Abstract.
25. Klijanienko J, El-Naggar A, Ponzio-Prion A, et al. Basaloid squamous carcinoma of the head and neck: immunohistochemical comparison with adenoid cystic carcinoma and squamous cell carcinoma. *Arch Otolaryngol Head Neck Surg* 1993; 119:887–890.
26. Seidman JD, Berman JJ, Yost BA, et al. Basaloid squamous carcinoma of the hypopharynx and larynx associated with second primary tumors. *Cancer* 1991; 68:1545–1549.
27. Shvili Y, Talmi YP, Gal R. Basaloid-squamous carcinoma of larynx metastatic to the skin of the nasal tip. *J Craniomaxillofac Surg* 1990; 18:322–324.
28. Luna MA, El Naggar A, Parichatikanond P, et al. Basaloid squamous carcinoma of the upper aerodigestive tract: clinicopathologic and DNA flow cytometric analysis. *Cancer* 1990; 66:537–542.
29. Tsang WYW, Chan JKC, Lee KC, et al. Basaloid-squamous carcinoma of the upper aerodigestive tract and so-called adenoid cystic carcinoma of the oesophagus: the same tumour type? *Histopathology* 1991; 19:35–46.
29a. Barnes L, Ferlito A, Altavilla G, et al. Basaloid squamous cell carcinoma of the head and neck: clinicopathological features and differential diagnosis. *Ann Otol Rhinol Laryngol*. In press.
30. Larner JM, Malcom RH, Mills SR, et al. Radiotherapy for basaloid squamous cell carcinoma of the head and neck. *Head Neck* 1993; 15:249–252.
30a. Ferlito A, Rinaldo A, Devaney KO. Malignant laryngeal tumors: phenotypic evaluation and clinical implications. *Ann Otol Rhinol Laryngol* 1995; 104:587–589.
31. Stanley RJ, Weiland LH, DeSanto LW, et al. Lymphoepithelioma (undifferentiated carcinoma) of the laryngohypopharynx. *Laryngoscope* 1985; 95:1077–1081.
32. Cumberworth VL, Narula A, MacLennan KA, et al. Mucoepidermoid carcinoma of the larynx. *J Laryngol Otol* 1989; 103:420–423.
33. Mitchell DB, Humphreys S, Kearns DB. Mucoepidermoid carcinoma of the larynx in a child. *Int J Pediatr Otorhinolaryngol* 1988; 15:211–215.
34. Ho K-J, Jones JM, Herrera GA. Mucoepidermoid carcinoma of the larynx: a light and electron microscopic study with emphasis on histogenesis. *South Med J* 1984; 77:190–195.
34a. Ferlito A, Recher G, Bottin R. Mucoepidermoid carcinoma of the larynx: a clinicopathological study of 11 cases with review of the literature. *ORL J Otorhinolaryngol Relat Spec* 1981; 43:280–299.
35. Ferlito A. Malignant epithelial tumors of the larynx. *In* Ferlito A (ed): *Cancer of the Larynx*, Vol I, pp 91–195. Boca Raton, CRC Press, 1985.
36. Hyams VJ, Heffner DK. Laryngeal pathology. *In* Tucker HM (ed): *The Larynx*, 2nd ed, pp 35–80. New York, Thieme, 1993.
37. El-Jabbour JN, Ferlito A, Friedmann I. Salivary gland neoplasms. *In* Ferlito A (ed): *Neoplasms of the Larynx*, pp 231–264. Edinburgh, Churchill Livingstone, 1993.
38. Irish JC, Gullane PJ, Cummings BJ, Pearson FG. Adenoid cystic carcinoma of the larynx: a 30-year review. Second World Congress on Laryngeal Cancer, Sydney, 1994. Abstract.
39. Matsunaga S, Tokushige E, Kohno M, et al. Adenoid cystic carcinoma of the larynx: report of a case. *Larynx Jpn* 1993; 5:76–79.
40. Irish JC. Adenoid cystic carcinoma: a 20-year review. *J Otolaryngol* 1993; 22(suppl 2):45.
41. Ferlito A, Barnes L, Myers EN. Neck dissection for laryngeal adenoid cystic carcinoma: is it indicated? *Ann Otol Rhinol Laryngol* 1990; 99:277–280.
42. Cohen J, Guillamondegui OM, Batsakis JG, et al. Cancer of the minor salivary glands of the larynx. *Am J Surg* 1985; 150:513–518.
43. Ferlito A. Neuroendocrine neoplasms of the larynx. Second World Congress on Laryngeal Cancer, Sydney, 1994. Abstract.
44. Ferlito A, Rosai J. Terminology and classification of neuroendocrine neoplasms of the larynx. *ORL J Otorhinolaryngol Relat Spec* 1991; 53:185–187.
45. Ferlito A, Friedmann I. Neuroendocrine neoplasms. *In* Ferlito A (ed): *Neoplasms of the Larynx*, pp 169–205. Edinburgh, Churchill Livingstone, 1993.
46. Wenig BM. Neuroendocrine tumors of the larynx. *Head Neck* 1992; 14:332–333. Letter.
47. Ferlito A, Friedmann I. Review of neuroendocrine carcinomas of the larynx. *Ann Otol Rhinol Laryngol* 1989; 98:780–790.
47a. Milroy CM, Ferlito A. Immunohistochemical markers in the diagnosis of neuroendocrine neoplasms of the head and neck. *Ann Otol Rhinol Laryngol* 1995; 104:413–418.
48. Salim SA, Milroy C, Rode J, et al. Immunocytochemical characterization of neuroendocrine tumours of the larynx. *Histopathology* 1993; 23:69–73.
49. Milroy CM. Paraganglioma of the larynx. *J Laryngol Otol* 1993; 107:664–665. Letter.
50. Wenig BM, Gnepp DR. The spectrum of neuroendocrine carcinoma of the larynx. *Semin Diagn Pathol* 1989; 6:329–350.
51. Andrews TM, Myer CM III. Malignant (atypical) carcinoid of the larynx occurring in a patient with laryngotracheal papillomatosis. *Am J Otolaryngol* 1992; 13:238–242.
52. Wenig BM. *Atlas of Head and Neck Pathology*. Philadelphia, WB Saunders, 1993.
53. Baugh RF, Wolf GT, Lloyd RV, et al. Carcinoid (neuroendocrine carcinoma) of the larynx. *Ann Otol Rhinol Laryngol* 1987; 96:315–321.
54. Woodruff JM, Senie RT. Atypical carcinoid tumor of the larynx: a critical review of the literature. *ORL J Otorhinolaryngol Relat Spec* 1991; 53:194–209.
55. Olofsson J, van Nostrand AWP. Anaplastic small cell carcinoma of larynx: case report. *Ann Otol Rhinol Laryngol* 1972; 81:284–287.

56. Ferlito A. Diagnosis and treatment of small cell carcinoma of the larynx: a critical review. *Ann Otol Rhinol Laryngol* 1986; 95:590–600.
57. Tabbara IA, Levine PA. Small-cell carcinoma of the head and neck: A novel treatment regimen. *Am J Clin Oncol (CCT)* 1991; 14:416–418.
58. Gnepp DR. Small cell neuroendocrine carcinoma of the larynx: a critical review of the literature. *ORL J Otorhinolaryngol Relat Spec* 1991; 53:210–219.
59. Stewart KL. Paragangliomas of the temporal bone. *Am J Otolaryngol* 1993; 14:219–226.
60. Ferlito A, Barnes L, Wenig BM. Identification, classification, treatment, and prognosis of laryngeal paraganglioma: review of the literature and eight new cases. *Ann Otol Rhinol Laryngol* 1994; 103:525–536.
61. Rüfenacht H, Mihatsch MJ, Jundt K, et al. PhU. Gastric epithelioid leiomyomas, pulmonary chondroma, non-functioning metastasizing extra-adrenal paraganglioma and myxoma: a variant of Carney's triad. Report of a patient. *Klin Wochenschr* 1985; 63:282–284.
62. Barnes L. Paragangliomas of the larynx. *J Laryngol Otol* 1993; 107:664. Letter.
62a. Ferlito A, Milroy CM, Wenig BM, et al. Laryngeal paraganglioma versus atypical carcinoid tumor. *Ann Otol Rhinol Laryngol* 1995; 104:78–83.
63. Barnes L. Paraganglioma of the larynx: a critical review of the literature. *ORL J Otorhinolaryngol Relat Spec* 1991; 53:220–234.
64. Martinez-Madrigal F, Bosq J, Micheau CH, et al. Paragangliomas of the head and neck: immunohistochemical analysis of 16 cases in comparison with neuroendocrine carcinomas. *Pathol Res Pract* 1991; 187:814–823.
65. Moisa II, Silver CE. Treatment of neuroendocrine neoplasms of the larynx. *ORL J Otorhinolaryngol Relat Spec* 1991; 53:259–264.
66. Silver CE, Moisa II. Treatment of neuroendocrine neoplasms of the larynx. Second World Congress on Laryngeal Cancer, Sydney, 1994. Abstract.
67. Bogdan CJ, Maniglia AJ, Eliachar I, Katz RL. Chondrosarcoma of the larynx: challenges in diagnosis and management. *Head Neck* 1994; 16:127–134.
68. Moran CA, Suster S, Carter D. Laryngeal chondrosarcomas. *Arch Pathol Lab Med* 1993; 117:914–917.
69. Nicolai P, Ferlito A, Sasaki CT, et al. Laryngeal chondrosarcoma: incidence, pathology, biological behavior, and treatment. *Ann Otol Rhinol Laryngol* 1990; 99:515–523.
70. Steurer M, Stiglbauer R, Zrunek N, et al. Chondromatöse Tumore des Larynx anhand dreier Kasuistiken unter besonderer Berücksichtigung der Magnetresonanztomographie. *Laryngorhinootologie* 1993; 72:256–260.
71. Traves F. A case of ossification and bony growth of the cartilages of the larynx. *Med Chir Trans* 1816; 7:150.
71a. New GB. Sarcoma of the larynx: report of two cases. *Arch Otolaryngol* 1935; 21:648–652.
72. Barnes L, Peel RL, Verbin RS, et al. Diseases of the bones and joints. *In* Barnes L (ed): *Surgical Pathology of the Head and Neck*, Vol 2, pp 883–1044. New York, Dekker, 1985.
73. Cheung W, Leong LLY, Chan FL. Case report: chondrosarcoma of the epiglottis. *Br J Radiol* 1993; 66:471–474.
74. Hasan S, Kannan V, Shenoy AM, et al. Chondrosarcoma of the hyoid. *J Laryngol Otol* 1992; 106:273–276.
75. Itoh K, Nobori T, Fukuda K, et al. Chondrosarcoma of the hyoid bone. *J Laryngol Otol* 1993; 107:642–646.
76. Kramer DS, Brown GP, Schuller DE. Proximal airway obstruction presenting as dyspnea: a case of chondrosarcoma of the larynx. *Postgrad Med* 1983; 5:133–135.
77. Shankar L, Hawke M. The CT appearance of cricoid chondrosarcoma. *J Otolaryngol* 1991; 20:297–298.
78. Munoz A, Penarrocha L, Gallego F, et al. Laryngeal chondrosarcoma: CT findings in three patients. *Am J Roentgenol* 1990; 154:997–998.
79. Brandwein M, Moore S, Som P, et al. Laryngeal chondrosarcomas: a clinicopathologic study of 11 cases, including two "dedifferentiated" chondrosarcomas. *Laryngoscope* 1992; 102:858–867.
80. Nakayama M, Brandenburg JH, Hafez GR. Dedifferentiated chondrosarcoma of the larynx with regional and distant metastases. *Ann Otol Rhinol Laryngol* 1993; 102:785–791.
81. Devaney K, Ferlito A. Cartilaginous and osteogenic neoplasms. *In* Ferlito A (ed): *Surgical Pathology of Laryngeal Neoplasms*, pp 393–424. London, Chapman & Hall, 1995.
82. Sztern J, Sztern D, Fonseca R, et al. Chondrosarcoma of the larynx. *Eur Arch Otorhinolaryngol* 1993; 250:173–176.
83. Silver CE. Chondrosarcoma of the larynx. Second World Congress on Laryngeal Cancer, Sydney, 1994. Abstract.
84. Barnes L, Peel RL. *Head and Neck Pathology: A Text/Atlas of Differential Diagnosis*. New York, Igaku-Shoin, 1990.
85. Neis PR, McMahon MF, Norris CW. Cartilaginous tumors of the trachea and larynx. *Ann Otol Rhinol Laryngol* 1989; 98:31–36.
86. Bleiweiss IJ, Kaneko M. Chondrosarcoma of the larynx with additional malignant mesenchymal component (dedifferentiated chondrosarcoma). *Am J Surg Pathol* 1988; 12:314–320.
87. Devaney KO, Ferlito A, Silver CE. Cartilaginous tumors of the larynx. *Ann Otol Rhinol Laryngol* 1995; 104:251–255.

Chapter 5

Conservation Surgery for Glottic Cancer

Carl E. Silver

BASIS AND DEFINITION OF CONSERVATION SURGERY

In Chapter 2 the anatomic compartmentation of the larynx and the connective tissue barriers to the spread of tumor from one compartment to another were described in detail. In chapter 3 the mode of spread of carcinoma within the larynx was discussed. In their earlier stages, glottic and supraglottic tumors tend to remain localized within their compartments because there is resistance to the spread of glottic tumors from one side of the larynx to the other, as well as to the spread of supraglottic tumors to involve the glottis. Transglottic and subglottic tumors, on the other hand, tend to spread deeply beyond the visible extent of tumor on the mucosal surface. These lesions often involve the laryngeal framework and extend beyond the confines of the larynx. Such lesions are unsuitable for conventional conservation surgery, although recent innovations have permitted extension of the indications to selected lesions with subglottic or transglottic involvement. The more confined glottic and supraglottic lesions can be adequately extirpated by removal of portions of the larynx, leaving a margin consisting of only a few millimeters of normal mucosa. Patients have a remarkable ability to adapt to the loss of considerable portions of the larynx and are able to retain the essential functions of speech, respiration, and deglutition.

Conservation surgery does not compromise the principles of adequate oncologic surgery. To be acceptable, cure rates obtained from a conservation operation must be comparable to the results that would be obtained by treatment of the same lesion with total laryngectomy. The smaller resection margins obtained with conservation surgery are compatible with this requirement. Batsakis[1] has noted that procedures that leave margins of more than 2 mm of uninvolved mucosa, as observed in histologic sections, produce results generally comparable to those procedures that leave widely clear margins. Indeed, Bauer et al.[2] found only 7 local recurrences among 39 patients with positive resection margins after hemilaryngectomy for vocal cord carcinoma, none of which led to fatality after subsequent treatment. Ogura et al.[3] listed the following reasons why wide margins are not necessary in treatment of carcinoma involving the true vocal cords or supraglottis: (1) the natural history of these lesions is one of slow growth, together with a tendency to remain localized to the primary site, (2) there is a paucity of lymphatics in the true vocal cord, (3) the lymphatic pathways above and below the cord are distinct, and (4) regional node metastases may be resected independently of the primary lesions if necessary.

In fact, satisfactory long-term cure and survival rates are obtained with conservation surgery. Good functional reconstruction of the larynx can be accomplished if one functioning arytenoid cartilage can be preserved. Ogura and Biller[4] estimated that 50% of all the laryngeal and laryngopharyngeal cancers evaluated by their service were treatable by conservation operations.

Depending on the location of the tumor, conservation surgery is carried out in the vertical or horizontal plane. Surgery for glottic tumors is performed in the vertical plane, as for laryngofissure and hemilaryngectomy. Supraglottic tumors are operated on in the horizontal plane, as for supraglottic subtotal laryngectomy. Because surgical exploration may reveal extension of tumor beyond the limits determined preoperatively, consent for total laryngectomy should be obtained prior to attempted conservation surgery.

SELECTION OF PATIENTS FOR CONSERVATION SURGERY

Age

The prevailing opinion, until recently, has been that conservation surgery should be avoided or approached with extreme caution in patients older than 65 years of age. The major problem after surgery in this age group has been the restoration of the sphincteric function of the larynx, permitting deglutition without aspiration of food. Conservation operations often involve loss of sensation, loss of function of one vocal cord, and loss of part of the anatomic barrier between the hypopharynx and the larynx. It is necessary for the patient to relearn the swallowing process and adapt to the loss of these various anatomic units. Obviously, a certain level of neuromuscular coordination and physical adaptability is required for this. The older the patients, the less capable they are of such adaptation, although this varies considerably among individuals. In general, conservation procedures should be considered with caution for older patients who may find adaptation difficult.[5]

Recent improvements in reconstruction have helped minimize the problems experienced by older patients after partial laryngectomy. Tucker[6] reported results of conservation surgery in 27 patients older than 65 years of age. The procedures were well tolerated, there was no mortality, and the overall complication rate was 11.1%. The results compared favorably with those in patients younger than 65 years of age. Our own experience in elderly patients has been similar to Tucker's and we agree that chronologic age alone need not be a contraindication to conservation surgery.

General Condition

The general condition of the patient is a more important consideration than age when selecting patients for conservation surgery. The ability of patients to compensate for the loss of portions of the larynx by reeducation of reflexes is related to their general physical condition. Patients suffering from chronic debilitating illnesses, including alcoholism, are not good candidates for conservation surgery. There are no absolute criteria for contraindications to conservation surgery. The judgment of the surgeon must be applied in each individual case. In doubtful instances the conservation procedure should be attempted because most patients will eventually adapt to the procedure if given proper postoperative care. Occasionally, conversion of a partial laryngectomy to a total laryngectomy may be necessary because of persistent aspiration or pulmonary infection.

Pulmonary Function

Chronic pulmonary disease is a greater deterrent to successful conservation surgery than is any other factor. The glottic narrowing and altered tussic function produced by conservation surgery contribute to pulmonary insufficiency. These patients cannot tolerate the inevitable aspiration of saliva, liquids, and food that occurs to a certain degree, at least temporarily, in almost all cases.

Previous Radiotherapy

Despite an initial reluctance to use conservation surgery in patients who have undergone high-dose radiotherapy, it has been shown that conservation surgery can be successfully used to salvage cases in which radiotherapy has failed.[7, 8] Complications, such as perichondritis and necrosis with resultant stenosis and fistula formation, occur more frequently in patients who have undergone radiotherapy. Conservation surgery can be used after radiotherapy only if the lesion was suitable for conservation surgery before radiologic treatment.[9] The evaluation of the extent of the tumor after radiotherapy by noting gross surface involvement is notoriously unreliable. Patients whose tumor status was unknown before radiotherapy present a problem. If conservation surgery is attempted in such cases, it is mandatory that the margins be carefully monitored by examining multiple frozen sections.

LARYNGOFISSURE (CORDECTOMY VIA THYROTOMY)

Laryngofissure is the oldest surgical procedure performed on the larynx for the extirpation of carcinoma and may be classified as a conservation operation. The development of this procedure through the nineteenth century and its gradual acceptance in the early twentieth century have been detailed in Chapter 1. Through the early years of its development the procedure was used for any lesion that could be grossly removed through the midline thyrotomy. As more sophisticated techniques of conservation surgery for glottic tumors developed, the indication for laryngofissure narrowed to the single instance of a T1 tumor of the true vocal cord limited to the membranous portion, with no limitation of motion, no involvement of the anterior commissure, and no extension onto the vocal process of the arytenoid. At the present time, laryngofissure is rarely used for treatment of carcinoma, even under the limited circumstances just described.

T1 tumors confined to the membranous portion of the cord respond well to radiation treatment, which is considered the treatment of choice by most surgeons.[10–17] The cure rates of 85% to 90% obtained by radiotherapy compare favorably with surgical results, and by avoiding resection of a vocal cord, radiotherapy has the advantage of preserving normal voice in a large percentage of patients. This opinion is not universal, however. In many centers laser surgery and minimally invasive endoscopic surgery are employed for treatment of suitable T1 tumors, supplanting both irradiation and laryngofissure.[18, 19] Radiotherapy is not without its disadvantages. Lawson[20] and Glanz[21] have presented convincing evidence that the incidence of second, presumably radiation-induced, primary tumors is significantly greater in patients with T1 glottic tumors treated by radiotherapy than in those treated with surgery alone.

There has been a loss of enthusiasm for laryngofissure, even among surgeons who prefer surgery to irradiation for treatment of T1 glottic cancer. Ogura and Biller[4] believe that surgery is preferable to irradiation for T1 lesions but advise hemilaryngectomy rather than laryngofissure. This is predicated from the belief that minor invasion of the vocal muscle by tumor may not be evident preoperatively and that hemilaryngectomy, with its wider field of resection, will ensure adequate margins. Daly[22] has noted that although the logic of this position is excellent, the 90% to 98% cure rates obtained with laryngofissure establish the effectiveness of this procedure in properly selected cases. DeSanto[19] has also affirmed the effectiveness of laryngofissure for T1 glottic cancer.

In most centers the failure of radiotherapy for unilateral T1 lesions remains the most frequent reason for the occasional laryngofissure that is done. In these cases, it is important to be sure that the original lesion, before radiotherapy, was suitable for laryngofissure. If that is not the case, then hemilaryngectomy should be performed.[22]

On our service most T1 lesions have been treated by radiotherapy, and either hemilaryngectomy or endoscopic laser surgery has been performed when surgery was thought advisable. Laryngofissure has not been used for treatment of cancer for a number of years. Nevertheless, as stated by Daly and Kwok,[23] "while specific indications for laryngofissure and cordectomy have declined, the procedure is an effective technique for the control of cordal cancer, when in the judgment of the surgeon, a simple surgical operation is called for."

Technique of Laryngofissure

Figure 5–1*A.* A transverse incision is made at the level of the midportion of the thyroid cartilage. The tracheostomy site is marked at the level of the thyroid isthmus, about one fingerbreadth below the cricoid cartilage.

Figure 5–1*B.* Skin flaps are elevated in the subplatysmal plane. If the procedure is performed under local anesthesia, only the inferior flap needs to be elevated at this stage. The superior flap will be raised after insertion of the tracheostomy tube and the induction of general anesthesia.

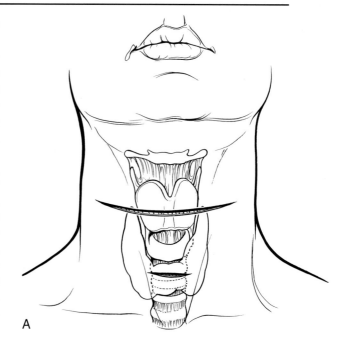

A

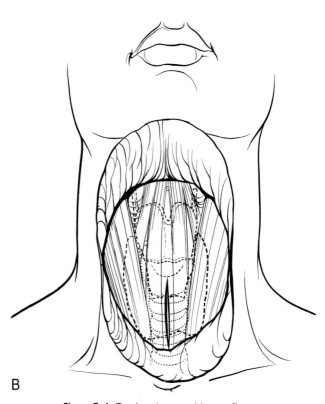

B

Figure 5–1. Tracheostomy and laryngofissure.
Illustration continued on following page

Figure 5–1C. A vertical incision is made in the midline between the sternohyoid muscles. The sternohyoid and sternothyroid muscles are retracted laterally, exposing the thyroid isthmus.

Figure 5–1D. A plane is established on the surface of the trachea deep to the thyroid isthmus. This is best done by dividing the subcricoid connective tissue between clamps (Fig. 5–1D_1), then dissecting on the tracheal surface with a right-angle clamp (Fig. 5–1D_2). Positive identification of the cricoid cartilage by palpation is essential before commencing this step.

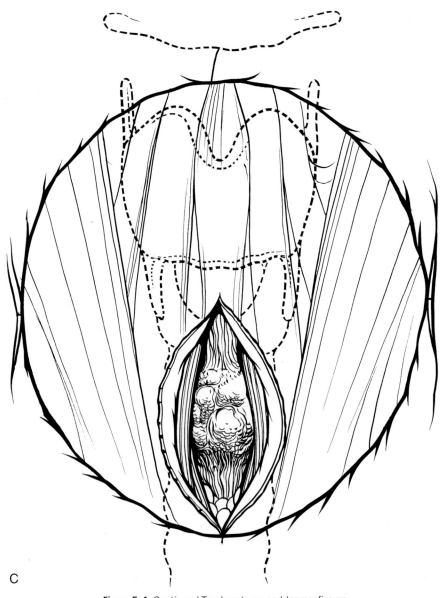

C

Figure 5–1 *Continued* Tracheostomy and laryngofissure.

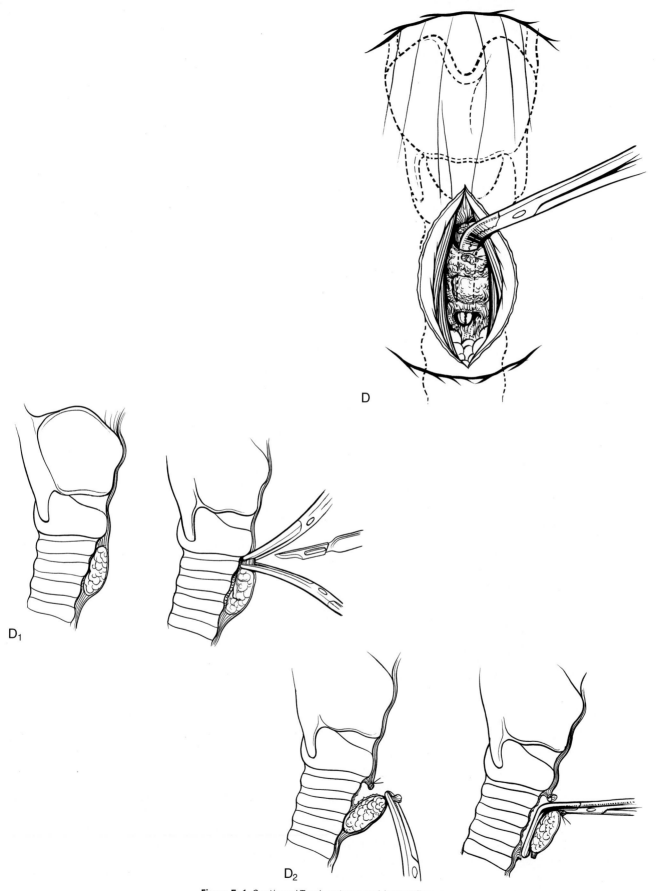

Figure 5–1 *Continued* Tracheostomy and laryngofissure.

Illustration continued on following page

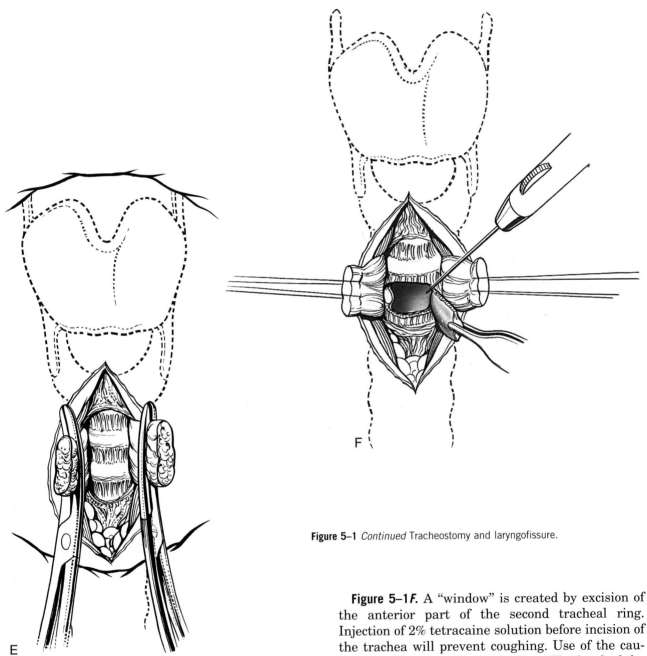

Figure 5–1 *Continued* Tracheostomy and laryngofissure.

Figure 5–1E. The thyroid isthmus is divided between the clamps and suture ligated. Routine division of the thyroid isthmus will ensure placement of the tracheostomy at the correct level.

Figure 5–1F. A "window" is created by excision of the anterior part of the second tracheal ring. Injection of 2% tetracaine solution before incision of the trachea will prevent coughing. Use of the cautery knife will minimize bleeding. The level of the second tracheal ring is appropriate for most laryngofissure and partial laryngectomy procedures. If there is subglottic extension, the tracheostomy is placed lower. In cases in which a subsequent total laryngectomy is anticipated, the tracheostomy should, if possible, be placed in the first ring without disturbing the tumor.

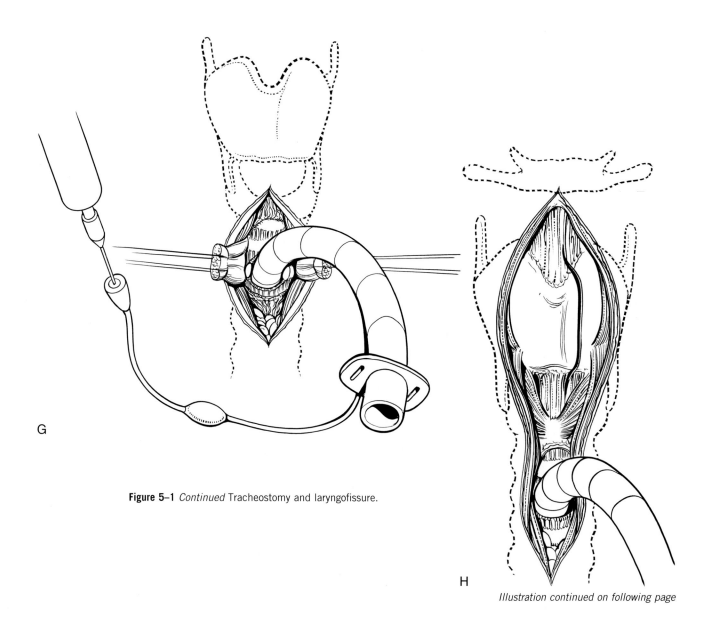

G

Figure 5–1 *Continued* Tracheostomy and laryngofissure.

H

Illustration continued on following page

Figure 5–1G. The tracheostomy tube is inserted. For laryngeal surgery, we prefer to use a kink-proof endotracheal tube (anode) temporarily during the operative procedure in order to minimize obstruction of the operative field by the flange of an ordinary tracheostomy tube. The endotracheal tube is connected to the anesthesia apparatus with appropriate sterile adapters and tubing.

Figure 5–1H. The vertical incision between the strap muscles is continued upward to the hyoid bone, and the muscles are retracted, exposing the thyroid cartilage in the midline. The thyrotomy incision is marked 1 to 2 mm lateral to the midline of the thyroid cartilage, on the left (contralateral) side.

Figure 5–1*I*. This transverse section shows the outline of the planned resection. This will include the true and false vocal cords anterior to the vocal process of the arytenoid cartilage, the underlying muscle, the internal perichondrium of the thyroid ala, the anterior commissure, and 2 to 3 mm of the opposite true vocal cord. The tumor, limited to the membranous portion of the right vocal cord, is shown.

Figure 5–1*J*. The thyroid cartilage is divided with an oscillating saw. The thyrohyoid membrane is incised along the superior border of the thyroid cartilage for about 1 cm on each side of the midline. The laryngeal interior is entered through a short transverse incision in the cricothyroid membrane, and a vertical incision is made just left of the midline, transecting the true and false cords. A special angulated blunt-tipped scissors facilitates this procedure by safely finding its way between the cords. Retraction of the thyroid alae exposes the laryngeal interior. A retractor placed in the superior angle of the thyrotomy facilitates exposure. The resection is indicated by the dotted line. The resection includes the entire false vocal cord and the subglottic mucosa to the lower border of the thyroid cartilage.

Figure 5–1*K*. This transverse section shows the relation of the thyrotomy incision to the tumor.

Figure 5–1*L*. The specimen is excised by sharp dissection. The injection of lidocaine-epinephrine solution between the thyroid cartilage and soft tissue minimizes bleeding and facilitates dissection. The mucosa and soft tissue are incised with a cautery knife. A small sharp separator is used to dissect beneath the thyroid ala. A curved scissors is convenient for the posterior vertical incision.

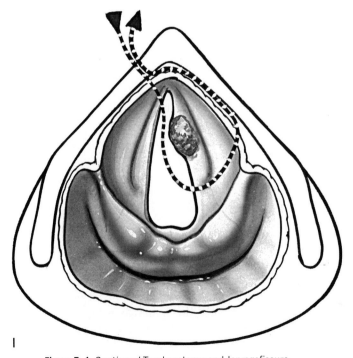

I

Figure 5–1 *Continued* Tracheostomy and laryngofissure.

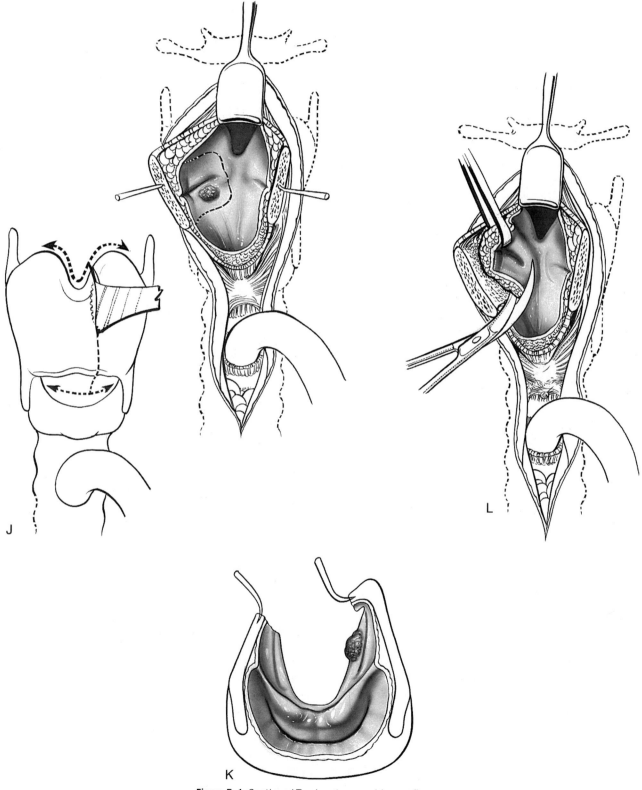

Figure 5–1 *Continued* Tracheostomy and laryngofissure.

Illustration continued on following page

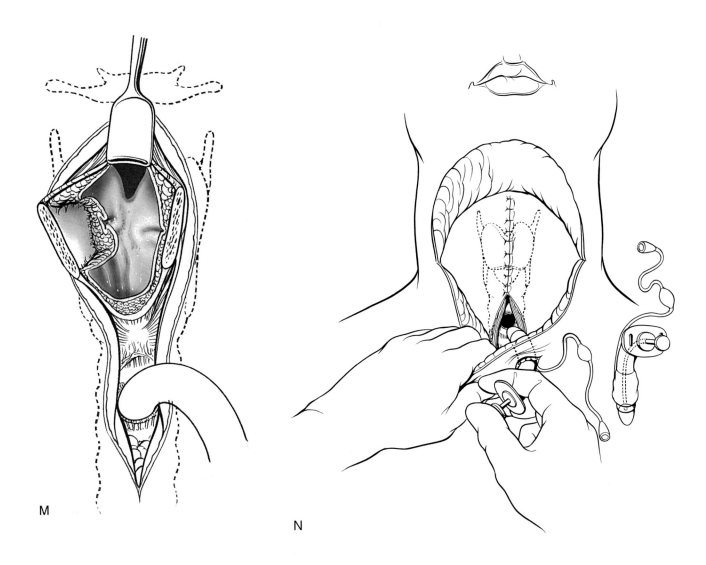

M

N

M₁

Figure 5–1 *Continued* Tracheostomy and laryngofissure.

Figures 5–1*M* **and 5–1***M₁***.** These views are of the completed resection. Resurfacing of the mucosal defect is not necessary. The thyrotomy is closed by the approximation of the overlying muscles and fascia.

Figure 5–1*N***.** The endotracheal tube is removed and a cuffed tracheostomy tube is inserted through the previously marked stab wound in the inferior flap. We prefer a plastic tube with an inner cannula and a high-volume, low-pressure cuff (Shiley-type). This routine is similar for all partial laryngectomy procedures with tracheostomy.

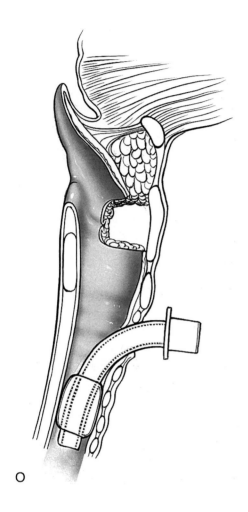

O

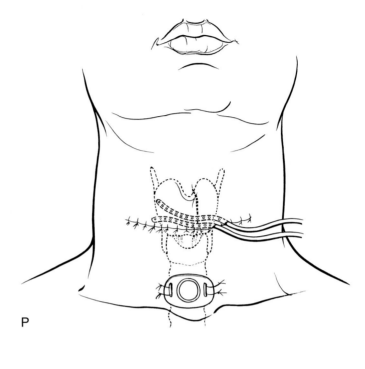

P

Figure 5–1 *Continued* Tracheostomy and laryngofissure.

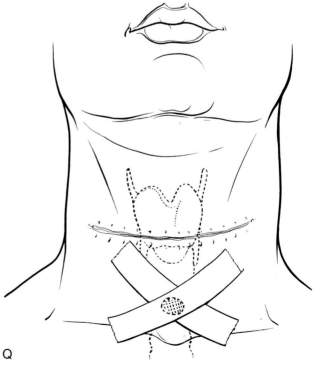

Q

Figure 5–1*O*. This sagittal view shows the relation of the tracheostomy tube to the surrounding structures.

Figure 5–1*P*. The skin incision is closed over wound suction drains (Jackson-Pratt). The tracheostomy tube is secured with sutures and tape.

Figure 5–1*Q*. When the wound has healed and the airway is satisfactory, the tracheostomy tube is decannulated. The tracheostomy site is occluded with tape. It will close spontaneously.

Results of Laryngofissure

Cure rates reported in the post–World War II literature have ranged from 60% to 98%.[19, 23–26] The differences are related to variations in the indications for the procedure and on whether the procedure was performed after radiotherapy failures. Cure rates greater than 90% should be consistently obtainable by limiting the procedure to the indications outlined earlier in this chapter, and especially, in cases of radiotherapy failure, by limiting the procedure to those patients who had surgically treatable lesions before radiologic treatment.

The quality of the voice obtained after laryngofissure varies. The standard technique does not provide for reconstruction or resurfacing of the site of the resected cord. The mucosal defect is permitted to granulate and eventually reepithelialize. Formation of scar tissue usually results in a band of tissue that replaces the resected cord. Because the bulk, smoothness, and flexibility of this band are not consistent from patient to patient, the quality of the voice obtained will also be variable. LeJeune and Lynch[24] reported comparatively good voice in 73% of patients, while Sessions et al.[26] reported good voice in 19 of 40 patients (48%) and only fair voice in another 19 patients (48%). In general, the voice obtained after laryngofissure is likely to be less satisfactory than the voice after radiotherapy.

The vertical subtotal laryngectomy and laryngoplasty described by Bailey[27, 28] and Bailey and Calcaterra[29] is an extended laryngofissure involving resection of all tissue within the thyroid ala, including the internal perichondrium and part or all of the arytenoid cartilage. The procedure can be used for T2 and T3 carcinomas with results that the authors report to be comparable to conventional hemilaryngectomy. A bipedicled sternohyoid muscle flap (see Fig. 5–9A) surfaced with external perichondrium is transposed into the laryngeal interior; this resurfaces the defect and provides bulk against which the opposite vocal cord can meet, thereby improving the voice. Canine experiments have revealed that the muscle undergoes considerable shrinkage subsequently, but the preservation of part of the arytenoid cartilage facilitates the formation of a ridge or "neocord" in the muscle flap.

A simpler method of improving the voice after laryngofissure may be the technique described by Jackson and Norris,[30] which involves resecting the anterior half of the ipsilateral thyroid cartilage, leaving the internal perichondrium intact. This permits some degree of collapse of the glottis, resulting in better approximation of the neocord and the remaining opposite cord during phonation.

VERTICAL PARTIAL LARYNGECTOMY

In Chapter 1, reference was made to Semon's definition of partial laryngectomy as a procedure requiring resection of at least an entire wing of the thyroid cartilage and also possibly an arytenoid cartilage and parts of the cricoid cartilage. Lesser resections are considered to be laryngofissures. This definition can still be used today to distinguish these procedures, with the exception that it be broadened to include procedures that involve substantial resection of the thyroid cartilage, rather than removal of an entire wing. The term "hemilaryngectomy" has also been broadened. Originally hemilaryngectomy, as performed by Gluck, involved resection of a true anatomic half of the larynx, including the cricoid. The modern vertical partial laryngectomies have usually consisted of lesser resections. Although partial laryngectomies and hemilaryngectomies were first described in the nineteenth century, the poor results discussed in the previous chapters precluded the general use of these procedures. In 1949, Goodyear[31] revived interest in hemilaryngectomy by describing an intralaryngeal obturator that could be used for simplified one-stage reconstruction, eliminating the need for multistaged reconstructive procedures that had formerly been required. Goodyear's use of the term "hemilaryngectomy" to describe the operation that involved resection of the thyroid ala and an arytenoid established its current meaning, although there are still variations in the procedure performed by different surgeons.

Reconstruction After Vertical Partial Laryngectomy

After removal of significant portions of laryngeal mucosa and cartilage, the resurfacing of the interior and the reconstruction of the framework and intralaryngeal bulk are of paramount importance in enabling the patient to regain normal laryngeal function. Thus, numerous reconstructive procedures have evolved, with more sophisticated methods developed as time passed. Resurfacing procedures were developed first, because the establishment of an intact airway was the primary objective in the development of partial laryngectomy. Later efforts were devoted to improving the voice and the deglutitory mechanism and in permitting more extended resection by replacement of glottic bulk, as well as replacement of the resected arytenoid and cricoid cartilages. The classification outlined in Table 5–1 is oversimplified because many of the procedures actually were designed to accomplish multiple pur-

Table 5–1. RESULTS OF ANTERIOR FRONTAL PARTIAL LARYNGECTOMY

Study	Follow-up (Years)	Tumor Stage	Survival No. Surviving/ Total No. (%)
Som and Silver[34]	3	T2	26/38 (68%)
Kirchner and Som[32]	4	T2	40/58 (69%)
Sessions et al.[33]	3	T1 and T2	111/157 (70%)

poses, and many may utilize more than one reconstruction technique.

Resurfacing Procedures

Intraluminal Prostheses. Goodyear[31] in 1949 initiated the modern era of partial laryngectomy by using an obturator after hemilaryngectomy. Goodyear's operation included resection of the thyroid and arytenoid cartilages and was used for unilateral lesions, including some with fixed vocal cords. The lumen was partially resurfaced by advancement of the hypopharyngeal mucosa, thereby anticipating later technical developments, but the resurfacing was incomplete. A solid acrylic tube, retained by the tracheostomy tube, was inserted to maintain the lumen in expectation of reepithelialization. The stent was left in place for 10 to 12 weeks. Goodyear's paper did not present data on the results of the procedure except to state his personal satisfaction with it.

Although the stent has been abandoned for most procedures for which Goodyear used it, the McNaught intralaryngeal keel (Fig. 5–2A) has been found useful by several authors[32–34] for reconstruction after anterior frontal vertical partial laryngectomy for carcinomas involving the anterior commissure. The keel, originally developed for treatment of anterior glottic webs,[35] partitions the larynx, permitting independent epithelialization of both sides.

Skin Flaps. Gluck[36, 37] used a cervical skin flap in his original hemilaryngectomy procedure to create a laryngostoma that was closed secondarily. A similar but more sophisticated and successful method with a skin flap and temporary laryngostoma was used by Meurman.[38] Conley[39–42] developed extensive experience with the use of skin flaps for resurfacing after various forms of partial laryngectomy and introduced many refinements of the technique. Conley's procedure consists of transposition of either unilateral or bilateral flaps into the laryngeal lumen, where they are meticulously sutured to the

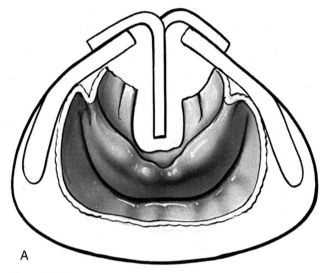

A

Figure 5–2. Laryngeal resurfacing procedures. *(A)* McNaught: intralaryngeal keel (Som and Silver procedure).

Illustration continued on following page

cut edges of the mucosa and the arytenoid (Fig. 5–2B). In nonirradiated cases, the incision may be closed in one stage by using an epithelial shave or by creating a new anterior commissure with a small epidermal flap. Originally, Conley created a new vocal cord by developing a secondary skin tube on the flap,[40] but this step was later abandoned as noncontributory.[42] Conley noted that the skin immediately over the larynx is not hair bearing in most males and is thus useful for laryngeal resurfacing.

Although skin flaps are usually not necessary in most nonirradiated patients undergoing initial surgery, Conley recommends their use in some cases where radiation therapy has failed, as well as in various specific conditions, including T2 anterior commissure lesions and lesions with "mild" subglottic extension and vocal cord fixation. I have found skin flaps to be useful in salvaging cases, usually after radiotherapy, that have undergone infection and necrosis. The use of skin flaps rather than a keel for reconstruction should be strongly considered for previously irradiated patients (see later discussion).

Skin and Mucosal Grafts. Figi[43, 44] used free skin grafts placed over a stent for laryngeal resurfacing (Fig. 5–2C). These procedures were often followed

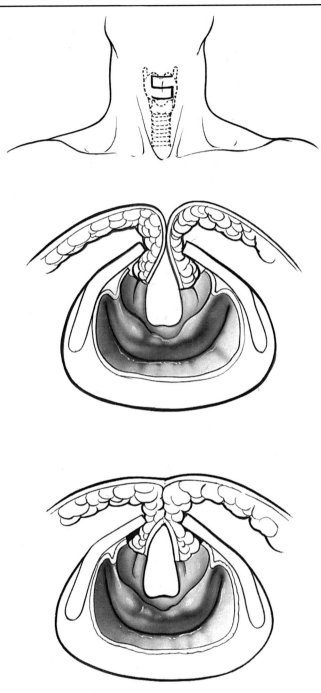

B

Figure 5–2 *Continued (B)* Skin flaps (Conley procedure).

by crusting and ozena. Norris[45] also used a free skin graft retained by a latex-covered foam rubber mold after extended frontolateral partial laryngectomy. Skin grafts were a useful step in the evolution of partial laryngectomy procedures, but they are not used much at present because relatively small areas can be left to reepithelialize spontaneously, and larger defects are repaired more satisfactorily with mucosal or skin flaps. Free mucosal grafts were used by Harpman,[46] eliminating some of the difficulties noted with skin grafts, but these have also been supplanted by other methods.

Mucosal Flaps. Som,[47] in 1951, described the procedure that has now become the standard method for resurfacing after hemilaryngectomy (extended frontolateral partial laryngectomy), namely, the advancement of the hypopharyngeal mucosa. The procedure, described in detail later, involves preservation of the hypopharyngeal and the piriform sinus mucosa on the side of the resection. The cut edge of the hypopharyngeal mucosa, corresponding to the aryepiglottic fold posteriorly, is thinned, removing the cuneiform and corniculate cartilages, and the mucosa is advanced to resurface the hemilarynx (Fig. 5–2D, D_1, D_2). A band of fibrous tissue develops beneath the mucosa, creating a structure that functions like a vocal cord. The new "cord" is located below the level of the opposite cord, causing the glottis to be somewhat "S" shaped. Although Som[47] originally used an acrylic obturator, this was subsequently found unnecessary when at least one side of the larynx was completely resurfaced.[16] In more recent procedures, when various structures are inserted for glottic and vestibular reconstruction, the hypopharyngeal mucosa is drawn over them and sutured in place.[48–50]

Conley[51] described modifications of advancement flaps of hypopharyngeal mucosa in 1959. Rotation flaps of hypopharyngeal mucosa have been used by Iwai[52] for extended hemilaryngectomy and "subtotal" laryngectomy and by Ogura and Dedo[53] after "subtotal" laryngectomy. ("Subtotal" laryngectomy is usually performed for supraglottic lesions and is discussed in Chapter 6.)

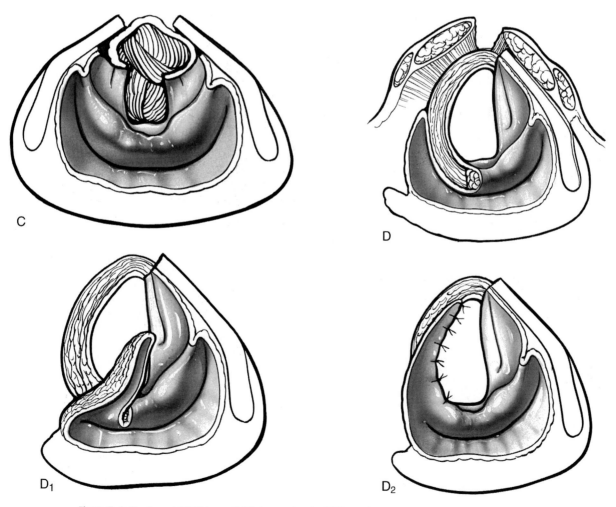

C

D

D_1

D_2

Figure 5–2 *Continued (C)* Skin graft (Figi procedure). *(D)* Hypopharyngeal mucosal flap (Som procedure).

Glottic and Vestibular Reconstruction

Resurfacing of the larynx enables restoration of the airway to a satisfactory degree. There will usually be vocal impairment because of the lack of sufficient bulk at the glottic level, with resultant "air wasting." Lack of glottic competence as well as deficiencies in the posterior wall of the vestibule may also impair the patient's ability to swallow without aspiration. Although most younger patients can adapt to the glottic and vestibular defects and will learn to swallow within a few weeks after surgery, elderly and chronically ill individuals may have great difficulty with this. In addition, because the indications for partial laryngectomy have been extended to include those lesions with a greater degree of posterior subglottic extension that necessitates resection of the cricoid cartilage, replacement of the laryngeal framework has become necessary to restore deglutition, even in active individuals.

Perichondrial and Muscle Flaps. Pressman[54] in 1954 described one of the earliest techniques of glottic reconstruction. His purpose was to achieve resurfacing, to maintain the lumen, and to provide rigidity of the laryngeal walls after extensive partial laryngectomy. With his technique, a subperichondrial hemilaryngectomy that includes resection of the arytenoid cartilage, the anterior commissure, and a portion of the opposite vocal cord is performed. Either one or both thyroid alae are resected separately and preserved, and the external perichondrium is reflected from the thyroid alae and sutured to the internal aspect of the deeper layer of the strap muscles. The external perichondrial flaps with the overlying muscles are now transposed inward to form a new lining, the muscles providing bulk for the new glottis. The thyroid alae are reinserted between the deep and superficial strap muscles as free grafts.

Bailey[27–29] modified Pressman's procedure to eliminate the removal of the thyroid alae except for a vertical midline segment in bilateral anterior commissure lesions. A subperichondrial unilateral or bilateral partial laryngectomy is performed, after which a bipedicled flap of sternohyoid muscle, covered on its inner aspect with external perichondrium, is transposed internal to the denuded thyroid ala (Fig. 5–3A). This is done either unilaterally or bilaterally, depending on the resection. As in Pressman's procedure, the external perichondrium forms the new lining, and the muscle provides bulk to buttress against the opposite true and false vocal cords.

Ogura and Biller[48] felt that bipedicled muscle flaps did not achieve the desired result in extended frontolateral hemilaryngectomy, including resection of the thyroid and arytenoid cartilages, because the muscle bulk obtained with the flap was located in the anterior glottis. After resection of the arytenoid

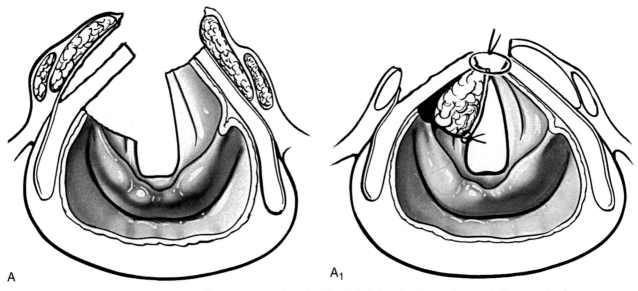

A   A₁

Figure 5–3. Glottic and vestibular reconstruction. *(A)* Bipedicled sternohyoid muscle flap (Bailey procedure).

cartilage, the major defect was in the posterior glottis. The authors described an inferiorly based single-pedicled sternohyoid muscle flap (Fig. 5–3B) transposed through an opening in the sternothyroid muscle into the larynx. The more mobile single pedicled flap, based at cord level, is placed posteriorly to fill the bed of the resected arytenoid cartilage, where it is secured by suture to the joint surface (Fig. 5–3B₁). A relaxing incision through the overlying fascia is made to relieve tension. The larynx is resurfaced, and the muscle flap is covered by advancement of the hypopharyngeal mucosa, as described previously (Fig. 5–3B₂).

Free Grafts. Similar procedures for glottic reconstruction have been described by Quinn,[50, 55] who used free transplants of muscle, and Dedo,[49] who used free transplants of fat and fascia. Both authors noted that the transplants tended to shrink; transplants, therefore, should be made larger than the volume of tissue they are intended to replace. Being unimpaired by a pedicle, these free transplants can be positioned at will and tailored exactly to the desired size and shape. The muscle transplant is obtained from the sternohyoid muscle, and the fat from the subcutaneous tissue in the hyoid area. When placed in the glottic defect, the free transplants are completely covered by the advancement of the hypopharyngeal mucosa, as described previously. Although they shrink, the transplants appear to be well tolerated, despite the absence of a blood supply, and they do not slough off. All of Dedo's patients had had previous radiotherapy.

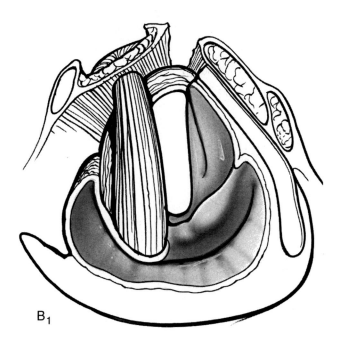

B₁

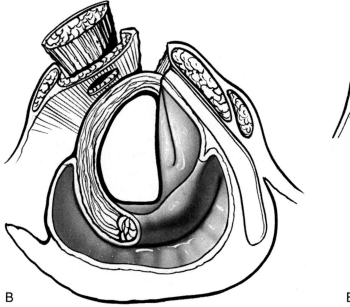

B

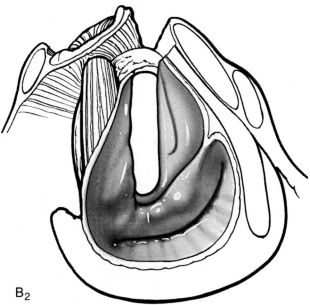

B₂

Figure 5–3 *Continued* Glottic and vestibular reconstruction. *(B)* Single-pedicled sternohyoid muscle flap (Ogura and Biller procedure).

Illustration continued on following page

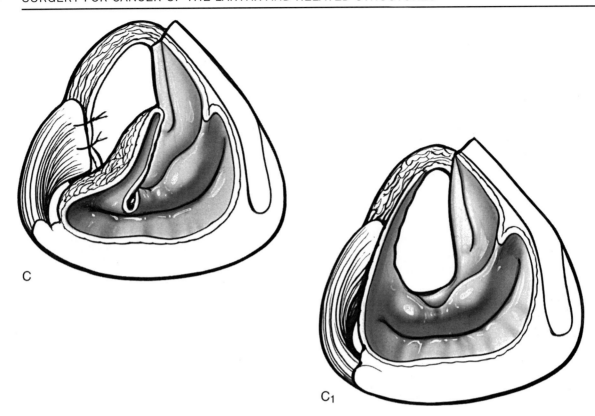

Figure 5–3 *Continued* Glottic and vestibular reconstruction. *(C)* Cartilage flap (Blaugrund and Kurland procedure).

Cartilage Flaps. The major objection to the soft tissue flaps and transplants used for glottic reconstruction has been the tendency for postoperative shrinkage, with the potential for developing recurrent glottic insufficiency. Cartilage provides a more consistent size and shape than does soft tissue. Free cartilage grafts have been used for glottic reconstruction after hemilaryngectomy, as well as for glottic augmentation in other situations.[56] The objection to free cartilage grafts is, of course, the absence of a blood supply and the possibility of necrosis.

Blaugrund and Kurland[57] described a muscle-pedicled cartilage flap that had the dual advantage of being of consistent size and of carrying its own blood supply. This procedure, which is now routinely performed on our service, is described in detail below. The cartilage, taken from the posterior third of the thyroid ala, is pedicled on the inferior constrictor muscle (Fig. 5–3C). The size and shape of the cartilage can be tailored according to need. If necessary, the bulk of the cartilage may be augmented by the attachment of a segment of free cartilage before rotation.

The pedicled thyroid cartilage flap proved suc-cessful early on in its use in the late 1970s[16, 57] and has subsequently been employed consistently for reconstruction of larger defects in the laryngeal framework. The possibility of using this muscle-based cartilage flap for replacement of both the cricoid and the arytenoid cartilages after extended hemilaryngectomy was suggested by Blaugrund and Kurland.[57] Biller and Som,[58] and subsequently Biller and Lawson,[59] reported the use of a similar but larger flap in five cases of hemilaryngectomy that was performed for glottic carcinoma with posterior subglottic extension and that necessitated resection of part of the cricoid lamina.

Iwai[52] employed a greenstick-fractured, preserved superior cornu of thyroid cartilage for reconstruction of the framework after extended hemilaryngectomy with cricoid resection and after subtotal laryngectomy. The cartilage was rotated into the defect, and the lumen was then resurfaced with an inferiorly based flap of mucosa from the lateral pharyngeal wall. Friedman et al.[60] described a similar procedure, in which they used the contralateral thyroid ala to maintain anteroposterior diameter and to reconstitute the glottis after subtotal laryngectomy.

Surgical Techniques for Vertical Partial Laryngectomy

Frontolateral Partial Laryngectomy

Lesions crossing the anterior commissure confounded the early advocates of laryngofissure and were regarded as a contraindication. In 1922, Chevalier Jackson, at the tenth International Congress of Otology in Paris,[61, 62] presented a technique for subperichondrial resection of anterior commissure tumors. The midline thyrotomy was made so as not to penetrate the internal perichondrium, and the involved anterior commissure and portions of both vocal cords were resected. In 1940, Louis Clerf[63] described a technique for resection of an inverted wedge of thyroid cartilage at the anterior commissure in continuity with the tumor and portions of both cords. Broyles,[64] in 1943, noted that the vocal cords inserted by a tendon directly into the cartilage at the anterior commissure, there being no true internal perichondrium at that region. Kemler,[65] in 1947, after confirming the difficulty of cutting through the thyroid cartilage in the midline without penetrating the underlying soft tissues, devised a technique of bilateral thyrotomy for resection of a vertical midline segment of thyroid cartilage en bloc with the anterior commissure and portions of both vocal cords. Leroux-Robert,[66–68] at the Curie Foundation in Paris, developed extensive experience in surgical treatment of laryngeal cancer over several decades from the 1930s on. His technique of frontolateral laryngectomy used the same principle of bilateral thyrotomy and resection of the midline vertical segment of thyroid cartilage. The degree of extension of the procedure laterally depended on the nature of the lesion. The extended frontolateral partial laryngectomy of Norris[45] was designed for lesions that involved both the anterior commissure and the posterior portions of the ipsilateral vocal cord.

Indications

Frontolateral laryngectomy is suitable for T1a and T1b lesions that approach or involve only 1 to 2 mm of the opposite vocal cord. Such lesions respond well to radiotherapy, and therefore, in our experience, we have had little occasion to use this technique. If no more than one third of the lesser involved vocal cord must be resected, postoperative stricture may be prevented by suturing the cut edge of the vocal cord mucosa to the external perichondrium[45] or by secondarily electrocoagulating the synechia that develop, as was done originally by Leroux-Robert.[67] If resection of more than one third of the contralateral cord is required, then a midline partition or reconstruction with epiglottis will be required (see the next section).

Technique (Repair with Bipedicled Sternohyoid Flap)

Figure 5–4A. Bilateral vertical thyrotomy incisions are placed about 8 to 9 mm on each side of the midline, with the greater amount of cartilage removed on the side of the tumor.

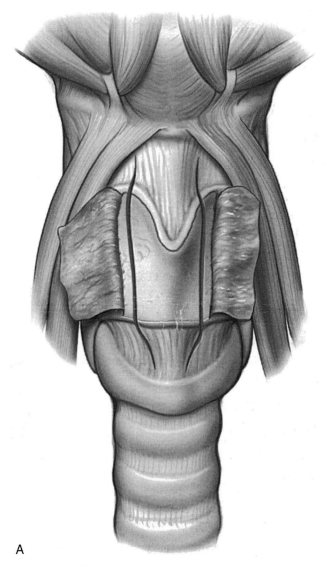

A

Figure 5–4. Frontolateral laryngectomy.
Illustration continued on following page

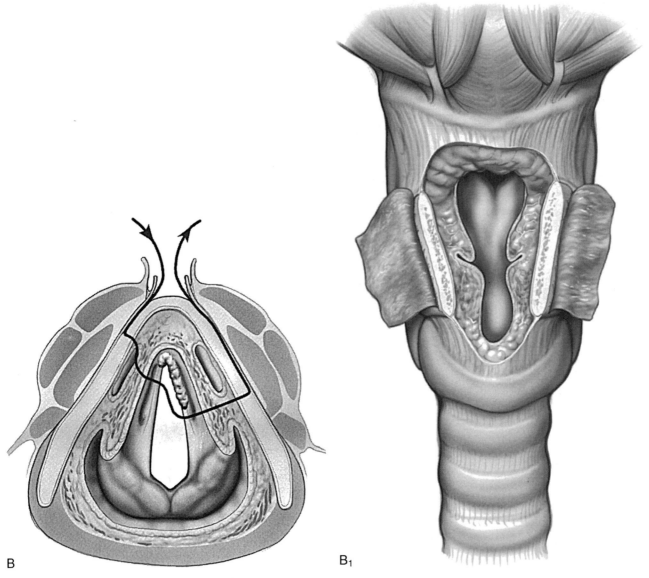

B

B₁

Figure 5–4 *Continued* Frontal laryngectomy.

Figure 5–4B. The area to be resected is outlined. On the ipsilateral (right) side, resection includes the anterior two thirds (the mobile portion) of the vocal cord. If resection of the arytenoid cartilage is required because of posterior extension, extended frontolateral laryngectomy (see discussion later in this chapter) will be required. On the contralateral (left) side, one third of the true vocal cord may be resected.

The larynx is entered on the side of lesser involvement, immediately deep to the thyrotomy incision. On the involved side, the laryngeal soft tissue, including the true and false cords and the ventricle, is separated subperichondrially from the inner aspect of the thyroid cartilage. The posterior line of excision may include the vocal process of the arytenoid cartilage, but it leaves the cricoarytenoid joint intact.

Figure 5–4C. For repair, the mucosa on the contralateral side is sutured to the external perichondrium in order to resurface one side of the larynx completely. The side of major resection may be left open to granulate, but a better result may be obtained by employing a muscle flap to replace the bulk of the resected vocal cord. For an anterior defect, a bipedicled flap of sternohyoid muscle is suitable. The muscle is transferred deep to the preserved perichondrium and sutured in place.

Figure 5–4D. The external perichondrium is closed over the muscle flap, restoring the glottic bulk and closing the larynx.

Figure 5–4E. This figure shows the relation of the muscle flap to the larynx.

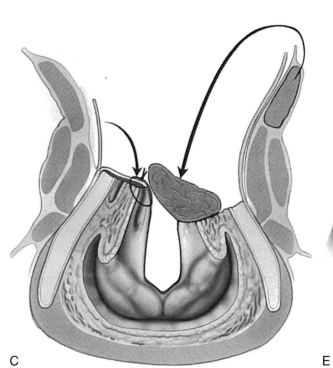

C

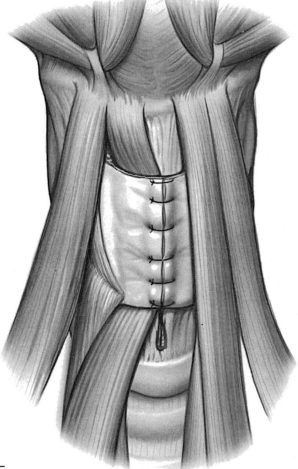

E

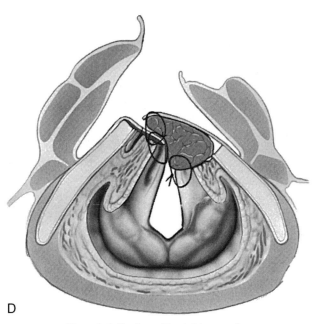

D

Figure 5–4 *Continued* Frontal laryngectomy.

Anterior Frontal Vertical Partial Laryngectomy

The frontolateral laryngectomy, described in the preceding section, is performed mainly for lesions that do not require resection of major portions of both vocal cords. Elaborate reconstruction is not necessary. For lesions traversing the anterior commissure and requiring resection of significant portions (one third or more) of both vocal cords, postoperative stricture formation is inevitable if bilateral raw surfaces are left to heal spontaneously. The techniques of Goodyear[31] (obturator), Meurman[38] (skin flap), Figi[43, 44] (skin graft), and Pressman[54] (external perichondrium and cartilage grafts) were employed to prevent this complication.

In 1968, Som and Silver[34] reported on the use of the McNaught keel for reconstruction after procedures that resulted in resection of major portions of both vocal cords. In nonirradiated patients, temporarily partitioning the larynx with a tantalum or silicone rubber (Silastic) keel provides a simple and effective means of preventing stricture formation.[32, 34] This technique has also been used in patients after radiotherapy, but complications, such as perichondritis, necrosis, stenosis, and fistula, are more likely to occur. In such patients it may be wise to consider a staged reconstruction with skin flaps rather than attempt primary closure and spontaneous epithelialization with the keel. Immediately covering the denuded irradiated cartilage with skin is safer than leaving it exposed within the laryngeal lumen.

Indications

This procedure is employed for T2 lesions that involve the membranous portions of both vocal cords and extend subglottically in the midline region. Lesions that involve as much as the anterior half of both vocal cords almost always extend subglottically beneath the anterior commissure.[32] Although some authors[10, 15, 69, 70] have reported satisfactory results in treatment of anterior commissure lesions with radiotherapy, others have concluded that T2 lesions do not respond well.[34, 71] Analysis of the papers written by some radiotherapy advocates[10, 69] indicates that when the cases are carefully analyzed according to tumor size, surgery has been felt to be more effective for the more extensive lesions.

Limitations

Posterior Extension. If the lesion extends onto the vocal process of the arytenoid on one side, extended frontolateral laryngectomy with resection of the arytenoid is required.

Subglottic Extension. The procedure may be used for lesions that extend 1 cm or less subglottically in the anterior region. The upper half of the anterior cricoid cartilage is included in the resected specimen for lesions that approach the cricothyroid membrane. Lesions that extend more than 1 cm below the anterior commissure involve the cricothyroid membrane and are associated with a high incidence of extralaryngeal spread and thyroid cartilage involvement. These tumors require total laryngectomy. Lesser degrees of subglottic extension are permissible laterally.

Vocal Cord Paralysis. If there is slight limitation of motion secondary to the bulk of the tumor, the limited resection described here may be used. Vocal cord fixation secondary to thyroarytenoid muscle invasion and associated with varying degrees of subglottic extension is not suitable for this limited resection, but it may be treatable by the more extensive hemilaryngectomy procedure according to the criteria already outlined.

Technique

Figure 5–5*A*. The preliminary steps including tracheostomy and separation of the strap muscles in the midline are the same as for laryngofissure and hemilaryngectomy. Bilateral vertical thyrotomy incisions are made 0.5 to 1.0 cm from the midline on both sides. The thyrotomy is placed farther laterally on the side of greater involvement.

Figure 5–5*B*. This transverse section demonstrates a lesion appropriate for the anterior commissure technique and the extent of resection. The lesion crosses the anterior commissure and involves significant portions of both vocal cords. Such lesions invariably have some degree of subglottic or supraglottic extension. The resection includes the membranous portions of both vocal cords with the underlying soft tissue and a midline vertical segment of thyroid cartilage.

Figure 5–5*C*. The laryngeal soft tissue is dissected subperichondrially from the inner aspect of the thyroid ala on either side, as far as the vocal processes.

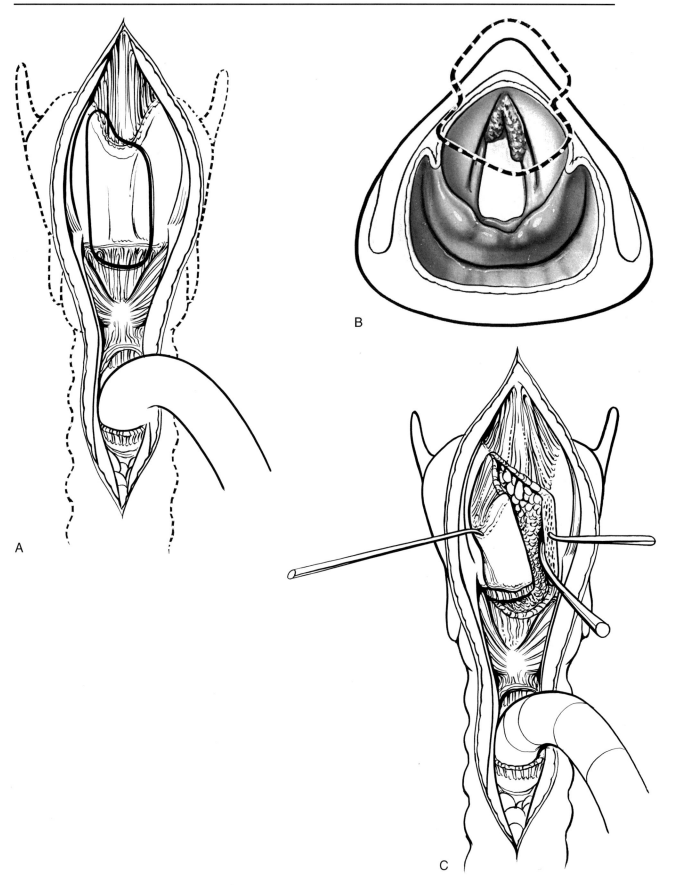

Figure 5–5. Anterior frontal partial laryngectomy.

Illustration continued on following page

Figure 5–5*D.* This transverse section demonstrates the above maneuver.

Figure 5–5*E.* The laryngeal lumen is entered through the cricothyroid membrane. This procedure should be done at a distance from the tumor. If there are more than 5 mm of subglottic extension,

the upper half of the cricoid cartilage should be included in the resection *(dotted line)*. By retracting the mucosa upward with a hook, it is possible to make certain that the mucosal incision does not encroach on the lesion. A vertical incision is made in the mucosa just anterior to the vocal process on the left (lesser involved) side.

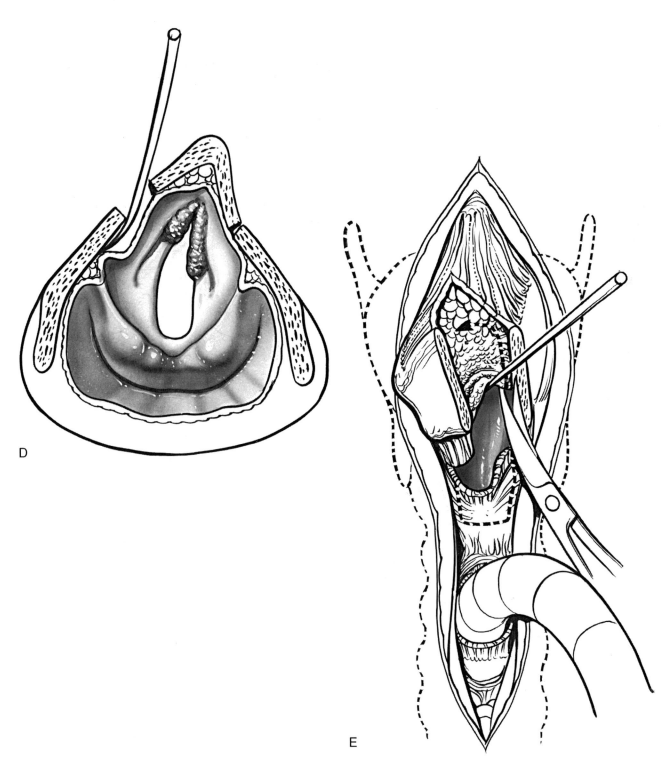

D

E

Figure 5–5 *Continued* Anterior frontal partial laryngectomy.

Figure 5–5F. The inferior, left lateral, and superior mucosal incisions have been made. The superior incision is through the thyrohyoid membrane. At this point the specimen is retracted outward, exposing the entire lesion.

Figure 5–5G. This transverse view shows the maneuver described in Figure 5–5F and the line of resection.

Figure 5–5H. The larynx is shown after removal of the specimen. Only the arytenoid cartilages, covered by a narrow band of mucosa, remain.

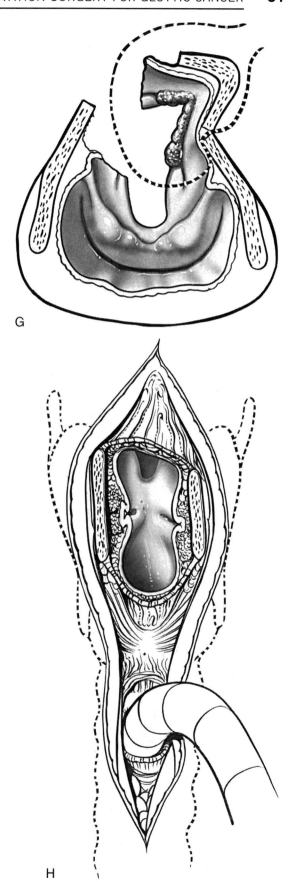

G

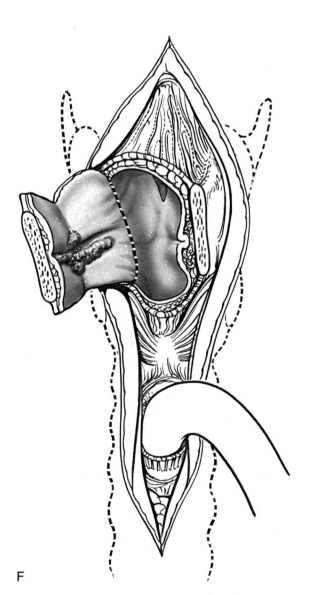

F

H

Figure 5–5 *Continued* Anterior frontal partial laryngectomy.

Illustration continued on following page

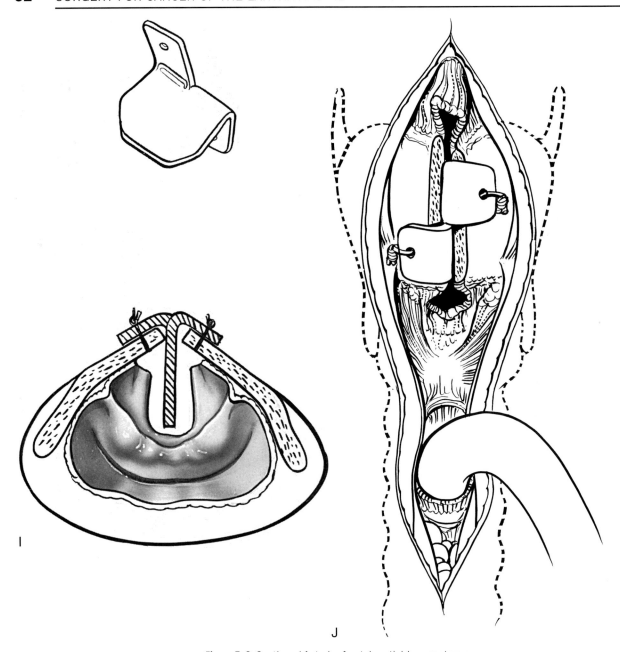

Figure 5–3 *Continued* Anterior frontal partial laryngectomy.

Figure 5–5*I*. This transverse section shows the relation of the Silastic keel to the laryngeal structures after placement. The keel should be trimmed if necessary. The keel should be deep enough to extend between the remaining stumps of the vocal cords, completely separating the raw surfaces on each side, but should not be so deep as to contact the posterior mucosa.

Figure 5–5*J*. The keel is fixed to the thyroid cartilage with wire or nonabsorbable synthetic sutures. The strap muscles are approximated, the tracheostomy tube is placed through a stab wound in the inferior skin flap, and the skin is sutured, as in Figures 5–1*N*, 5–1*O*, and 5–1*P*. The tracheostomy is not decannulated between the first and second stages of the operation.

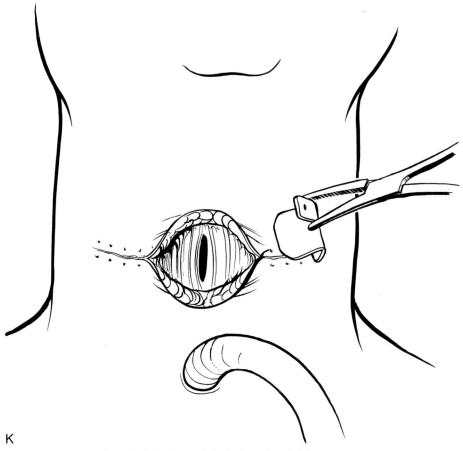

K

Figure 5–5 *Continued* Anterior frontal partial laryngectomy.

Figure 5–5K. In 6 to 8 weeks the keel is removed by reentering the central portion of the wound, raising skin flaps a short distance, and separating the strap muscles. The keel is exposed and removed by dividing the sutures holding it in place. The wound is closed tightly. The tracheostomy is decannulated within a few days. The second-stage procedure can be performed under local anesthesia.

It is possible to eliminate the second stage by using a sheet of Silastic instead of a keel to partition the larynx. The Silastic sheet is retained in place with sutures placed through the skin and can be removed endoscopically after cutting the sutures.

Results

The anterior commissure technique described here was originally reported by Som and Silver[34] in 1968 in a series of 38 patients. Twenty-six (68%) were cured by the initial conservation surgery, and an additional five patients were cured by secondary procedures, thus producing an overall cure rate of 81%. Of the 38 patients, 7 had recurrent or persis-tent lesions after radiotherapy, and 5 of these were cured by the anterior commissure technique. In Kirchner and Som's series of 58 patients,[32] 40 survived 4 or more years without recurrence, but 3 of these subsequently required total laryngectomy for salvage. Of 11 cases of radiotherapy failure, 5 were cured by the anterior commissure technique. All the lesions reported in these series were T2 glottic carcinomas with a maximum subglottic extension of 1 cm at the anterior commissure. Sessions et al.[33] reported a cure rate of 74% in 61 patients with T1 and T2 anterior commissure lesions.

Extended Frontolateral Laryngectomy (Vertical Hemilaryngectomy)

Lesions with sufficient posterior extension to require resection of the arytenoid cartilage require resection of the ipsilateral thyroid ala, the arytenoid cartilage, the mucosa from the aryepiglottic fold to the upper border of the cricoid cartilage, and the underlying muscle from the posterior midline to just beyond the anterior midline. The procedure, described by Som[47] in 1951, was a major influence in establishing widespread acceptance of hemilaryngectomy. The outstanding feature of the procedure was the use of a flap of hypopharyngeal mucosa that was advanced into the larynx for primary reconstruction. This eliminated the need for skin grafts, stents, or temporary laryngostomas, thus simplifying the management of these patients.

Norris,[45] in 1958, extended the concept of Leroux-Robert of including the anterior commissure with its overlying cartilage in the resected specimen, along with resection of the vocal cord and arytenoid cartilage for lesions extending posteriorly to or beyond the tip of the vocal process. Norris employed a skin graft for resurfacing the side of major resection. Ogura and his colleagues at Washington University in St. Louis were instrumental in developing vertical hemilaryngectomy.[4, 49, 72, 73] Resections varied according to the lesion but usually included the ipsilateral thyroid ala with the exception of a 3-mm-wide posterior vertical strip and part or all of the arytenoid cartilage. Because this group preferred to use hemilaryngectomy for T1 lesions confined to the mobile vocal cord, in many of their cases only the vocal process was resected along with the thyroid cartilage. The extent of resection of the opposite vocal cord varied with the lesion. For reconstruction, if the arytenoid had been resected, a hypopharyngeal flap was used for resurfacing, usually in conjunction with a single-pedicled sternohyoid muscle flap (see Fig. 5–3*B*) placed beneath the mucosa to provide bulk in the resected area. The McNaught[35] type of keel was employed for lesions requiring resection of significant portions of the contralateral vocal cord.

Indications

T1 Tumors. As discussed earlier, T1 tumors confined to the membranous part of the vocal cord can be extirpated by radiotherapy, endoscopic removal, or laryngofissure. Some surgeons prefer to use hemilaryngectomy for these lesions, feeling that only by resecting the overlying thyroid ala can complete removal of possibly unrecognized deeply infiltrating tumor be achieved. The choice of hemilaryngectomy versus laryngofissure for these lesions is more a matter of preference than of scientific necessity. If hemilaryngectomy is preferred, it is not necessary to resect the arytenoid cartilage unless there is extension onto the vocal process, which is unusual with T1 tumors. The posterior line of resection may transect the vocal process, leaving the arytenoid intact and mobile. The external perichondrium and strap muscles can be sutured to the opposite thyroid ala without requiring intralaryngeal resurfacing.

T2 Tumors. The major indication for hemilaryngectomy with arytenoid cartilage resection is for carcinoma extending either posteriorly onto the arytenoid cartilage or laterally into the floor of the ventricle.[16] The posterior extension may involve the vocal process or the anterior surface of the arytenoid cartilage, but not the cricoarytenoid joint or the posterior (hypopharyngeal) surface of the arytenoid cartilage.

Lesions involving the floor of the ventricle laterally often infiltrate the vocal muscle and limit its motion to varying degrees. These lesions are amenable to hemilaryngectomy. However, extension of the lesion to the ventricular surface of the false cord indicates that it is a transglottic tumor and has a high probability of cartilaginous invasion. Hemilaryngectomy should not be attempted in such a case.[74]

Whereas radiotherapy is highly effective for treatment of T1 vocal cord lesions, it is far less effective in treatment of T2 and T3 lesions.[10, 16, 75] Partial laryngectomy is the treatment of choice for suitable lesions.

T3 Tumors. Complete fixation of a vocal cord was originally thought to be a contraindication to hemilaryngectomy by surgeons in North America,[45, 73, 76] although Meurman[38] and Leroux-Robert[77] performed hemilaryngectomy in some cases of this type in Europe. In 1971, Kirchner and Som,[74] after evaluating a series of total laryngectomy specimens resected because of vocal cord fixation, concluded that most of them could have been adequately resected by hemilaryngectomy. A set of criteria for resection of T3 lesions by hemilaryngectomy was established, and 22 patients with fixed vocal cords underwent that procedure. Of the 22 patients, 13 (60%) survived 2 years or more; 3 of 9 recurrences were treated successfully by total laryngectomy.

The criteria of these authors for selection of patients with T3 lesions for hemilaryngectomy are as follows:

1. The tumor may have 8 to 9 mm of subglottic extension from the anterior to the midportion of the true cord but no more than 3 to 4 mm of subglottic extension posteriorly, where the cricoid lamina is immediately below the arytenoid and likely to be invaded.
2. The lesion must be restricted to the true cord at the anterior commissure. Upward or downward extension at this level is often associated with thyroid cartilage involvement or extension beyond the larynx.
3. The lesion must not extend across the ventricle to the inferior surface of the false cord.
4. The arytenoid cartilage itself should not be involved.

Technique (Reconstruction with Pedicled
Thyroid Cartilage Flap)

Figure 5–6A. The preliminary tracheostomy is performed in the same manner as for laryngofissure. The infrahyoid muscles are separated in the midline, exposing the larynx. The thyrotomy incision is made slightly to the left (contralateral side) of the midline.

Figure 5–6B. This transverse view shows a lesion of the right vocal cord that is suitable for hemilaryngectomy. Note the extension onto the vocal process of the arytenoid. The extent of resection is outlined, including the anterior two thirds of the right thyroid ala, the entire right vocal cord including the arytenoid, the anterior commissure, and 2 to 3 mm of the opposite vocal cord.

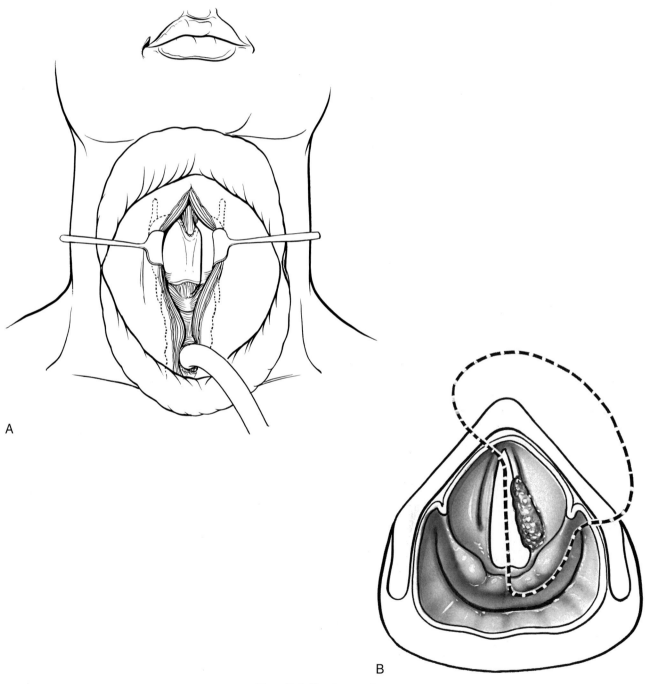

A

B

Figure 5–6. Hemilaryngectomy.

Illustration continued on following page

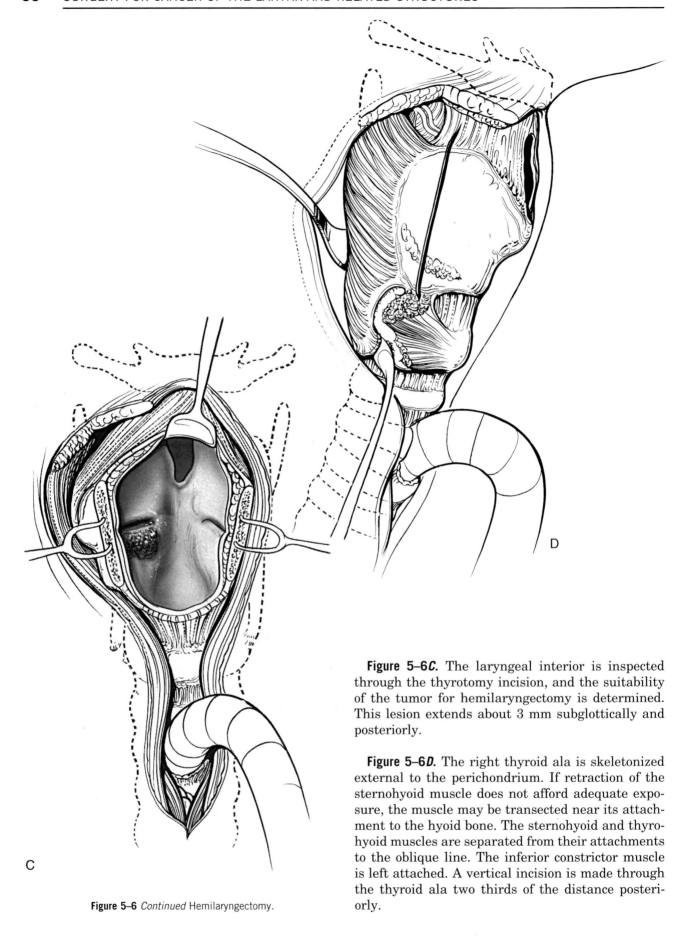

Figure 5–6*C.* The laryngeal interior is inspected through the thyrotomy incision, and the suitability of the tumor for hemilaryngectomy is determined. This lesion extends about 3 mm subglottically and posteriorly.

Figure 5–6*D.* The right thyroid ala is skeletonized external to the perichondrium. If retraction of the sternohyoid muscle does not afford adequate exposure, the muscle may be transected near its attachment to the hyoid bone. The sternohyoid and thyrohyoid muscles are separated from their attachments to the oblique line. The inferior constrictor muscle is left attached. A vertical incision is made through the thyroid ala two thirds of the distance posteriorly.

C

Figure 5–6 *Continued* Hemilaryngectomy.

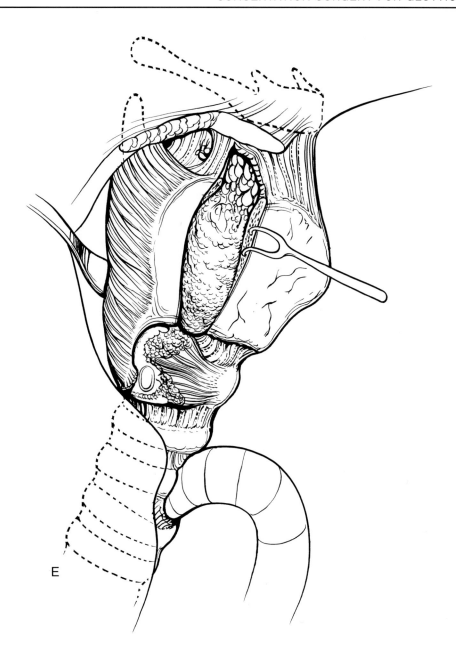

Figure 5–6E. The posterior third of the thyroid ala will be used for reconstruction, and it is separated from the portion to be resected. It is dissected posteriorly, leaving it attached to the inferior constrictor muscle, while preserving the internal and external perichondrium. The external aspect of the right pyriform sinus mucosa is seen bulging deep to the posterior third of the thyroid ala. The separation of the inferior cornu of the thyroid from the cricoid cartilage through the joint releases this portion of the cartilage, permitting lateral retraction. The superior laryngeal blood vessels and nerve are divided and ligated.

Figure 5–6 *Continued* Hemilaryngectomy.
Illustration continued on following page

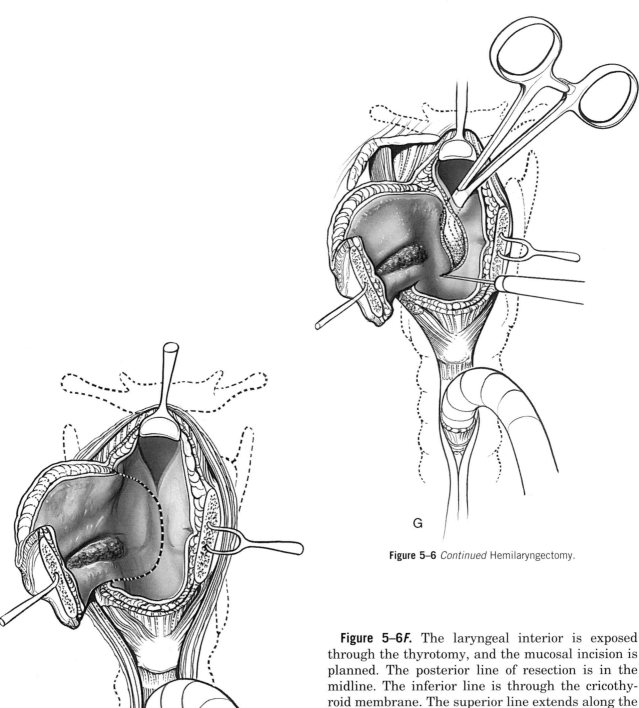

G

Figure 5–6 *Continued* Hemilaryngectomy.

Figure 5–6F. The laryngeal interior is exposed through the thyrotomy, and the mucosal incision is planned. The posterior line of resection is in the midline. The inferior line is through the cricothyroid membrane. The superior line extends along the aryepiglottic fold and continues anteriorly through the thyrohyoid membrane. The anterior line is at the thyrotomy site through the opposite vocal cord, about 2 to 3 mm from the midline. If the anterior commissure is infiltrated by tumor, a greater portion of the opposite cords is resected. It is wise to outline the entire resection with the cautery knife before making deeper incisions.

Figure 5–6G. The placement of a right-angle clamp in the hypopharynx between the arytenoid cartilages facilitates the division of the interarytenoid

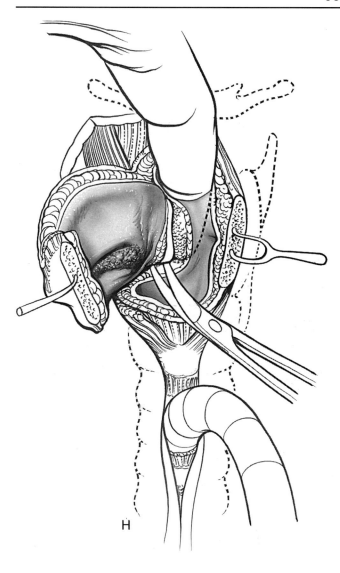

H

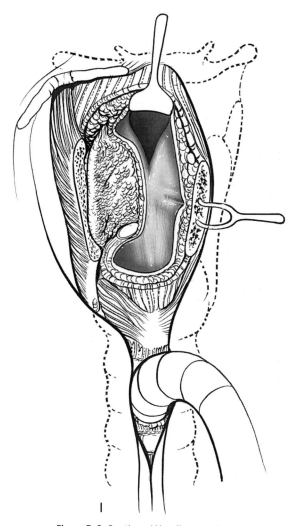

I

mucosa and the muscle by permitting traction on the tissues as they are incised. It is important not to carry this posterior vertical incision through the mucosa of the anterior hypopharynx, which is deep to the interarytenoid muscle.

Figure 5–6*H.* The cricoarytenoid joint is separated with scissors. Placement of a finger into the pyriform sinus facilitates this maneuver by permitting palpation and fixation of the arytenoid cartilage. With the finger still in place, the arytenoid cartilage is separated from the outer aspects of the pyriform sinus mucosa, and the specimen is liberated while the pyriform sinus is preserved.

Figure 5–6*I.* The laryngeal structures that remain after removal of the tumor are shown.

Figure 5–6 *Continued* Hemilaryngectomy.
Illustration continued on following page

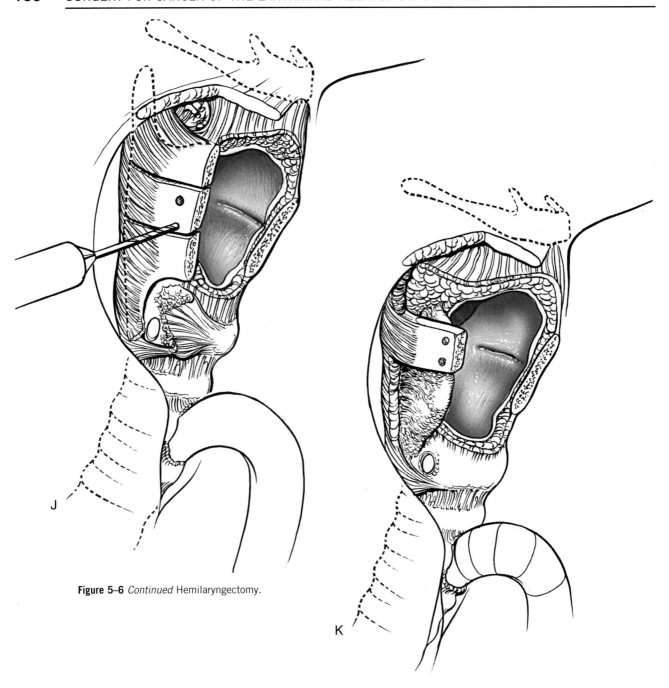

Figure 5–6 *Continued* Hemilaryngectomy.

Figure 5–6J. The cartilage flap is prepared. The upper and lower portions of the posterior third of the thyroid ala are removed, whereas the central portion, left attached to the inferior constrictor muscle and the perichondrium, is preserved. The size and shape of the remaining portion of cartilage should roughly correspond to the resected arytenoid cartilage. Holes are drilled in the cartilage for placement of sutures.

Figure 5–6K. The fully mobilized and prepared cartilage flap is shown.

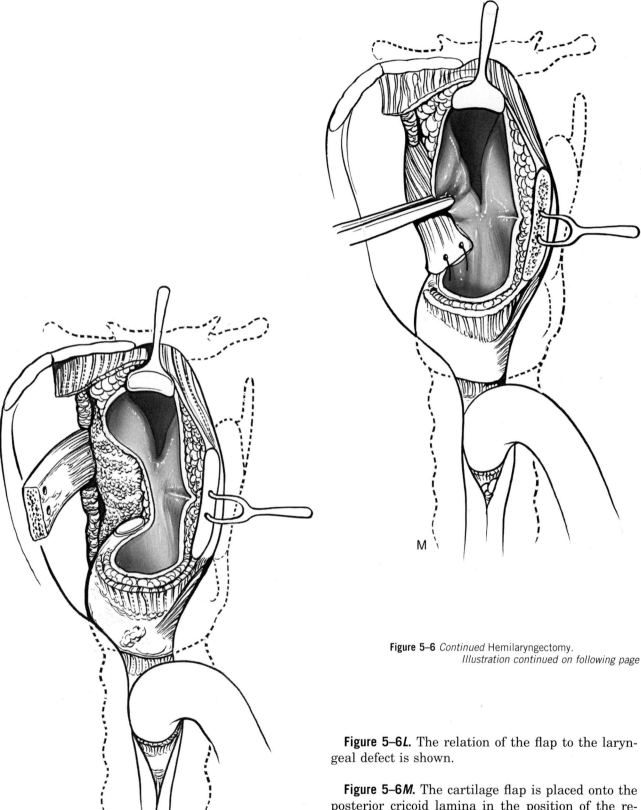

Figure 5–6 *Continued* Hemilaryngectomy.
Illustration continued on following page

Figure 5–6*L.* The relation of the flap to the laryngeal defect is shown.

Figure 5–6*M.* The cartilage flap is placed onto the posterior cricoid lamina in the position of the resected arytenoid cartilage. It does not matter which aspect of the cartilage flap is placed on the cricoid. This should be determined by the best fit. Holes are drilled in the cricoid cartilage, and the cartilage flap is fixed with 2–0 or 3–0 polyglactin sutures.

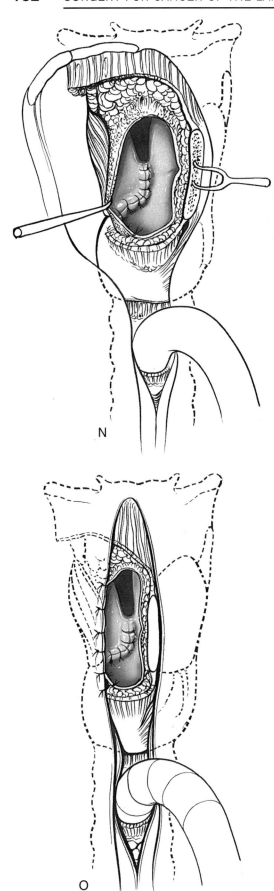

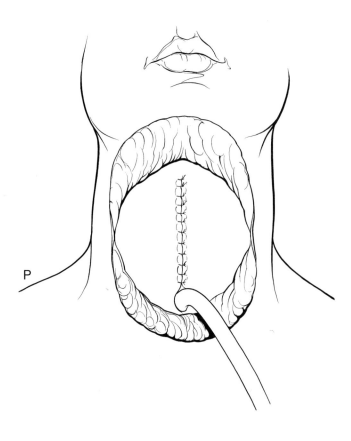

Figure 5–6 *Continued* Hemilaryngectomy.

Figure 5–6N. The pyriform sinus mucosa is advanced over the cartilage flap and sutured to the cut edge of the laryngeal mucosa. The flap is first sutured to the interarytenoid mucosa and is continued across the cut edge of the mucosa overlying the cricoid cartilage.

Figure 5–6O. The anterior edge of the hypopharyngeal mucosa is sutured to the sternohyoid muscle in the midline. It is not possible to resurface the anterior portion of the larynx completely, particularly over the cricoid.

Figure 5–6P. Approximation of the strap muscles in the midline completes the closure of the reconstructed larynx. The remaining steps in the procedure are identical to those in Figures 5–1N, 5–1O, 5–1P, and 5–1Q.

Results

Although the techniques used in the various studies differ somewhat, all of these procedures involve resection of a substantial portion of the thyroid cartilage and an arytenoid cartilage, performed for removal of T2 or T3 glottic tumors. The results, as summarized in Table 5–2,[2, 16, 72, 78–82] show an overall cure rate of 82% (382 patients out of a total of 446) for T2 vocal cord carcinoma and 64% (112 patients out of a total of 176) for the T3 tumors that were amenable to this type of surgery. The results in this latter group of patients compare favorably with the results of total laryngectomy for T3 glottic carcinoma and are considerably better than those previously reported with radiotherapy.[11, 17] The question of choice of treatment for T3 glottic carcinoma has been discussed in some detail in Chapter 5. It is fairly clear that hemilaryngectomy is the treatment of choice for glottic tumors that are amenable to this procedure.

Extended Hemilaryngectomy with Cricoid Excision

As discussed above, Biller and Som[58, 83] have extended the indications for hemilaryngectomy to include lesions with greater degrees of posterior subglottic extension, which require resection of part of the cricoid lamina. The thyroid cartilage flap is used to replace the resected portion of the cricoid and arytenoid cartilages. The upper 75% of the lateral portion of the cricoid may be resected and extended posteriorly to the midline. Patients requiring this type of resection have either marked limitation of motion or fixation of the vocal cord because of thyroarytenoid muscle involvement, usually with subglottic extension of the tumor.

Indications

Partial excision of the cricoid cartilage is required for tumors that extend 5 mm or more subglotically. These patients have either marked limitation of motion or complete fixation of the vocal cord.

Technique

Figure 5–7A. The cartilage cuts are shown. The vertical incisions through the thyroid cartilage are similar to those shown for conventional vertical hemilaryngectomy (extended frontolateral). The posterior third of the thyroid ala is detached from the anterior two thirds and left pedicled on the inferior constrictor muscle. The vertical cartilage cut on the contralateral (left) side is extended through the upper two thirds or three fourths of the cricoid cartilage and is then carried posteriorly to the midline. Often the decision to include the cricoid cartilage in the resection is not made until the initial thyrotomy has been made. This may partly disrupt the continuity of the mucosal surface, but care must be taken to avoid transection of the tumor.

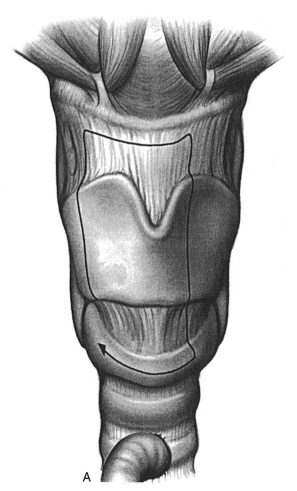

Figure 5–7. Extended hemilaryngectomy with cricoid excision.
Illustration continued on following page

Table 5–2. RESULTS OF EXTENDED FRONTOLATERAL LARYNGECTOMY			
			Cure Rate
Study	Follow-up (Years)	Tumor Stage	No. Tumor-Free/ Total No (%)
Ogura et al.[78]	3	T2	45/55 (82%)
Som[16]	3	T2	70/105 (74%)
	3	T3	15/26 (58%)
Mohr et al.[79]	5	T2	25/27 (94%)
	5	T3	5/5 (100%)
Bauer et al.[2]	5	T3	12/18 (67%)
Leroux-Robert[80]	5	T2	187/215 (87%)
	5	T3	55/95 (58%)
Biller et al.[72]	5	T2	23/33 (69%)
Skolnik et al.[81]	5	T2	23/32 (72%)
	5	T3	2/5 (40%)
Kessler et al.[82]	2	T3	23/27 (85%)
Total		T2	382/466 (82%)
		T3	112/176 (64%)

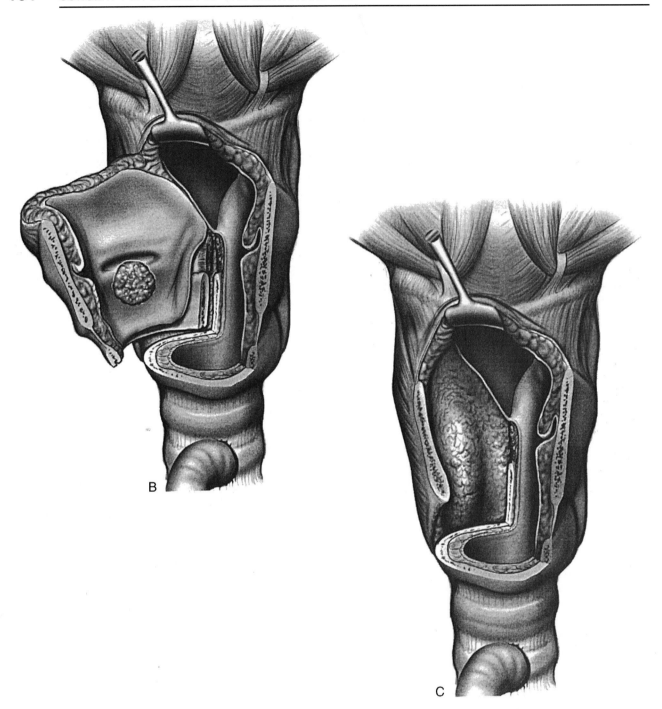

B

C

Figure 5–7 *Continued* Extended hemilaryngectomy with cricoid excision.

Figure 5–7B. The hemilarynx is rotated outward. The cricoid cartilage is divided vertically in the posterior midline, and the arytenoid is included in the specimen and dissected from the aryepiglottic fold and the pyriform sinus.

Figure 5–7C. The specimen has been removed, revealing the pyriform sinus, which will be used for mucosal resurfacing.

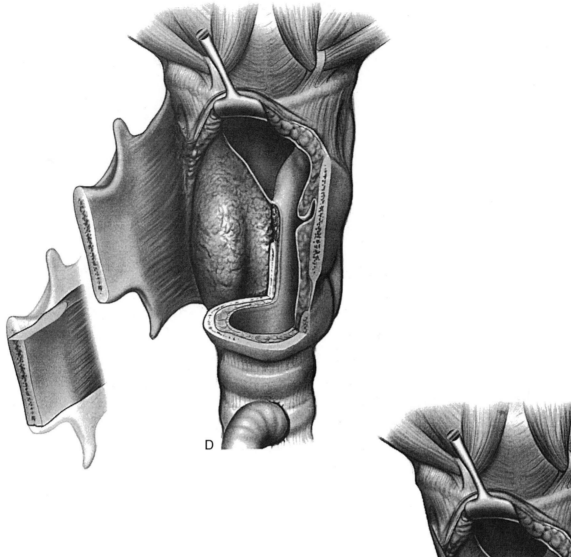

D

Figure 5–7 *Continued* Extended hemilaryngectomy with cricoid excision.

Figure 5–7D. The posterior thyroid cartilage, pedicled on the inferior constrictor muscle, will be used to replace the arytenoid and cricoid cartilages. The cartilage is trimmed only slightly by removing the superior and inferior cornua.

Figure 5–7E. The cartilage flap is positioned on the upper edge of the partly resected cricoid cartilage in its posterior portion. It is secured to the cricoid cartilage with polyglactin sutures.

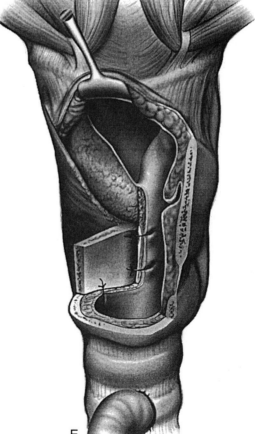

E

Illustration continued on following page

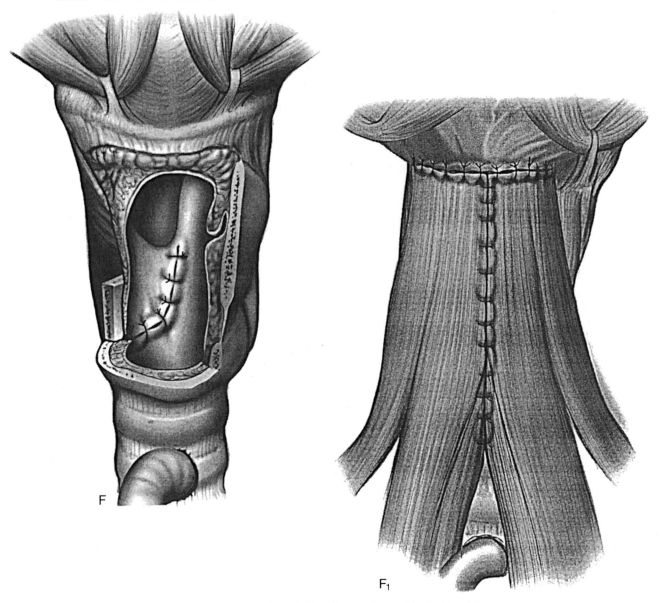

Figure 5–7 *Continued* Extended hemilaryngectomy with cricoid excision.

Figure 5–7F. The pyriform sinus mucosa is advanced to cover the cartilage flap. The mucosa is sutured to the cut edge of the laryngeal mucosa in the posterior midline and is continued anteriorly to the subglottic mucosa.

Results

Biller and Som[58] reported five cases of hemilaryngectomy for glottic carcinoma with posterior subglottic extension necessitating resection of part of the cricoid lamina. Initial functional results in all five patients were good. One patient subsequently required a total laryngectomy, and another developed laryngeal stenosis after postoperative radiotherapy. Three patients retained good laryngeal function, and all patients were free of tumor after 2 years or more. Biller and Lawson[84] reported their experience with 18 patients who had considerable limitation of motion or fixation of the vocal cord with subglottic involvement. Fifteen of their patients had tumors with subglottic extensions of 5 mm or more and underwent extended hemilaryngectomy with cricoid excision. Ten of the 15 patients (66%) remained free of local recurrence at 24 months. Four had local recurrence, and 1 died of a pulmonary tumor. The authors noted a higher incidence of complications compared to standard hemilaryngectomy and concluded that the cartilage flap reconstruction did not withstand postoperative irradiation. Three of the 15 patients were not totally rehabilitated. Two developed stenosis requiring permanent tracheostomy, and 1 developed persistent aspiration requiring gastrostomy.

Extended Hemilaryngectomy with Epiglottic Reconstruction

Glottic lesions involving at least one half of each vocal cord lead to major defects requiring extensive reconstruction. The anterior frontal partial laryngectomy, described earlier, is suitable for lesions involving only the anterior halves. In these cases, reconstruction may be accomplished with a midline partition, as described, or with skin grafts or flaps. These reconstructive methods prove to be insufficient for restoring adequate laryngeal lumen and competence after resection of bilateral glottic lesions that extend far enough posteriorly on one side to require removal of the arytenoid cartilage. The use of the epiglottis for reconstruction of glottic defects was first reported in the European literature by Bouche et al.[85] Tucker's adaptation[86] of this procedure for very large glottic defects was introduced in the United States in 1979.

The epiglottis provides several reconstructive advantages. Its mucosal lining is similar to that of the larynx, enhancing mucus transport and voice production. Its cartilaginous structure provides rigidity in order to maintain the anterior-posterior diameter of the larynx but still remains flexible enough to allow for movement of the remaining arytenoid cartilage and the pseudocord. It provides tissue bulk for glottic competence, and reconstruction may be accomplished in one stage.

Several unique rehabilitative problems are created by the use of the epiglottis, particularly after resections involving an arytenoid cartilage. The normally positioned epiglottis can no longer divert the food bolus during deglutition. Its new position tethers the tongue base, and the surgical manipulation may produce some degree of superior laryngeal denervation. The neoglottis, after epiglottic reconstruction, tends to be abnormally wide, encouraging aspiration and poor voice. Nong et al.[87] have described modifications to solve these problems. These modifications include the creation of a new anterior commissure by subperichondrial vertical incision of the displaced epiglottis. Nevertheless, patient selection must be stringent, and only highly motivated individuals with good pulmonary function are suitable candidates for this procedure.

This procedure may be performed in selected patients after radiation failure, as may other conservation operations. The major criterion for suitability for postirradiation conservation surgery is that the lesions should have been suitable for the same resection before irradiation. A higher incidence of complications and greater difficulty with adaptation may be expected.

Technique

Figure 5–8A. Extended hemilaryngectomy with epiglottic reconstruction is most useful when 60% to 70% of the glottis has been resected, including the anterior halves of both thyroid cartilages. In the example shown here neither of the arytenoid cartilages has been resected, but the epiglottiplasty may be employed for reconstruction after resection of all glottic structures except for one arytenoid cartilage.

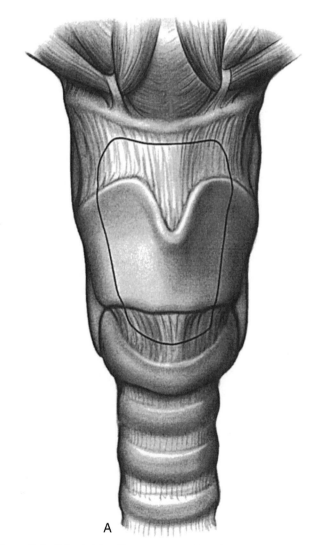

Figure 5–8. Extended hemilaryngectomy with epiglottic reconstruction.

Illustration continued on following page

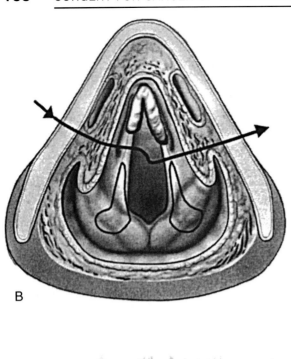

B

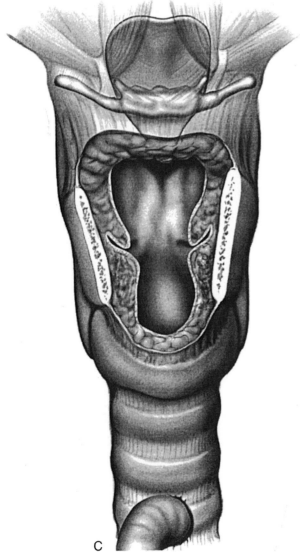

C

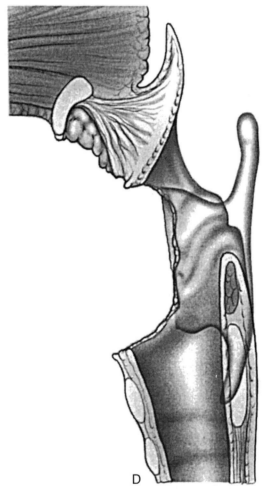

D

Figure 5–8 *Continued* Extended hemilaryngectomy with epiglottic reconstruction.

Figure 5–8*B*. The cartilage cuts and external incisions in the larynx are shown. The upper half of the anterior cricoid cartilage may be included in the resection when required.

Figure 5–8*C, D*. After resection only the posterior thirds of the vocal cords remain.

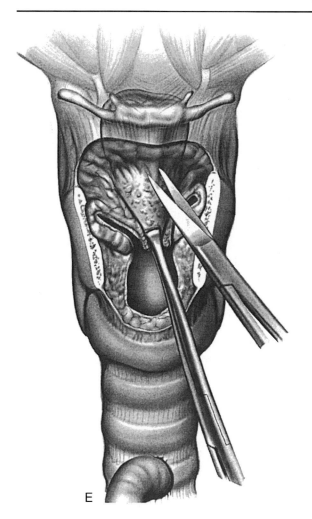

E

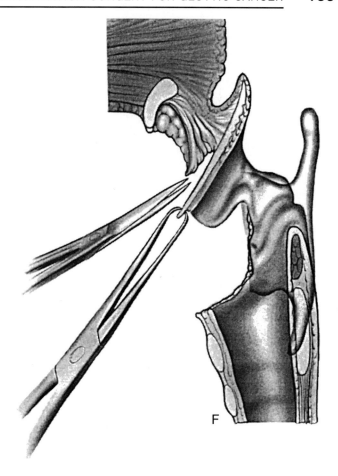

F

Figure 5–8*E*. The epiglottis must be freed from all anterior attachments. The petiole is grasped with a tenaculum, and the overlying soft tissue attachments are severed by sharp dissection until the cartilage of the external surface is exposed. This is developed in the subperichondrial plane with a Freer elevator.

Figure 5–8*F*. The perichondrium is incised with a knife or scissors at the points in the infrahyoid epiglottis where it inserts into the lacunae.

Figure 5–8*G*. The dissection is carried to the tip of the epiglottis. Traction sutures are employed to pull the epiglottis to the level of the cricoid cartilage without tension. Flexion of the neck facilitates this maneuver. Schechter[88] observed that placement of only a few sutures through the cartilage, but not the mucosa, results in a prominent pseudocord and more masculine voice, whereas the placement of many sutures through both the cartilage and the intraluminal mucosa produces a smoother surface and a more "feminine" voice.

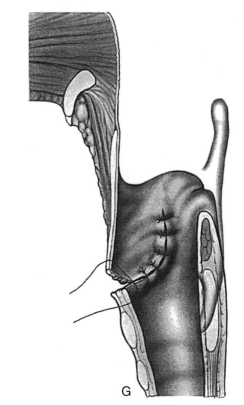

G

Figure 5–8 *Continued* Extended hemilaryngectomy with epiglottic reconstruction.

Results

Tucker[89] recently reported his experience with 48 patients, with a 2-year survival rate of 96%. Five patients required total laryngectomies for recurrence; one of these five patients died of disease. All patients were decannulated, but nine required minor surgical procedures (that is, laser surgery) prior to decannulation. All experienced some degree of aspiration. Nine patients required feeding supplementation beyond 2 months; only one of these required assistance after 6 months. Approximately one third of the patients had good voices, while two thirds had "functional" voices. Schechter[88] reported a 3-year survival rate of 71% in 38 patients. All deaths occurred in patients with previous radiotherapy. Four of the surviving patients required total laryngectomy for treatment. All patients were decannulated by the 6th week after operation. Although all experienced some degree of aspiration for the first few postoperative weeks, only four patients required feeding tubes for longer than 3 months, and all were free of feeding tubes by 6 months. Voice quality was generally "satisfactory." Zanaret et al.[90] reported the long-term results of near-total laryngectomy with epiglottic reconstruction in 57 patients. Resection included both the true and the false vocal cords, and one arytenoid cartilage. Tumor control was obtained in 93% of the patients with T1 lesions and 79% of the patients with T2 lesions. All patients tolerated decannulation, and all were able to swallow after a mean of 12 days. While slightly more than one half of the patients had less than completely satisfactory voices, all were able to speak with lung-powered voices.

Supracricoid Laryngectomy with Cricohyoidoepiglottopexy

All of the vertical partial laryngectomies described earlier share a similar approach, which consists of vertical entry into the laryngeal lumen through the thyroid cartilage. An inherent difficulty of this approach is the "blind" entry into the larynx. The surgeon must estimate a "safe" point of entry on the basis of preoperative evaluation. This may result in an unsafe margin at the point of entry. Another difficulty that these procedures share is that with partial resection of the thyroid cartilage, there is only partial resection of the paraglottic space. An approach to partial laryngectomy that avoids these pitfalls has been developed and employed for the past two decades. Supracricoid laryngectomy with cricohyoidoepiglottopexy (CHEP) was first developed by Piquet et al.[91] based on a technique described by Majer and Rieder[92] in 1959. The procedure was modified by Laccourreye et al.[93] and has been used extensively in Europe, particularly in France, although it has not been popular in the United States. Modifications of the approach have been employed for supraglottic[94] and pyriform sinus[95] carcinomas.

The basic concept of CHEP is a sleeve-like resection of the laryngeal structures including both thyroid cartilages, from the cricoid cartilage to the hyoid bone and the base of epiglottis. One or preferably both arytenoid cartilages are preserved, with intact innervation and mobility. This procedure avoids entry into the larynx in proximity to the tumor and results in complete removal of the paraglottic space. Preservation of the epiglottis with supraglottic innervation and mobile arytenoids results in physiologic speech and deglutition, and saving the cricoid cartilage maintains a patent airway and permits decannulation. The large laryngeal defect is repaired by mobilizing the trachea anteriorly along its length and impacting the cricoid and epiglottis onto the cricoid, using heavy retention sutures.

Indications

Piquet and Chevalier[96] listed the indication for CHEP as follows: "a tumor of the anterior two-thirds of the vocal cord extending to the anterior commissure; a tumor of the entire vocal cord with limited mobility; an early ventricular tumor; an early anterior commissure tumor; and a tumor involving both vocal cords." An immobile arytenoid cartilage and a subglottic extension greater than 7 mm were considered to be contraindications. The authors distinguished between vocal cord immobility due to bulk or invasion of the thyroarytenoid muscle anteriorly, which was not considered a contraindication, and immobility due to fixation of the arytenoid cartilage with tumor, which rendered the lesion unsuitable for CHEP. Other authors have employed similar indicators; the majority of patients operated on have T2 glottic carcinomas.

Technique

Figure 5–9A. A transverse of U-shaped incision may be employed. The skin flap should be raised at least 1 cm above the hyoid bone to prevent skin retraction at the time of closure. The sternohyoid and thyrohyoid muscles are transected at the level of the superior border of the thyroid cartilage, and the thyrohyoid muscles are transected along the inferior border.

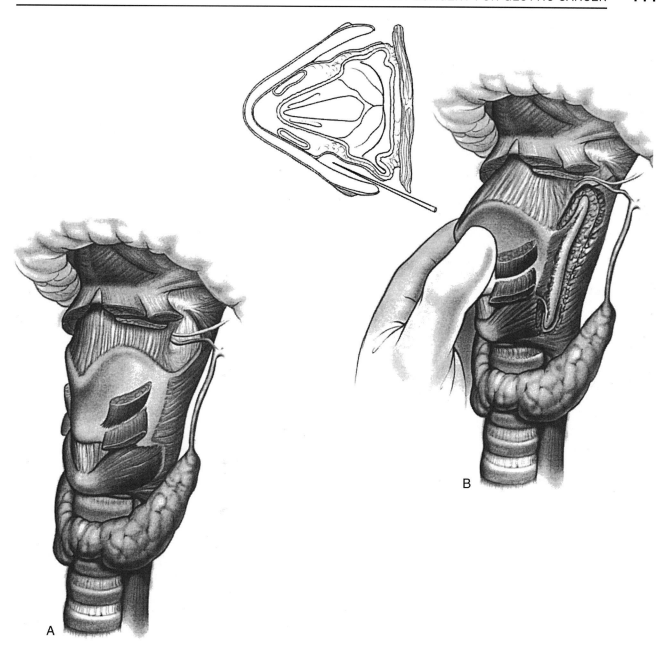

Figure 5–9. Supracricoid laryngectomy with cricohyoidoepiglottopexy (CHEP).

Illustration continued on following page

Figure 5–9*B.* The inferior constrictors are incised along the posterior border of the thyroid cartilage, and the pyriform sinuses are dissected from the internal aspect of the posterior thyroid alae. The cricothyroid joint is separated on the ipsilateral side. Piquet[99] suggests that rather than separating the joint, the contralateral inferior cornu should be divided to avoid injury to the recurrent laryngeal nerve. In any case, it is important to be aware of the presence of the nerve, immediately posterior to the joint.

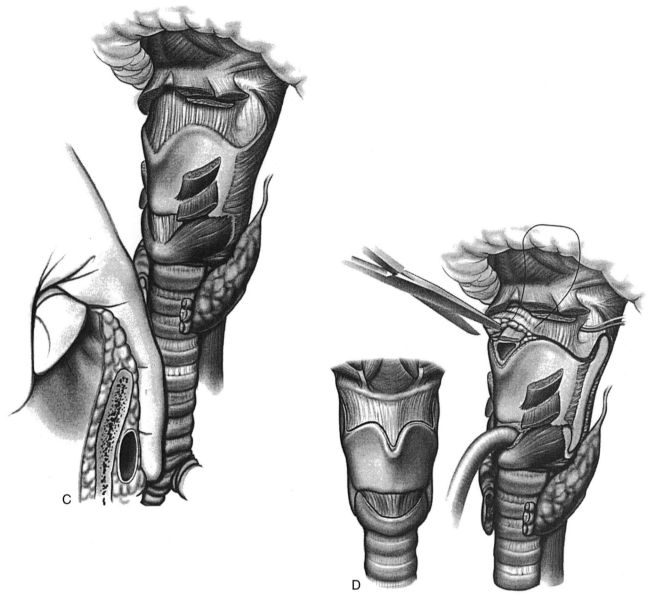

Figure 5–9 *Continued* Supracricoid laryngectomy with cricohyoidoepiglottopexy (CHEP).

Figure 5–9C. The thyroid isthmus is divided and blunt dissection performed with a finger along the anterior wall of trachea to the level of the carina. This will permit upward displacement of the trachea at the time of laryngeal closure.

Figure 5–9D. The larynx is entered inferiorly through the inferior cricothyroid membrane, and the incision is extended posterolaterally in either direction. The oroendotracheal tube is removed and replaced with an endotracheal tube inserted through the cricothyrotomy for temporary maintenance of ventilation. An incision is made through the thyrohyoid membrane at the upper level of the

thyroid cartilage, and the laryngeal lumen is entered at that level by sharply transecting the epiglottis just above the petiole. Care is taken during these maneuvers to avoid injury to the superior laryngeal nerves.

Figure 5–9E. The incision in the thyrohyoid membrane and the supraglottic mucosa is extended posteriorly on one side. This incision, which follows the contour of the upper edge of the thyroid cartilage, transects the aryepiglottic fold and continues posteriorly through the lateral pharyngeal wall to a point posterior to the arytenoid. With the glottic structures retracted anteriorly and the supraglottic

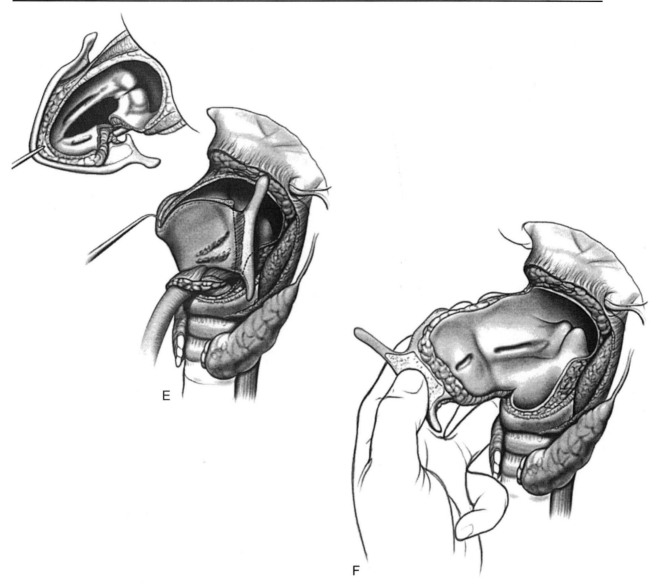

Figure 5–9 *Continued* Supracricoid laryngectomy with cricohyoidoepiglottopexy (CHEP).

Illustration continued on following page

structures retracted posteriorly, the surgeon can visualize and assess the tumor from the head of the table. A vertical incision is made through the aryepiglottic fold, directly anterior to the arytenoid cartilage on the contralateral side. This is carried inferiorly to the level of the cricoid cartilage, where it joins the previously made transverse cricothyroidotomy incision.

Figure 5–9F. The vertical incision traverses the cricothyroid and cricoarytenoid muscles. The endolarynx has now been entered posteriorly on the contralateral side, although access is limited by the overlying thyroid cartilage. At this point the surgeon grasps the thyroid ala manually and fractures it forward along the midline, as though "opening a book." This maneuver allows complete visualization of the endolarynx. The tumor-bearing side has not been incised, and is now completely accessible. The tumor is directly visible and can now be excised by cutting the remaining mucosa at a safe margin around the lesion. If appropriate, the posterior vertical incision is made through the vocal process of the arytenoid cartilage, leaving the body of the cartilage in place. If necessary, the entire arytenoid cartilage can be included with the specimen. Resection can be extended inferiorly to include the upper portion of the anterior cricoid cartilage.

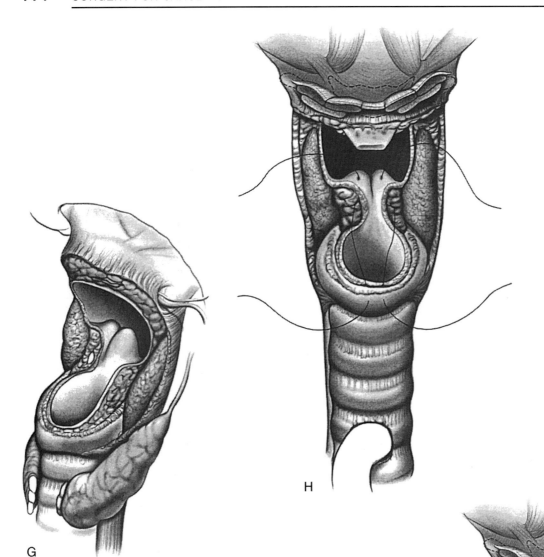

Figure 5–9 *Continued* Supracricoid laryngectomy with cricohyoido-epiglottopexy (CHEP).

Figure 5–9*G*. The structures remaining after resection are shown. These include both arytenoid cartilages (in the case demonstrated), the cricoid cartilage, the epiglottis above the petiole, the hyoid bone, and both pyriform sinuses.

Figure 5–9*H*. The mucosa over the upper portions of the arytenoid cartilages is sutured to the cut edge of the subglottic mucosa anteriorly.

Figure 5–9*I*. When these sutures are tied, the arytenoid cartilages are oriented anteriorly and prevented from rotating posteriorly. If necessary, the sutures extend through the empty space between the arytenoid cartilage and the anterior cricoid cartilage.

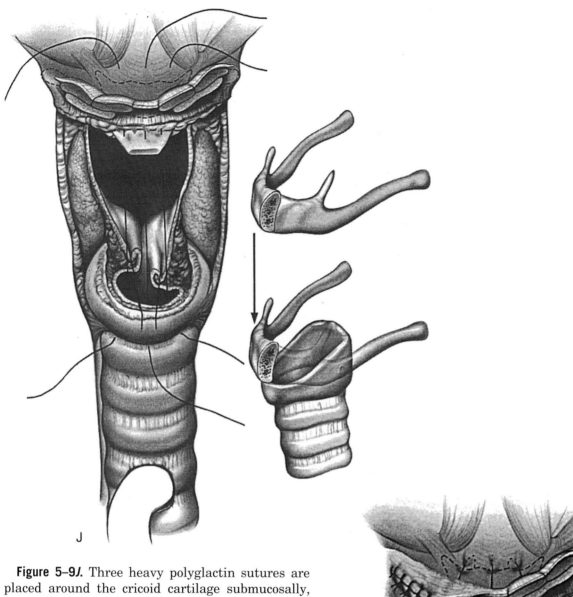

J

K

Figure 5–9J. Three heavy polyglactin sutures are placed around the cricoid cartilage submucosally, passed through the epiglottis, and looped around the hyoid bone. The first suture is placed in the midline. The other two are placed on each side, about 0.5 cm from the midline. Symmetric placement of the sutures is important, and when pulled together, the anterior borders of the hyoid bone and the cricoid cartilage must be carefully aligned. With the cricoid and the trachea pulled upward to approximate their final position, a tracheostomy is created in the anterior tracheal wall at a point that will be at the level of the skin closure.

Figure 5–9K. The sutures are tied, impacting the hyoid bone over the cricoid cartilage. The sternohyoid muscles are reapproximated and the tracheostomy tube is placed through the skin incision. The supraglottic mucosa will heal to the subglottic mucosa, and the aryepiglottic folds and pseudocords will form during the healing process.

Figure 5–9 *Continued* Supracricoid laryngectomy with cricohyoido-epiglottopexy (CHEP).

Results

Piquet et al.[96] reported results of 104 patients with stage T2 and T3 lesions of the glottis, treated between 1972 and 1985 with CHEP. Eighty-six percent of the patients survived 3 years, and 75% survived 5 years. There were only 5 instances (5%) of local recurrence. Seven patients had neck recurrence and 8 developed a second primary tumor. Thirteen patients developed intercurrent disease or were lost to follow-up. Normal deglutition was achieved in all patients, except 2 who aspirated occasionally. Eighty-five patients (81.5%) were decannulated before the 28th day. Three patients developed stenosis, requiring surgical reconstruction. The voice, produced by vibration of the arytenoid mucosa against the epiglottis, was satisfactory in all the patients. Laccourreye et al.[93] reported a 3-year actuarial survival of 86.5% in 36 patients operated on from 1974 through 1986. In 2 cases (5.6%) there was a local recurrence of tumor. All 36 patients were decannulated between 3 and 57 days postoperatively. All patients recovered normal deglutition; 35 of the 36 patients achieved deglutition within the first postoperative month. Physiologic phonation was achieved by all patients. Vocal quality allowed for normal social interaction.

Postoperative Management After Vertical Partial Laryngectomy

Maintenance of Airway

The surgeon should anticipate functional occlusion of the glottic airway after most vertical partial laryngectomy procedures. Such occlusion can persist for 2 weeks or longer postoperatively. A patent tracheostomy cannula is essential for survival during this period. A cuffed tracheostomy tube is used for surgery, and the cuff is kept inflated for the first 12 hours (with periodic decompression to protect the tracheal mucosa) in order to minimize aspiration of blood. The tracheostomy tube is changed on or before the sixth postoperative day and at 48-hour intervals thereafter. As glottic swelling decreases, the patient becomes able to tolerate intervals of plugging of the cannula. Before decannulation, the patient should be able to tolerate 24 to 48 hours of continuous occlusion of the tracheostomy cannula. It is wise before decannulating the tracheostomy to wait until the patient is swallowing food reasonably well and to be sure that the wound has healed completely, although in some instances, decannulation will help with swallowing. If a prosthesis has been inserted in the larynx, the tracheostomy is not decannulated until the prosthesis has been removed.

Use of Antibiotics

Antibiotic administration is commenced 12 to 24 hours before surgery and continued for the first 5 postoperative days. This is done to minimize microbial load during the intraoperative and immediate postoperative periods. First- or second-generation cephalosporins with metronidazole are the drugs favored by our service.

Recovery of Deglutition

The sphincteric function of the larynx is the most difficult function to recover after partial laryngectomy. The degree of difficulty varies with the extent of the resection and the particular structures removed. Problems occur most often after procedures involving resection of an arytenoid cartilage. Patients may be permitted to attempt swallowing on about the fifth postoperative day. We usually do not use a nasogastric tube in the immediate postoperative period following vertical partial laryngectomy but will insert a tube subsequently if persistent aspiration prevents adequate nutrition. For initial attempts at swallowing, semisolids rather than liquids should be given, because liquids are more readily aspirated. Gelatin dessert and custard are usually offered first. The colored gelatin is readily detectable when it is coughed up from the tracheostomy. The patient should be instructed to lean to the unoperated side when swallowing. Plugging the tracheostomy is often helpful. Patience and persistence are often required, particularly with elderly individuals. The patient should "practice" swallowing small amounts at frequent intervals throughout the day. Although most patients will "learn" to swallow within a few days, some may require several weeks of persistent effort before they can eat well enough to be safely decannulated and discharged.

Complications After Vertical Partial Laryngectomy

Ogura and Biller[4] reported an overall complication rate of 11.6% (occurring in 11 of 95 patients) after hemilaryngectomy. These complications included laryngeal stenosis, aspiration and pneumonia, wound infection, pulmonary embolus, and laryngeal granulations. Sessions et al.[60] have described the nature of long-term functional disability following partial laryngectomy. This postsurgical "glottic insufficiency" occurs either as glottic incompetence, with aspiration, inability to cough or strain, and weak voice, or as stenosis, with stridor and respiratory distress. The authors noted 21 cases

Table 5–3. FUNCTIONAL DISABILITY AFTER HEMILARYNGECTOMY*		
	Minor	Major
Aspiration	1	7
Respiratory distress	6	8
Weak voice	2	1
Recurrent pneumonia	0	2

*Data from Sessions DG, Ogura JH, Ciralsky RH. Late glottic insufficiency. *Laryngoscope* 1975; 85:950–959, with permission.

of late glottic insufficiency among their large number of partial laryngectomies for glottic cancer. The distribution of functional problems is listed in Table 5–3. Respiratory obstruction is slightly more prevalent than aspiration after vertical hemilaryngectomy, unlike the situation after supraglottic laryngectomy, where aspiration occurs more frequently. Krespi and Khetarpal,[97] in a literature review, quantified the incidence of persistent laryngeal edema and stenosis with delayed decannulation or late recannulation as varying from 2% to 15% after horizontal partial laryngectomy and from 1% to 20% after vertical partial laryngectomy, with or without irradiation.

Glottic Stenosis

Respiratory obstruction in the early postoperative period may be due to excessive intralaryngeal granulation tissue or to prolapse of redundant supraglottic mucosa into the glottis. The latter problem may result from insufficient thinning of the edge of the hypopharyngeal mucosa before advancement into the laryngeal defect and may be corrected endoscopically, particularly with use of the carbon dioxide laser. Diabetes, radiation, nonabsorbable suture material, infection, and inadequate reconstruction all may contribute to granuloma formation, most commonly at the anterior commissure and the anterior third of the neocord.[97] Most granulomas develop a few months after surgery and regress spontaneously. Granulomas that persist beyond a reasonable follow-up period should be examined by endoscopic biopsy to rule out tumor recurrence and should be removed with the carbon dioxide laser. Treatment with topical or systemic steroids may be employed briefly in the conservative management of granuloma or in the effort to prevent subsequent scarring.

Chronic glottic stenosis is frequently preceded by infection, which causes cartilage necrosis and loss of mucosa, most often occurring after previous radiation therapy. Stenosis may be due to web formation, intraluminal scarring, or an inadequate residual laryngeal framework. Preservation of the cricoid cartilage, meticulous reconstruction and resurfacing of the framework and lumen, and immediate treatment of postoperative infection are the most effective means of preventing postoperative glottic stenosis. Planned radiation therapy is associated with a lower incidence of postoperative complications than when surgery is performed for salvage of a radiation failure.[98]

Simple webs may be treated by endoscopic division, using a laser if desired, and insertion of a midline partition such as a McNaught-type keel. Sessions et al.[60] reported good results of treatment of more complicated strictures with a midline thyrotomy and a stented skin graft. We have favored a staged repair, exteriorizing the larynx after a midline thyrotomy by advancing the cervical skin into the larynx. The temporary laryngostoma is secondarily closed, and the cervical skin used to resurface the laryngeal interior. Rigidity of the skin flap can be enhanced by a subcutaneous cartilage or polyethylene implant. The use of microsurgically revascularized bone or cartilage with skin or mucosa for single-stage reconstruction has not been reported to date but is theoretically possible. Supraglottic obstructive rings or bands may be resected.

Often, complicated reconstruction cannot be accomplished without loss of glottic competence, and many patients may simply continue tracheostomy cannulation, with preservation of voice and deglutition, rather than risk the loss of the swallowing function.

Glottic Incompetence

Persistent aspiration after partial laryngectomy, unlike stenosis, results from factors other than just anatomic problems. Many patients, after vertical partial laryngectomy, have some degree of anatomic glottic incompetence, yet most manage to adapt to the deficiency and swallow without aspiration. Age, chronic debilitating illness, chronic lung disease, and radiotherapy are factors that detract from the ability to regain laryngeal sphincteric function after partial laryngectomy. Glottic incompetence after vertical hemilaryngectomy occurs mainly in cases in which the arytenoid cartilage has been resected. It results from the loss of the structure of the posterior laryngeal vestibule, so that a "trough" is created where food and saliva in the hypopharynx may spill into the glottis. Inadequate glottic closure because of lack of bulk of the pseudocord also leads to glottic incompetence. Biller et al.[99] concluded that approximately 50% of patients will experience significant aspiration unless adequate reconstructive measures are employed. These methods of primary glottic and vestibular reconstruction have been discussed above and are helpful in preventing postoperative aspiration, particularly in patients with less favorable conditions for conservation surgery.

Various nonsurgical techniques may be helpful in minimizing postoperative aspiration or hastening the return of adequate deglutition. Decannulation of the tracheostomy and removal of the nasogastric feeding tube prior to offering the patient semisolid food appears to help with deglutition in the immediate postoperative period. A "three swallow" technique has been described by Tucker.[100] While holding a deep breath, the patient takes a small bolus of semisolid material, swallows twice, coughs, and swallows a third time. Leaning to the unoperated side may help some patients. It is generally easier to swallow semisolid material than free liquids, and the latter should be withheld until adequate deglutition has been restored. Patients will often find certain foods easy and other foods difficult to swallow and must learn to adjust their diet accordingly.

Secondary surgical correction of glottic incompetence after vertical partial laryngectomy is a more difficult problem than correction of stenosis. In order to correct the insufficiency it is necessary to augment the "pseudocord" mass. Teflon injection has been used since 1962 for vocal cord augmentation to correct dysphonia after vocal cord paralysis[101, 102] and has been applied to correction of glottic insufficiency after laryngeal surgery. Its use for this purpose has been generally ineffective for several reasons. Scarification of the laryngeal sphincter, lack of potential space in the pseudocord for augmentation, and the high viscosity of Teflon prevent dispersal of the material to the location where augmentation may be most required. In addition, a strong inflammatory reaction may be elicited by the injected Teflon. Injectable collagen has been shown to be useful for vocal and laryngeal rehabilitation and appears to be more useful for correction of glottic incompetence after partial laryngectomy.[103, 104] Gax collagen is a purified, soluble bovine collagen that is integrated into host tissues, has low viscosity, and is relatively inert. Remacle et al.[104] reported improvement in all eight patients treated with Gax collagen for aspiration problems after subtotal laryngectomy. The authors noted that the material is useful only when aspiration is due to anatomic rather than neurologic factors.

Sessions et al.[60] and Biller et al.[99] have reported good results with submucosal implantation of cartilage for surgical correction of aspiration following partial laryngectomy.

Infection and Necrosis

Subcutaneous wound infections may occur in these "clean-contaminated" cases, despite prophylactic antibiotics and wound drainage. Usually there is communication with the interior of the larynx. In addition to the usual measures of establishing drainage by packing the wound open and administering appropriate antibiotics, as determined by culture and sensitivity studies, the most important element in the management of wound infections after partial laryngectomy is the tracheostomy. Decompression of the wound site by a patent tracheostomy cannula will permit rapid healing in most cases.

More serious infections are associated with perichondritis and cartilage necrosis. These occur most often in patients after radiotherapy and are rare in nonirradiated cases.[32, 33] Treatment consists of débridement of necrotic soft tissue and removal of obviously necrotic fragments of cartilage. Denuded intact portions of the thyroid and cricoid cartilages should be preserved but must be completely covered with healthy soft tissue. Exteriorization of the larynx with advancement of cervical skin into the laryngostoma, in a manner similar to the procedure described for glottic stenosis, is an effective way of dealing with this problem. The laryngostoma, when healed, is closed by incising and turning in the skin around its margins and rotating a local flap for coverage. Failure to manage perichondritis and necrosis of cartilage adequately after partial laryngectomy can lead to stenosis and persistent laryngeal fistula.

Voice After Vertical Partial Laryngectomy

The true incidence of phonatory problems is difficult to determine because of the lack of standardized criteria for comparing voice results. Thus, Neel et al.[105] have reported the incidence of poor voice after partial laryngectomy or cordectomy at as low as 3.3%, whereas Moore[106] found that almost all cases of vertical partial laryngectomy and supraglottic laryngectomy had suboptimal postoperative voice. The ability of a patient to generate an adequate voice depends on the ability to develop adequate subglottic pressure, to resonate the vocal cords, and to develop adequate sphincteric activity of the supraglottic strictures. After cordectomy, compensatory hyperkinesia of the supraglottis may result in supraglottic hypertrophy or constriction. Krespi[97] concluded that in an attempt to preserve the vibratory mechanism in the glottic area, the supraglottic sphincter may act as a generator of noise, thus distorting the phonatory effect. Less subtle effects on voice are caused by glottic defects producing "air wasting" in many patients following vertical partial laryngectomy with resection of portions of one or both vocal cords. In addition, postoperative granulation tissue, scar formation, glottic incompetence, and paralysis of laryngeal nerves will adversely affect voice quality.

Voice difficulties have been prevented and treated by the same procedures employed to prevent or treat aspiration, by providing bulk to enhance glottic closure (see previous section). During the past decade, interest in the original work of Isshiki[107, 108] has led to the increasing application of laryngeal framework surgery for functional voice problem.[109–112] Medialization of the neocord, vocal fold tightening, and implantation of cartilage grafts or Silastic prostheses have proven to be effective methods for vocal improvement in various problems and may be employed in selected cases after conservative laryngeal surgery.

REFERENCES

1. Batsakis JG. *Tumors of the Head and Neck.* Baltimore, Williams & Wilkins, 1974.
2. Bauer WC, Lesinski SG, Ogura JH. The significance of positive margins in hemilaryngectomy specimens. *Laryngoscope* 1975; 85:1–13.
3. Ogura JH, Sessions DG, Spector GJ, et al. Roles and limitations of conservation surgical therapy for laryngeal cancer. *In* Alberti PW, Bryce DP (eds): *Workshops from the Centennial Conference on Laryngeal Cancer.* New York, Appleton-Century-Crofts, 1976.
4. Ogura JH, Biller H. Conservation surgery in cancers of the head and neck. *Otolaryngol Clin North Am* 1969; 2:641–665.
5. Alajmo E, Fini-Storchi O, Agostini V, et al. Conservation surgery for cancer of the larynx in the elderly. *Laryngoscope* 1985; 95:203–205.
6. Tucker HM. Conservation laryngeal surgery in the elderly patient. *Laryngoscope* 1977; 87:1995–1999.
7. Biller H, Barnhill F, Ogura J, et al. Hemilaryngectomy following radiation failure for carcinoma of the vocal cords. *Laryngoscope* 1970; 80:249–253.
8. Som ML. Limited surgery after failure of radiotherapy in the treatment of carcinoma of the larynx. *Ann Otol Rhinol Laryngol* 1951; 60:695–703.
9. Strauss M. Hemilaryngectomy rescue surgery for radiation failure in early glottic carcinoma. *Laryngoscope* 1988; 98:317–320.
10. Boles R, Komorn R. Carcinoma of the laryngeal glottis: a five-year review at a university hospital. *Laryngoscope* 1969; 79:909–920.
11. Lederman M. Place of radiotherapy in treatment of cancer of the larynx. *Br Med J* 1961; 1:1639–1646.
12. Lederman M. Radiotherapy of cancer of the larynx. *J Laryngol Otol* 1970; 84:867–896.
13. Lederman M, Dalley VM. The treatment of glottic cancer: the importance of radiotherapy to the patient. *J Laryngol Otol* 1965; 79:767–770.
14. Perez C, Holtz S, Ogura JH, et al. Radiation therapy of early carcinoma of the true vocal cords. *Cancer* 1968; 21:764–771.
15. Perez C, Mill W, Ogura JH, et al. Irradiation of early carcinoma of the larynx. *Arch Otolaryngol* 1971; 93:465–472.
16. Som ML. Cordal cancer with extension to vocal process. *Laryngoscope* 1975; 85:1298–1307.
17. Vermund H. Role of radiotherapy in cancer of the larynx as related to the TNM system of staging. *Cancer* 1970; 25:485–504.
18. Vaughan CW, Strong MS, Jako GJ. Laryngeal carcinoma: transoral treatment utilizing the CO_2 laser. *Am J Surg* 1978; 136:490–493.
19. DeSanto LW. Selection of treatment for in situ and early invasive carcinoma of the glottis. *In* Alberti PW, Bryce DP (eds): *Workshops from the Centennial Conference on Laryngeal Cancer.* New York, Appleton-Century-Crofts, 1976.
20. Lawson W, Som ML. Second primary cancer after irradiation of laryngeal cancer. *Ann Otol Rhinol Laryngol* 1975; 84:771–775.
21. Glanz H. Late recurrence of radiation induced cancer of larynx. *Clin Otolaryngol* 1976; 1:123–129.
22. Daly J. Limitations of cordectomy. *In* Alberti PW, Bryce DP (eds): *Workshops from the Centennial Conference on Laryngeal Cancer.* New York, Appleton-Century-Crofts, 1976.
23. Daly JF, Kwok FN. Laryngofissure and cordectomy. *Laryngoscope* 1975; 85:1290–1297.
24. LeJeune FE, Lynch MG. The value of laryngofissure. *Ann Otol Rhinol Laryngol* 1955; 64:256–262.
25. McGavran MH, Spjut H, Ogura J. Laryngofissure in the treatment of laryngeal carcinoma: a critical analysis of success and failure. *Laryngoscope* 1959; 69:44–53.
26. Sessions DG, Maness GM, McSwain B. Laryngofissure in the treatment of carcinoma of the vocal cord: a report of forty cases and a review of the literature. *Laryngoscope* 1965; 75:490–502.
27. Bailey BJ. Partial laryngectomy and laryngoplasty: a technique and review. *Trans Am Acad Ophthalmol Otolaryngol* 1966; 70:559–574.
28. Bailey BJ. Glottic reconstruction after hemilaryngectomy: bipedicle muscle flap laryngoplasty. *Laryngoscope* 1975; 85:960–977.
29. Bailey BJ, Calcaterra TC. Vertical subtotal laryngectomy and laryngoplasty. *Arch Otolaryngol* 1971; 93:232–237.
30. Jackson CL, Norris CM. Evolution of surgical technique in the treatment of carcinoma of the larynx. *Laryngoscope* 1956; 66:1034–1040.
31. Goodyear HM. Hemilaryngectomy, method of maintaining satisfactory airway and voice. *Ann Otol Rhinol Laryngol* 1949; 58:581–585.
32. Kirchner J, Som ML. The anterior commissure technique of partial laryngectomy: clinical and laboratory observations. *Laryngoscope* 1975; 85:1308–1317.
33. Sessions DG, Ogura JH, Fried MP. The anterior commissure in glottic carcinoma. *Laryngoscope* 1975; 85:1624–1632.
34. Som ML, Silver CE. The anterior commissure technique of partial laryngectomy. *Arch Otolaryngol* 1968; 87:138–145.
35. McNaught RC. Surgical correction of anterior web of the larynx. *Laryngoscope* 1950; 60:264–272.
36. Gluck T. A discussion on the operative treatment of malignant diseases of the larynx. *Br Med J* 1903; 2:1119.
37. Kirschner M, Lautenschlager A, Kleinschmidt O. *Operative Surgery.* Philadelphia, JB Lippincott, 1937.
38. Meurman Y. Extended cordectomy for intrinsic laryngeal cancer. Application and results. Plastic covering of excision surface. Proceedings of the Fifth Int Cong Otol Rhinol Laryngol. Amsterdam, 1973.
39. Conley J. The use of regional flaps in head and neck surgery. *Ann Otol Rhinol Laryngol* 1960; 69:1223–1234.
40. Conley J. Glottic reconstruction and wound rehabilitation: procedures in partial laryngectomy. *Arch Otolaryngol* 1961; 74:239–242.
41. Conley J. Rehabilitation of the airway system by neck flaps. *Ann Otol Rhinol Laryngol* 1962; 71:404–410.

42. Conley J. Regional skin flaps in partial laryngectomy. *Laryngoscope* 1975; 85:942–949.

43. Figi FA. Removal of carcinoma of the larynx with immediate skin graft for repair. *Ann Otol Rhinol Laryngol* 1950; 59:474–486.

44. Figi FA. Hemilaryngectomy with immediate skin graft for removal of the larynx. *Trans Am Acad Ophthalmol Otolaryngol* 1954; 58:22.

45. Norris CM. Technique of extended fronto-lateral partial laryngectomy. *Laryngoscope* 1958; 68:1240–1250.

46. Harpman JA. Management of raw areas in the larynx. *Arch Otolaryngol* 1961; 73:678–680.

47. Som ML. Hemilaryngectomy: a modified technique for cordal carcinoma with extension posteriorly. *Arch Otolaryngol* 1951; 54:524–533.

48. Ogura JH, Biller H. Glottic reconstruction following extended frontolateral hemilaryngectomy. *Laryngoscope* 1969; 79:2181–2184.

49. Dedo HH. A technique for vertical hemilaryngectomy to prevent stenosis and aspiration. *Laryngoscope* 1975; 85:978–984.

50. Quinn HJ. A new technique for glottic reconstruction after partial laryngectomy. *Laryngoscope* 1969; 79:1980–2011.

51. Conley J. The use of mucosal flaps for wound rehabilitation in partial laryngectomy. *Arch Otolaryngol* 1959; 69:700–703.

52. Iwai H. Limitations of conservation surgery in carcinoma involving the arytenoid. *In* Alberti PW, Bryce DP (eds): *Workshops from the Centennial Conference on Laryngeal Cancer.* New York, Appleton-Century-Crofts, 1976.

53. Ogura JH, Dedo HH. Glottic reconstruction of following subtotal glottic-supraglottic laryngectomy. *Laryngoscope* 1965; 75:865–878.

54. Pressman JJ. Cancer of the larynx: laryngoplasty to avoid laryngectomy. *Arch Otolaryngol* 1954; 59:395–412.

55. Quinn HJ. Free muscle transplant method of glottic reconstruction after hemilaryngectomy. *Laryngoscope* 1975; 85:985–986.

56. Sessions DG, Ogura JH, Ciralsky RH. Late glottic insufficiency. *Laryngoscope* 1975; 85:950–959.

57. Blaugrund S, Kurland S. Arytenoid replacement following hemilaryngectomy. *Laryngoscope* 1975; 85:935–941.

58. Biller HF, Som ML. Vertical partial laryngectomy for glottic carcinoma with posterior subglottic extension. *Ann Otol Rhinol Laryngol* 1977; 86:715–718.

59. Biller HF, Lawson WL. Partial laryngectomy for transglottic cancers. *Ann Otol Rhinol Laryngol* 1984; 93:297–300.

60. Friedman WH, Katsantonis GP, Siddoway JR, et al. Contralateral laryngoplasty after supraglottic laryngectomy with vertical extension. *Arch Otolaryngol* 1981; 107:742–745.

61. Jackson C. The results of operative methods in the treatment of cancer of the larynx. Symposium. *Ann Mal Oreille Larynx* 1922; 41:1221.

62. Jackson C, Jackson CL. *Cancer of the Larynx.* Philadelphia, Saunders, 1939.

63. Clerf LH. Cancer of the larynx; analysis of 250 operative cases. *Arch Otolaryngol* 1940; 32:484–498.

64. Broyles EN. The anterior commissure tendon. *Ann Otol Rhinol Laryngol* 1943; 52:342–345.

65. Kemler JL. Bilateral thyrotomy for carcinoma of the larynx. *Laryngoscope* 1947; 7:704–718.

66. Leroux-Robert J. Formes anatomo-cliniques et indications thérapeutiques des épithéliomas intra-laryngés. *Ann Otolaryngol* 1937; 1003–1044.

67. Leroux-Robert J. Indications for radical surgery, radiotherapy and combined surgery and radiotherapy for cancer of the larynx and hypopharynx. *Ann Otol Rhinol Laryngol* 1956; 65:137–153.

68. Leroux-Robert J. Les possibilités thérapeutiques du cancer du larynx par la chirurgie et les associations radio-chirurgicales. A propos d'une statistique personelle de 1,000 cas opérés depuis plus de 5 ans. *Presse Med* 1965; 73:1031–1036.

69. Jesse RH, Lindberg R, Horiot JC. Vocal cord cancer with anterior commissure extension. *Am J Surg* 1971; 122:437–439.

70. Olofsson J, Williams G, Rider W, et al. Anterior commissure carcinoma. *Arch Otolaryngol* 1972; 95:230–239.

71. Kirchner J. Cancer at the anterior commissure of the larynx. *Arch Otolaryngol* 1970; 91:524–525.

72. Biller H, Ogura J, Pratt L. Hemilaryngectomy for T_2 glottic cancers. *Arch Otolaryngol* 1971; 93:238–243.

73. Ogura JH, Biller H, Calcaterra TC, et al. Surgical treatment of carcinoma of the larynx, pharynx, base of tongue and cervical esophagus. *Int Surg* 1969; 52:29–40.

74. Kirchner J, Som ML. Clinical significance of fixed vocal cord. *Laryngoscope* 1971; 81:1029–1044.

75. Kirchner J, Owen JR. Five hundred cancers of the larynx and pyriform sinus: results of treatment by radiation and surgery. *Laryngoscope* 1977; 87:1288–1303.

76. Bryce DP, Ireland PI, Rider WD. Experience in the surgical and radiological treatment of 500 cases of carcinoma of the larynx. *Ann Otol Rhinol Laryngol* 1963; 72:416–430.

77. Leroux-Robert J. La chirurgie conservatrice par laryngofissure ou laryngectomie partielle dans le cancer du larynx. *Ann Otolaryngol* 1957; 74:40.

78. Ogura JH, Sessions DG, Spector GJ. Analysis of surgical therapy for epidermoid carcinoma of the laryngeal glottis. *Laryngoscope* 1975; 85:1522–1530.

79. Mohr RM, Quenelle DJ, Shumrick DA. Vertio-frontolateral laryngectomy (hemilaryngectomy): indications, technique and results. *Arch Otolaryngol* 1983; 109:384–395.

80. Leroux-Robert J. A statistical study of 620 laryngeal carcinomas of the glottic region personally operated upon more than five years ago. *Laryngoscope* 1975; 85:1440–1452.

81. Skolnik EM, Yee KF, Wheatley MA, et al. Carcinoma of the laryngeal glottis: therapy and end results. *Laryngoscope* 1975; 85:1453–1466.

82. Kessler DJ, Trapp TK, Calcaterra TC. The treatment of T_3 glottic carcinoma with vertical partial laryngectomy. *Arch Otolaryngol Head Neck Surg* 1987; 113:1196–1199.

83. Biller HF, Blaugrund SM, Som ML. Decreasing limitations of partial laryngectomy for vocal cord cancer. *In* Alberti PW, Bryce DP (eds): *Workshops from the Centennial Conference on Laryngeal Cancer.* New York, Appleton-Century-Crofts, 1976.

84. Biller HF, Lawson W. Partial laryngectomy for vocal cord cancer with marked limitation or fixation of the vocal cord. *Laryngoscope* 1986; 96:61–64.

85. Bouche J, Frecje CH, Husson U. L'hemilaryngectomie avec epiglottoplastie: nouvelle application de l'epiglottoplastie. *Ann Otolaryngol Chir Cervicofac* 1965; 82:421–428.

86. Tucker HM, Wood BG, Levine H, Katz R. Glottic reconstruction after near-total laryngectomy. *Laryngoscope* 1979; 89:609–619.

87. Nong HU, Huang GW, Chen L, Guo YC. Epiglottic laryngoplasty after hemilaryngectomy for glottic cancer. *Otolaryngol Head Neck Surg* 1991; 104:809–813.

88. Schechter GL. Subtotal laryngectomy with epiglottic reconstruction. *In* Silver CE (ed): *Laryngeal Cancer,* pp 193–196, New York, Thieme, 1991.

89. Tucker HM, Benninger MS, Roberts JK, et al. Near-total laryngectomy with epiglottic reconstruction: long-term results. *Arch Otolaryngol Head Neck Surg* 1989; 115:1341–1344.

90. Zanaret M, Giovanni A, Gras R, et al. Near total laryngectomy with epiglottic reconstruction: long term results in 57 patients. *Am J Otolaryngol* 1993; 14:419–425.

91. Piquet JJ, Desaulty A, Decroix G. Crico-hyoido-épiglotto-pexie: technique opératoire et résultats fonctionnels. *Ann Otolaryngol Chir Cervicofac* 1974; 91:681–690.

92. Majer H, Rieder A. Technique de la laryngectomy permettant de conserver la perméabilité respiratoire: la crico-hyoido-pexie. *Ann Otolaryngol Chir Cervicofac* 1959; 76:677–683.

93. Laccourreye H, Laccourreye O, Weinstein G, et al. Supra-

cricoid laryngectomy with cricohyoidoepiglottopexy: a partial laryngeal procedure for glottic carcinoma. *Ann Otol Rhinol Laryngol* 1990; 99:421–426.

94. Laccourreye H, Laccourreye O, Weinstein G, et al. Supracricoid laryngectomy with cricohyoidopexy: a partial laryngeal procedure for selected supraglottic and transglottic carcinomas. *Laryngoscope* 1990; 100:735–741.

95. Laccourreye O, Merite-Drancy A, Brasnu D, et al: Supracricoid hemilarygopharyngectomy in selected pyriform sinus carcinoma staged as T₂. *Laryngoscope* 1993; 103:1373–1379.

96. Piquet JJ, Chevalier D. Subtotal laryngectomy with cricohyoido-epiglotto-pexy for the treatment of extended glottic carcinomas. *Am J Surg* 1991; 162:357–361.

97. Krespi YP, Khetarpal U. Laryngeal Surgery. *In* Krespi YP, Ossoff R (eds): *Complications in Head and Neck Surgery,* pp 215–231. Philadelphia, Saunders, 1992.

98. Thawley SE. Complications of combined radiation therapy and surgery for carcinoma of the larynx and inferior hypopharynx. *Laryngoscope* 1981; 91:677–700.

99. Biller HF, Lawson W, Sacks S. Correction of posterior glottic incompetence following partial laryngectomy. *Ann Otol Rhinol Laryngol* 1982; 91:448–449.

100. Tucker H. Deglutition following partial laryngectomy. *In* Silver CE (ed): *Laryngeal Cancer,* pp 197–200. New York, Thieme, 1991.

101. Arnold G. Vocal rehabilitation of paralytic dysphonia. IX Techniques of intracordal injection. *Arch Otolaryngol* 1962; 76:358–368.

102. Lewy RB. Glottic reformation with voice rehabilitation in vocal cord paralysis. *Laryngoscope* 1963; 73:547–555.

103. Ford CN, Bless DN. Clinical experience with injectable collagen for vocal fold augmentation. *Laryngoscope* 1986; 96:863–869.

104. Remacle M, Hamoir M, Marbaix E. Gax-Collagen injection to correct aspiration problems after subtotal laryngectomy. *Laryngoscope* 1990; 100:663–669.

105. Neel HB, Devine KD, De Santo LW. Laryngofissure and cordectomy for early cordal carcinoma: outcome in 182 patients. *Otolaryngol Head Neck Surg* 1980; 88:79–84.

106. Moore GP. Voice problems following limited surgical excision. *Laryngoscope* 1975; 85:619–625.

107. Isshiki N, Okamura H, Ishikawa T. Thyroplasty Type I (lateral compression) for dysphonia due to vocal cord paralysis or atrophy. *Acta Otolaryngol* 1975; 80:465–473.

108. Isshiki N, Tanabe M, Sawada M. Arytenoid adduction for unilateral vocal cord paralysis. *Arch Otolaryngol* 1978; 104:555–558.

109. Tucker HM. Anterior commissure laryngoplasty for adjustment of vocal fold tension. *Ann Otol Rhinol Laryngol* 1985; 94:547–549.

110. Koufman JA. Laryngoplasty for vocal cord medialization: an alternative to Teflon. *Laryngoscope* 1986; 96:726–731.

111. Maves MD, McCabe BF, Gray S. Phonosurgery: indications and pitfalls. *Ann Otol Rhinol Laryngol* 1989; 98:577–580.

112. Tucker HM, Wanamaker J, Trott M, Hicks D. Complications of laryngeal framework surgery (phonosurgery). *Laryngoscope* 1993; 103:525–527.

Chapter 6

Conservation Surgery for Supraglottic Cancer

Carl E. Silver

BASIS OF SUPRAGLOTTIC CONSERVATION SURGERY

Chapter 3 discussed the surgical pathology of supraglottic carcinoma. The majority of these lesions are at least moderately well differentiated, with pushing margins. The tumors have little tendency to extend inferiorly to the glottis or laterally to the thyroid cartilage, but they have a marked propensity for invasion of the preepiglottic space. Only the less frequently encountered anaplastic carcinomas, which most often present as ulcerative rather than exophytic lesions, will extend downward and invade the cartilage. Such extension usually occurs at the anterior commissure. Supraglottic tumors must be distinguished from tumors originating primarily in the ventricle, which penetrate readily into the paraglottic space, from which extensive submucosal spread, cartilage invasion, and extralaryngeal spread occur. Ventricular tumors are transglottic, a term that has some ambiguity as it may be applied to supraglottic carcinomas that cross anterior or posterior to the ventricle to involve the glottic level, as well as to the true transventricular tumors just described. Conservation surgery has been employed for supraglottic tumors with glottic involvement, as well as for transventricular ("transglottic") carcinomas that extend into the paraglottic space, but results of treatment are considerably better for the supraglottic than for the transglottic lesions (see below).

Frazier,[1] in 1909, noted that the supraglottic structures are embryonically derived from the buccopharyngeal anlage, whereas the glottic and infraglottic portions of the larynx are derived from the pulmonary anlage. The supraglottic structures thus emanate from primitive branchial arches III and IV, and the glottic and subglottic structures develop from branchial arch VI.[2, 3] The larynx has two independent lymphatic systems that correspond to these separate embryologic components.[4] Although numerous authors[3, 5, 6] have pointed to this embryologic duplicity as the basis for the behavior of supraglottic tumors, as well for the anatomic compartmentation of the larynx discussed in Chapter 2, it is nevertheless difficult to define the exact points of embryologic demarcation for the entire larynx.[2]

Anatomically the entire preepiglottic space is confined above the true vocal cords. Thus, a resection that includes the epiglottis, the hyoid bone, and the upper half of the thyroid cartilage above a plane through the ventricles should completely excise a primary supraglottic tumor together with its potential extension into the preepiglottic space. The epiglottis cannot be adequately excised for cancer treatment by transhyoid pharyngotomy or by laryngofissure because the preepiglottic space cannot be totally removed by these approaches.[3] Supraglottic subtotal laryngectomy (SSL) meets all the requirements for adequate resection of supraglottic tumors confined to above the vocal cords.

RADIOTHERAPY

Radiotherapy as an Alternative to Supraglottic Subtotal Laryngectomy

The purpose of this book is to discuss the technical aspects of surgical procedures performed on the larynx, rather than to debate the relative merits of radiation and surgery in the selection of treatment. Nevertheless, it would appear myopic indeed to disregard the controversies or the role of radiation therapy in treatment of supraglottic cancer. Radiation alone may be employed in the treatment of supraglottic carcinoma amenable to conservation surgery, and it is an important adjuvant to surgical therapy, particularly in patients with lymph node metastasis.

The older literature emphasized the superiority of surgery over primary irradiation for supraglottic lesions, particularly those that were bulky and in more advanced stages. Vermund,[7] in a literature review covering 544 supraglottic tumors staged T2, T3, or T4N0, reported a 5-year survival of 32% for lesions treated with primary irradiation as opposed to 64% for those treated with primary surgery. Other studies have reported surgical cure rates that are almost double those for radiotherapy.[8–10]

In 1975, Goepfert et al.,[11] at the M.D. Anderson Cancer Center, reported that the results with radiotherapy for supraglottic lesions, that would have been amenable to partial laryngectomy were equivalent to those obtained with surgery. Initial control of the primary tumor, with retention of normal voice was achieved with a range of 88.5% for T1 lesions to 60% for T4 lesions. This group felt that most T2 and many T3 lesions could be treated effectively with primary irradiation. The main contraindications to treatment with irradiation were bulky or infiltrative tumors with cord fixation, marked edema, or extensive preepiglottic space invasion. Since 1984, the M.D. Anderson group has employed hyperfractionated therapy of 110 or 120 cGy two times a day for all patients with T2 or T3 supraglottic tumors who have been selected for primary radiation treatment. The actuarial 2-year local control rate was 90%, with an 84% local-regional control rate. Five of the six failures were successfully salvaged with surgery, yielding total 2-year local-regional control in 96% of the patients.[12]

Mendenhall et al.[13] have reported local control in 100% of T1, 81% of T2, 61% of T3, and 50% of T4 supraglottic tumors.

The advent of the sophisticated imaging techniques of computed tomography (CT) and magnetic resonance imaging (MRI) has provided a better means of distinguishing which supraglottic tumors can be satisfactorily managed by radiation therapy. In general, successful radiation treatment of primary supraglottic carcinoma is correlated with the volume of the tumor, with the best results being obtained with superficial and small-volume tumors.[14, 15] Studies at the University of Florida have indicated an overall local control rate of 83% for lesions less than 6 cc in volume, and a control rate of 46% for lesions 6 cc or larger.[15, 16]

A major disadvantage of primary radiotherapy treatment for supraglottic carcinoma is that subsequent conservation surgery for salvage becomes most difficult in cases of radiation failure. Som[17] reported on five cases of supraglottic laryngectomy after high-dose primary radiotherapy. One patient developed flap necrosis with rupture of the carotid artery, and three others developed perichondritis with elevation of skin flaps and prolonged postoperative courses. One of these patients had persistent laryngeal stenosis. DeSanto et al.[18] studied a large number of radiation failures treated at the Mayo Clinic. They noted that tumor recurrence is often recognized too late to utilize conservation surgery and concluded that the concept of "radiate and watch," which had been designed to save larynges, had resulted in more total laryngectomies than would have been necessary had the patients been treated by conservation surgery in the first place.

Radiotherapy as Adjuvant Treatment

Radiotherapy may be used as an adjunct to surgical treatment in an effort to increase cure rates, either as planned preoperative low-dose radiation or as postoperative radiotherapy. Ogura and Biller's group[19, 20] found no significant difference between patients with supraglottic carcinoma treated surgically with and without preoperative radiotherapy of 1500 to 3000 cGy over a 2- to 3-week period. Som[17] found little justification for assuming the additional hazards of radiation for lesions that, treated by surgery alone, had 70% curability with preservation of laryngeal function. Ogura et al.,[10] however, reported better results in patients with clinically positive lymph nodes who were treated with preopera-

tive radiotherapy than in those treated by surgery alone.

The current trend is to employ postoperative rather than preoperative irradiation, most often in cases with extralaryngeal spread of tumor, extensive preepiglottic and paraglottic space involvement and in patients with positive lymph nodes. Nevertheless, postoperative irradiation presents a significant risk after supraglottic subtotal laryngectomy. Bocca et al.[5] reported chondronecrosis, laryngeal edema, and severe respiratory stenosis in patients treated with radiotherapy after this procedure. A modified irradiation protocol consisting of 5500 cGy delivered in 30 fractions over a period of 6 weeks, with an increased dose of electron beam therapy to the neck, when indicated, has been employed at the M.D. Anderson Cancer Center to minimize these problems.[21]

SUPRAGLOTTIC SUBTOTAL LARYNGECTOMY

Conventional Supraglottic Subtotal Laryngectomy

Excision of carcinoma of the epiglottis by lateral pharyngotomy was first performed by Trotter in 1913.[22–24] As discussed in Chapter 1, development of this procedure was continued by College[25] and Orton,[26, 27] but the procedure remained obscure until the work of Alonso[28, 29] in Uruguay. Alonso used a temporary pharyngostoma because of difficulty in approximating the base of the tongue to the cut surface of the larynx after resection. The attendant discomfort and need for secondary plastic closure hampered popular acceptance of this operation.

In 1958, Ogura[3] published his technique for SSL and radical neck dissection, with primary closure using a muscle flap and skin graft. He reported the results of treatment of 15 patients with epiglottic carcinoma, with no local recurrence and with preservation of the larynx in all cases. This paper was instrumental in stimulating interest in the procedure. In 1959, Som[30] described a similar procedure, with primary closure obtained by direct approximation of local tissues, without a skin graft. Sixteen patients were treated, with only one local recurrence.

Following these two reports, work by some groups proceeded, experience was gained, techniques for closure were improved, and indications for the operation were broadened. Surgeons in many major cancer centers, however, were troubled by the narrow inferior margins of resection obtained by SSL and continued to advocate total laryngectomy for supraglottic carcinomas. By 1968, supraglottic surgery for vestibular cancer was still not widely accepted, and many total laryngectomies were performed for tumors that were suitable for conservation surgery. In that year, Bocca et al.[5] reported results of 124 supraglottic laryngectomies, with 72.7% survival in the 33 cases studied 5 years or longer. By the 1970s, because of favorable results reported in an increasingly large number of patients, supraglottic laryngectomy had become widely accepted in the United States.

Indications

It is difficult to relate the surgical indications for SSL to the TNM system of tumor staging because, according to the TNM system, any supraglottic lesion that involves the preepiglottic space is considered to be a stage T3 tumor regardless of the area of mucosal involvement. Infrahyoid carcinomas staged as T1 or T2 are frequently found to invade the preepiglottic space.[31]

The use of modern imaging techniques may facilitate more accurate staging in this regard. Although it is difficult to detect clinically, the gross spread of the tumor to the preepiglottic space can be readily assessed by CT and MRI. Microscopic involvement of the preepiglottic space may defy preoperative detection by any method. As 60% to 80% of supraglottic tumors involve the preepiglottic space, such involvement must be assumed in all cases that are treated surgically.

The "conventional" supraglottic laryngectomy consists of resection of the epiglottis, the hyoid bone, the thyrohyoid membrane, the upper half of the thyroid cartilage, and the supraglottic mucosa, with lines of transection going through both aryepiglottic folds, the valleculae, and the ventricles. Thus, lesions confined to the laryngeal surface of the epiglottis or to the false vocal cords, without extension onto the lingual surface of the epiglottis, the aryepiglottic folds, or the arytenoid region, are amenable to this resection.

A major consideration has been the inferior extent of the tumor. As previously stated, the early practitioners of this technique were reluctant to use this procedure for tumors extending below the petiole. As the major barrier to spread of supraglottic tumor to the vocal cords was better understood, surgeons became willing to accept narrower inferior resection margins. Indeed, it has become apparent that lesions arising low in the vestibule are more suitable for supraglottic laryngectomy than lesions involving the suprahyoid portion of the epiglottis. Although suprahyoid lesions appear easier to resect

and provide wider inferior margins, they are more likely to extend superiorly and laterally beyond the confines of conventional supraglottic laryngectomy and can thus lead to recurrence because of inadequate resection. Inferiorly, however, a margin of only 2 to 3 mm of normal mucosa is adequate to prevent recurrence at the glottic level.[4, 17]

In evaluating supraglottic tumors for partial laryngectomy, the bulk of the tumor may completely obscure the inferior margin of the tumor as viewed from above by indirect or direct laryngoscopy. Fiberoptic laryngoscopy or endoscopic examination with a small right-angle telescope as well as thin axial CT sections may be helpful in determining the lower limit and also in ruling out cartilage involvement or extralaryngeal spread. There is a great tendency for even bulky supraglottic tumors to spare the ventricle, although it may be quite difficult to visualize this structure with the tumor in situ. Demonstration of mobile uninvolved vocal cords will provide assurance in most cases that there is a reasonable margin of normal ventricular mucosa inferior to the tumor, which is thus amenable to supraglottic laryngectomy.

The greatest difficulty in evaluating the inferior extension of the tumor occurs with lesions that extend to the anterior commissure. At this point the apparent barrier to the downward spread of the tumor seems to be ineffective. Once the anterior commissure is penetrated, thyroid cartilage involvement (in the midline) and extralaryngeal spread occur readily. Although extension to the anterior commissure may be demonstrated by CT, occasionally cartilaginous involvement may be inapparent until the perichondrium is elevated at surgery, revealing the underlying thyroid cartilage to be invaded by tumor. This finding makes total laryngectomy mandatory.

Vocal cord fixation is usually a contraindication to supraglottic laryngectomy. Fixation from supraglottic lesions is usually due to invasion of the cricoarytenoid joint or to extension of the tumor into the paraglottic space. These situations require total laryngectomy. In some instances fixation of the cord may simply result from the bulkiness of the tumor. We have successfully resected lesions with fixed vocal cords for which examination revealed no extension beyond the limits defined for supraglottic laryngectomy. Exploratory lateral pharyngotomy with the option of converting to total laryngectomy is worthwhile in questionable cases.

Because it is often impossible to establish preoperatively, with certainty, the suitability of a given lesion for conservation surgery, consent for possible total laryngectomy should be obtained in all cases.

Technique of Supraglottic Subtotal Laryngectomy for a Lesion on the Laryngeal Surface of the Epiglottis with Extension to the False Vocal Cord

Figure 6–1A. Incisions are made for SSL with right neck dissection in continuity. The transverse portion of the incision is made somewhat higher than for total laryngectomy. If a complete neck dissection is to be done, the single trifurcate incision is preferred. Bilateral neck dissections are often performed in conjunction with supraglottic laryngectomy. With palpable lymph nodes, a functional neck dissection of levels I through V is usually performed on the ipsilateral side, with selective dissection of levels II, III, and IV ("lateral neck dissection") on the contralateral side. For patients with clinically negative necks, bilateral selective lateral neck dissections are usually performed.

Figure 6–1B. This sagittal view shows the extent of resection. The line of resection transects the aryepiglottic fold and extends through the ventricle, thus excising the entire epiglottis, the upper half of the thyroid cartilage, the thyrohyoid membrane, and the body of the hyoid bone. Note that the preepiglottic space is completely excised. The resection may be extended to include an arytenoid cartilage if indicated.

Figure 6–1C. The neck dissection is completed. The specimen may be left attached to the hyoid bone by the omohyoid muscle or by the fascia surrounding the upper portion of the strap muscles. It is not possible to maintain broad continuity of the neck specimen to the larynx, and the surgeon should not hesitate to detach and remove the neck specimen if it proves cumbersome.

A tracheostomy is performed through the second tracheal ring. The infrahyoid muscles are transected as far superiorly as possible.

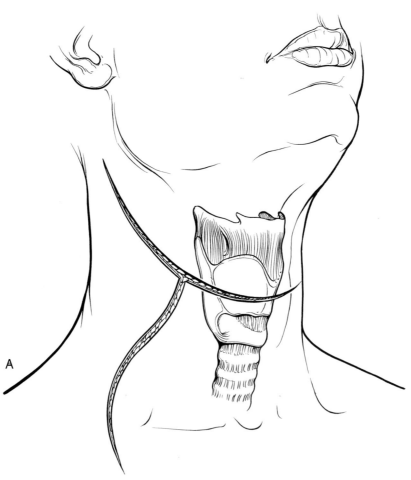

Figure 6–1. Supraglottic subtotal laryngectomy.

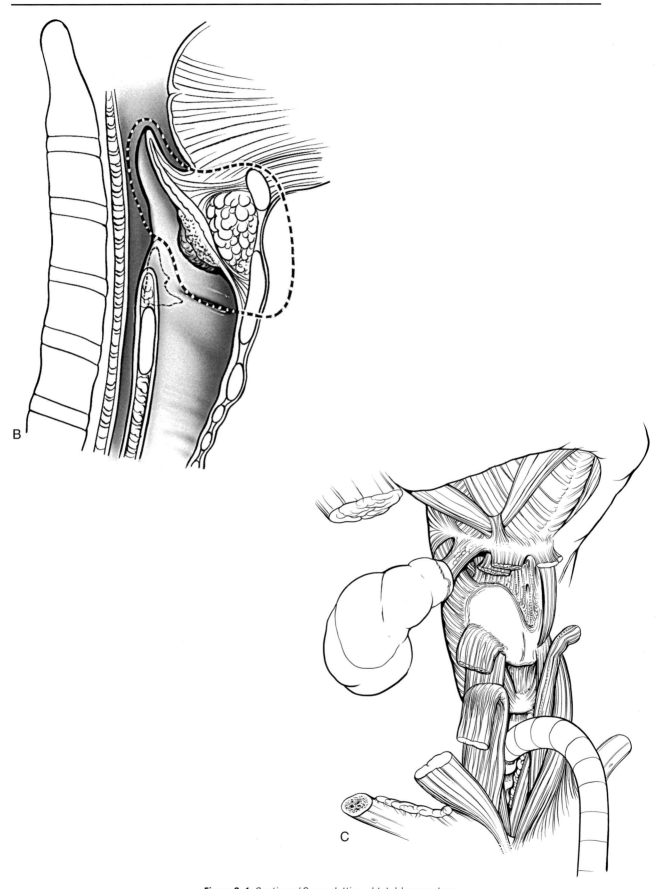

B

C

Figure 6–1 *Continued* Supraglottic subtotal laryngectomy.

Illustration continued on following page

Figure 6–1 *D.* The suprahyoid muscles are detached from the body and the right greater cornu of the hyoid.

Figure 6–1 *E.* The inferior constrictor muscle is incised over the posterior edge of the thyroid ala, and the external aspect of the pyriform sinus is exposed. The superior cornu of the thyroid cartilage is excised for convenience. The superior thyroid vessels and nerve are divided. An incision is made through the perichondrium along the upper border of the thyroid cartilage, and a flap of perichondrium is reflected inferiorly to the level of the vocal cord.

Figure 6–1 *F.* The perichondrial flap is completely reflected, exposing the portion of the thyroid cartilage to be resected.

Figure 6–1 *G.* The bone and cartilage cuts are shown. Resection will include the body and the right greater cornu of the hyoid bone, the upper half of the right thyroid ala, and an oblique anterior portion of the left thyroid ala.

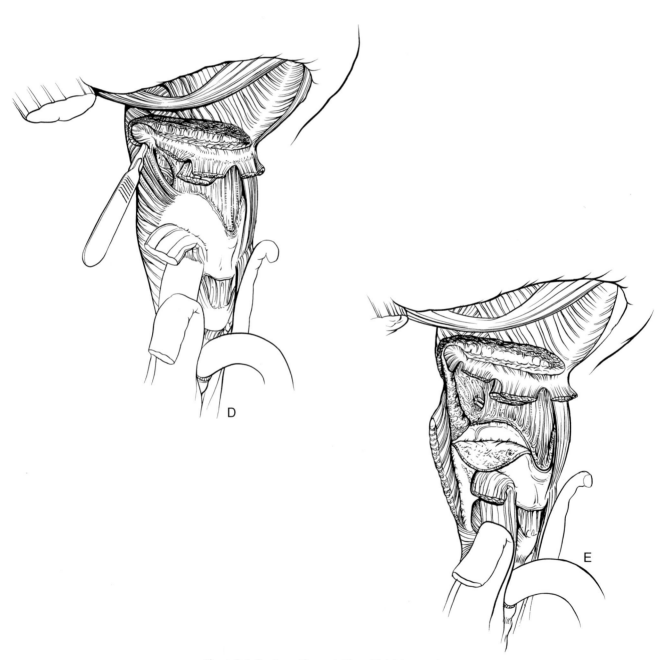

Figure 6–1 *Continued* Supraglottic subtotal laryngectomy.

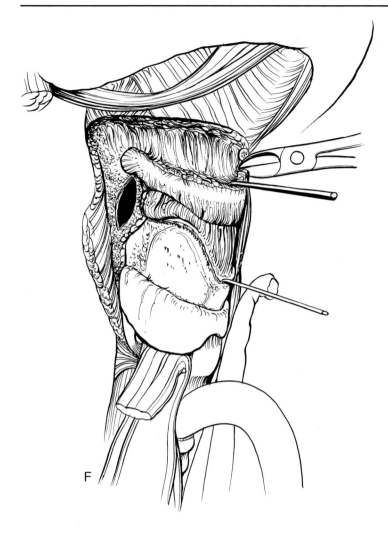

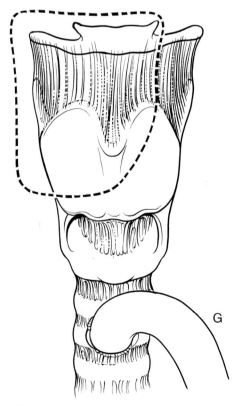

Figure 6–1 *Continued* Supraglottic subtotal laryngectomy.

Illustration continued on following page

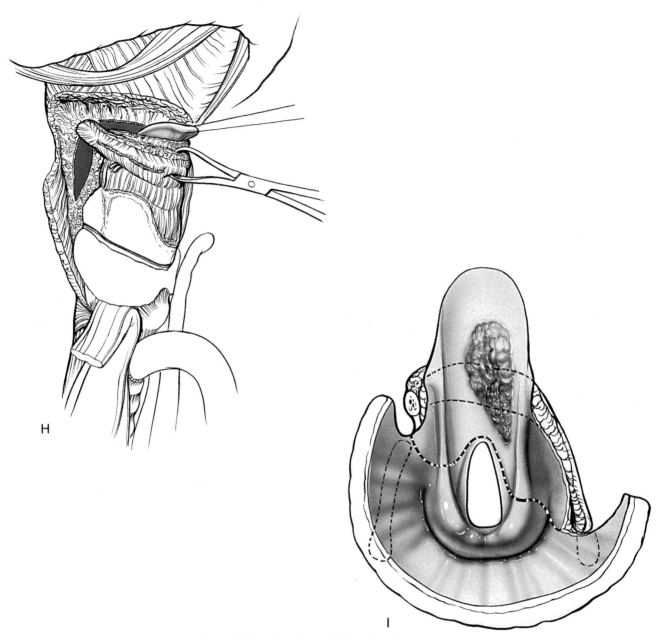

Figure 6–1 *Continued* Supraglottic subtotal laryngectomy.

Figure 6–1*H.* The hypopharynx is entered through the right pyriform sinus, and the incision extended through the vallecula. As the mucosa is incised, it must be carefully inspected to be certain it is not involved with tumor. The epiglottis is delivered through the mucosal incision with the aid of a traction suture.

Figure 6–1*I.* By retraction of the mucosal edges and traction on the epiglottis, the laryngeal introitus is visualized. It is usually not possible to visualize the glottis as well, as shown here at this stage of the procedure. The aryepiglottic folds on both sides are incised, anterior to the arytenoid, well away from the tumor.

Figure 6–1*J.* The incision in the left aryepiglottic fold has been carried through the posterior part of the false cord into the ventricle and continued anteriorly through the ventricle to the anterior midline. The same procedure is being performed on the right side. As these incisions progress, exposure of the tumor and the glottis improves. As wide a margin of normal mucosa as possible is maintained, although inferiorly this may be no more than a few millimeters.

If preferred, the side of greater involvement may be incised first, rather than the less involved side, as shown here. In either case, the inferior incision should be made through the ventricle, thus resecting most of both false vocal cords, even if they are uninvolved. Residual portions of the false vocal cords tend to become edematous and may obstruct the glottis postoperatively, requiring endoscopic removal.

Figure 6–1*K.* Completed resection. Note the relation of the resected soft tissue to bone and cartilage cuts.

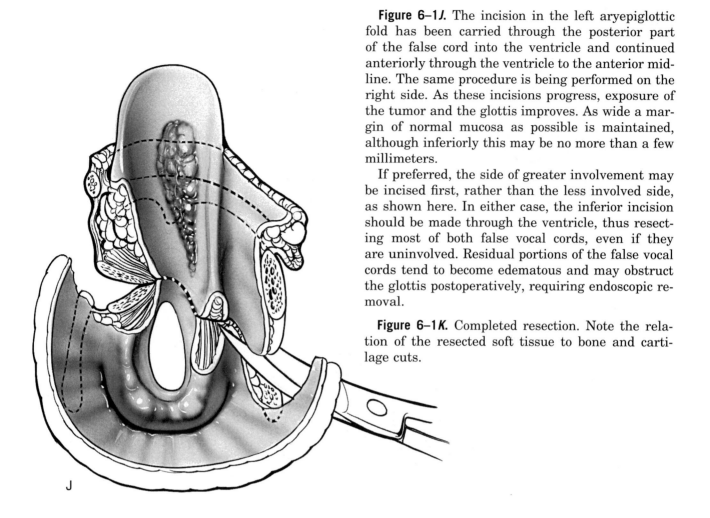

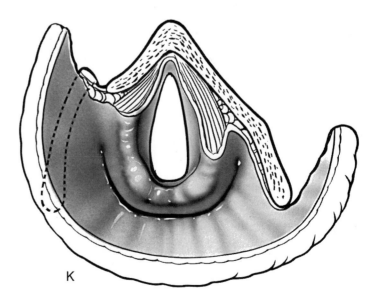

Figure 6–1 *Continued* Supraglottic subtotal laryngectomy.

Illustration continued on following page

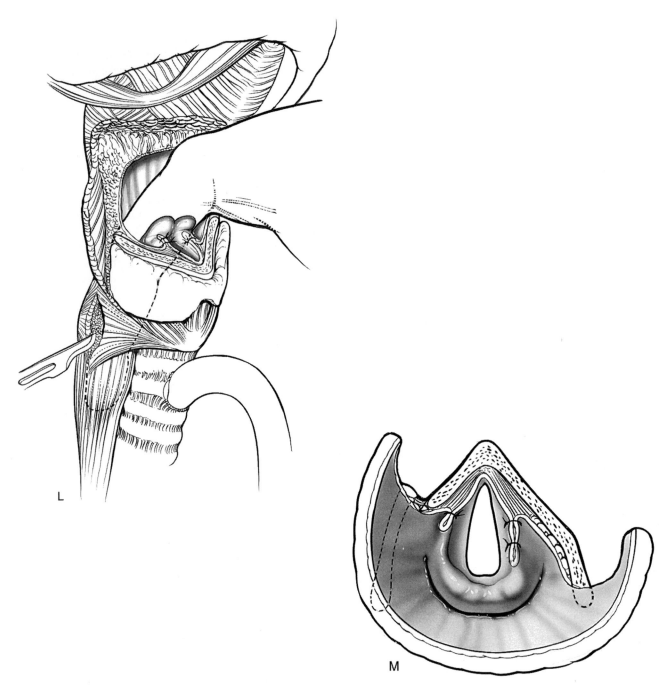

Figure 6–1 *Continued* Supraglottic subtotal laryngectomy.

Figure 6–1*L.* A myotomy of the cricopharyngeal muscle is performed by inserting a finger through the sphincter and incising the muscle fibers in the posterior midline.

Figure 6–1*M.* Closure is performed by suturing the cut edges of the false vocal cords to the pyriform sinus mucosa on each side, as far as possible, thus creating new aryepiglottic folds.

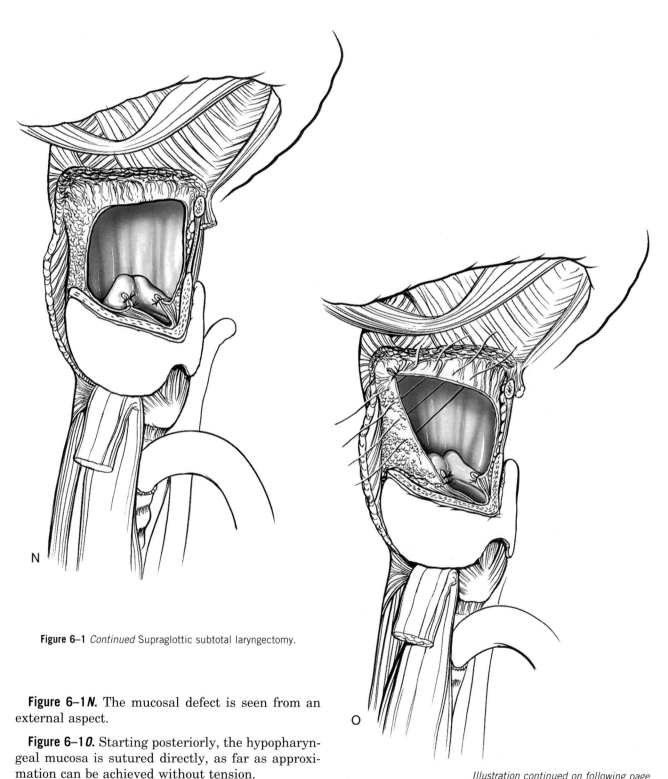

Figure 6–1 *Continued* Supraglottic subtotal laryngectomy.

Figure 6–1N. The mucosal defect is seen from an external aspect.

Figure 6–1O. Starting posteriorly, the hypopharyngeal mucosa is sutured directly, as far as approximation can be achieved without tension.

Illustration continued on following page

Figure 6–1*P.* This will leave a defect anteriorly, where the cut edge of ventricular mucosa cannot be approximated to the base of the tongue.

Figure 6–1*Q.* The defect is closed by suturing the perichondrial flap to the base of the tongue. The resultant nonmucosal surfaces in the hypopharynx will epithelialize spontaneously.

Figure 6–1*R.* The cut edges of the infrahyoid muscles are sutured to the edges of the suprahyoid muscles, providing a second layer of closure. Sutures are placed appropriately to cover the larynx as well as possible. The tracheostomy tube will be reinserted through a stab wound in the inferior skin flap. Skin sutures are placed. Note the muscle flap covering the carotid artery.

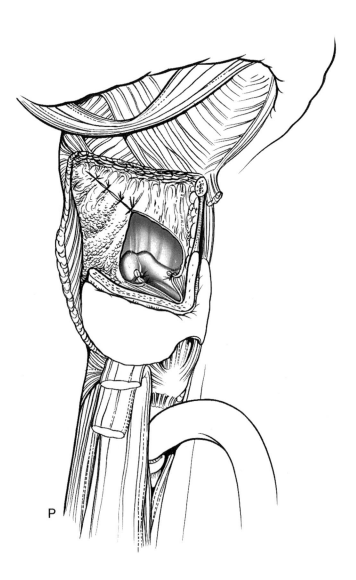

P

Figure **6–1** *Continued* Supraglottic subtotal laryngectomy.

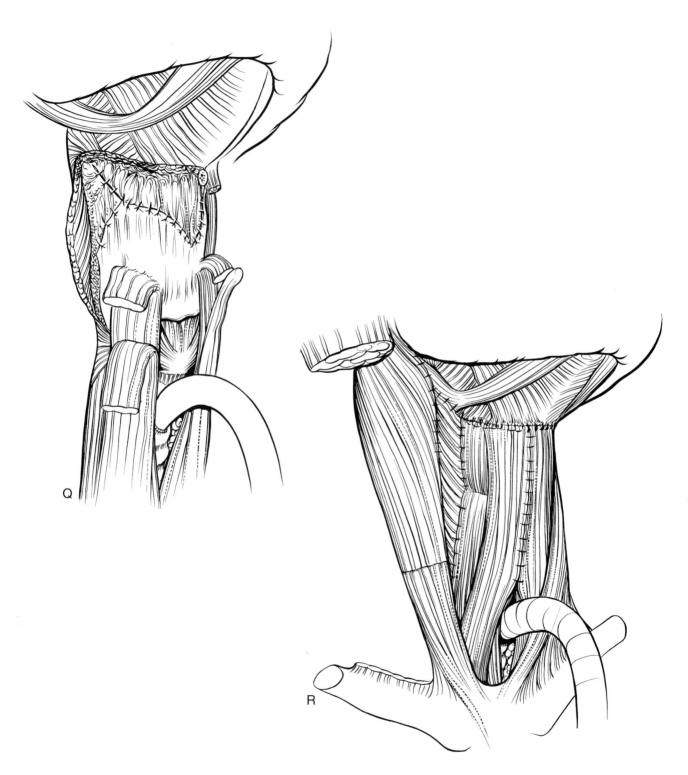

Figure 6–1 *Continued* Supraglottic subtotal laryngectomy.

Results of Conventional Supraglottic Subtotal Laryngectomy

SSL is one of the most successful surgical procedures available for the treatment of cancer. Satisfactory cure rates, even in fairly advanced lesions, are obtained, with the added benefit of preservation of laryngeal function. The results of a number of the largest recently published series are summarized in Table 6–1.[10, 17, 32–35] Cure rates consistently ranging from 70% to 80% are obtained in the treatment of primary supraglottic carcinoma.

The success of salvage procedures after failure of SSL is questionable. Som[17] was unable to salvage any of five local recurrences, all occurring within the first year, by combined total laryngectomy and postoperative radiotherapy. Ogura et al.[10] reported five cases with local recurrence, all successfully salvaged—two by total laryngectomy and three by irradiation. The experience in our service has indicated that failure resulting from lymph node metastases is far more common than failure resulting from local recurrence. Local recurrence is more common in lesions that involve the hypopharynx than in lesions confined to the supraglottic structures. Local recurrences almost always involve the base of the tongue and the pharyngeal structures and rarely involve the vocal cords.[5, 17] They are often difficult to manage by any combination of modalities.

Extended Supraglottic Laryngectomy

Som[30] and Ogura[3] were originally stringent in their indications for supraglottic laryngectomy. They were reluctant to perform this surgery on lesions extending below the petiole or on lesions extending superiorly or laterally from the epiglottis itself. Involvement of the true vocal cords, the valleculae, the arytenoid cartilages, or the base of the tongue were considered contraindications to the procedure.

Nevertheless, it became evident that, within limits, SSL could be extended to include various contiguous parts of the hypopharynx. Cure rates would not be as high as for lesions confined to the endolaryngeal part of the vestibule but would be comparable to results of treatment of the same tumors by total laryngectomy. Thus, the operation was extended, first by Alonso[28, 29] and then by Ogura and his colleagues at Washington University[36–40] to include the ipsilateral arytenoid cartilage and various portions of the hypopharynx. "Partial laryngopharyngectomy" could be used for resection of suitable primary hypopharyngeal tumors or for supraglottic laryngeal tumors with extension into the hypopharynx.

Supraglottic Subtotal Laryngectomy with Resection of Arytenoid Cartilage

Indications

The conventional supraglottic resection may be extended posteriorly to include resection of the arytenoid cartilage. The line of resection traverses the cricoarytenoid joint and the vocal process of the arytenoid. This procedure is used for lesions that grow posteriorly along the vestibular fold or along the aryepiglottic fold to involve the mucosa over the arytenoid cartilage or, occasionally, the upper portion of the cartilage itself. Lesions with extensive arytenoid cartilage or cricoarytenoid joint involvement require total laryngectomy, as do lesions that extend across the posterior commissure to the opposite arytenoid cartilage.

Technique of Supraglottic Subtotal Laryngectomy with Resection of Arytenoid Cartilage

Figure 6–2A. The procedure is identical to that shown in Figures 6–1A through 6–1H. If the ipsilateral (right) arytenoid cartilage is to be resected, the endolaryngeal mucosal incisions should be made through the contralateral (left) side first. Incision of the contralateral aryepiglottic fold and false cord will provide good exposure of the tumor and of the ipsilateral arytenoid cartilage.

Series	Follow-up (Years)	Number of Patients	Percentage of Patients Tumor Free
Ogura et al.[10]	3	177	76
Som[17]	5	75	68
Bocca et al.[32]	5	467	75
Burnstein and Calcaterra[33]	2	41	90
Maceri et al.[34]	2	25	80
Robbins et al.[35]	5	34	89

Table 6–1. RESULTS OF CONVENTIONAL SUPRAGLOTTIC SUBTOTAL LARYNGECTOMY

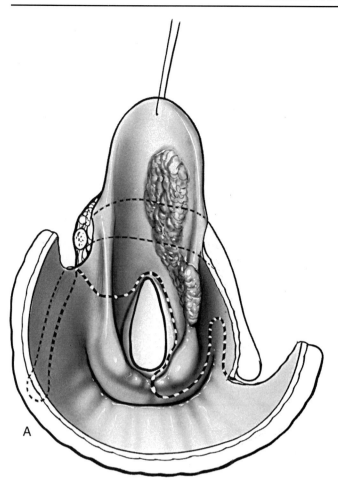

Figure 6–2B. The ipsilateral mucosa is incised through the interarytenoid region rather than through the aryepiglottic fold. This incision is carried through the cricoarytenoid joint and then through the vocal process of the arytenoid cartilage into the ventricle. Transection of the ventricular mucosa continues anteriorly to the midline, completing the resection.

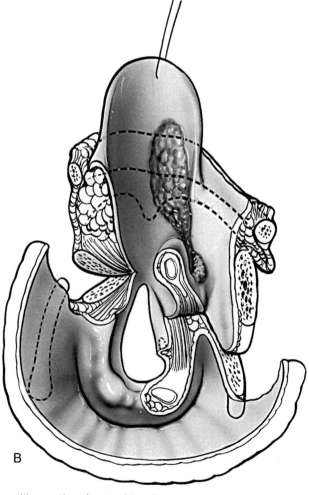

Figure 6–2. Supraglottic subtotal laryngectomy with resection of arytenoid cartilage.

Illustration continued on following page

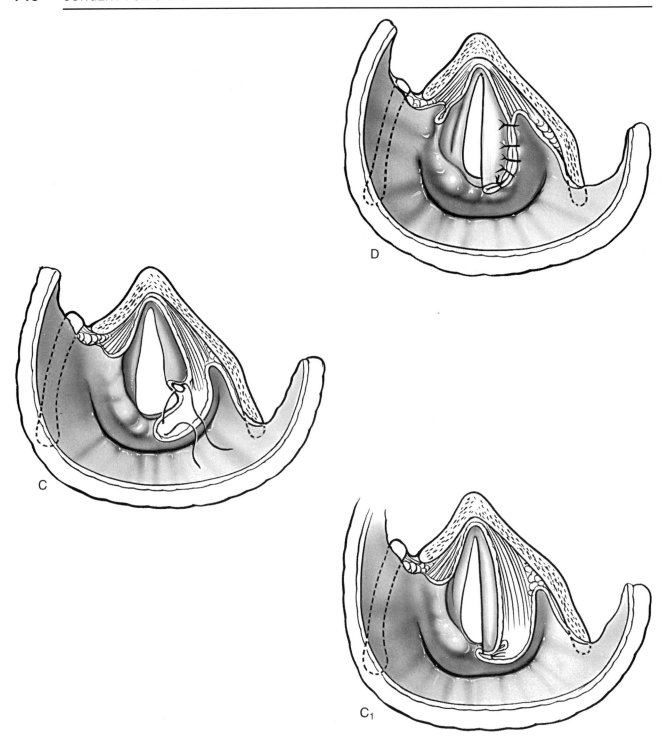

Figure 6–2 *Continued* Supraglottic subtotal laryngectomy with resection of arytenoid cartilage.

Figure 6–2*C.* After removal of the specimen, the right vocal cord must be fixed in the midline to avoid glottic incompetence. Small holes are drilled in the cricoid lamina in the midline and through the vocal process remaining on the right vocal cord. A suture of 2–0 polyglactin is passed through the drill holes and tied, fixing the cord in the midline (Fig. 6–2*C₁*).

Figure 6–2*D.* The posterior glottis is resurfaced by suturing the medial (interarytenoid and ventricular) mucosa to the pyriform sinus mucosa. The remainder of the closure procedure is identical to that in Figures 6–1*O* and 6–1*R*.

Results

Ogura et al.[39] reported 3-year disease-free survival in 44 of 59 patients (75%) treated by SSL extended to include resection of the arytenoid cartilage because of posterior extension. Bocca et al.[41] reported similar results, with 5-year disease-free survival in 56 of 74 patients (75%) treated by extended SSL. These results are comparable to those that would be obtained with total laryngectomy for the same lesions.

Supraglottic Subtotal Laryngectomy with Extension to the Hypopharynx

The SSL may be extended for adequate resection of tumors of the hypopharynx. These procedures are similar to those described in detail and illustrated in Chapter 8.

Superior Hypopharyngeal Extension

The resection can be expanded to include the valleculae and the base of the tongue. For lesions involving the lingual surface of the epiglottis, the valleculae, or the base of the tongue, the resection can be extended upward to include the superior hypopharynx. The limitations imposed on resection of the base of the tongue are due to functional and reconstructive problems. It is not feasible to attempt resection of lesions that will require sacrifice of both lingual arteries. In addition, if too much of the bulk of the base of the tongue is resected, deglutition will become impossible. The superior margin of transection of the base of the tongue should be well below the circumvallate papillae. Generally an area about 3 cm above the valleculae is the maximum that can be safely included with a supraglottic resection. This must provide a margin of resection of at least 1 cm.

Involvement of the Pyriform Sinus

Lesions may spill over the laryngeal vestibule laterally onto the aryepiglottic fold or the medial wall of the pyriform sinus. The supraglottic resection may be extended to include the entire aryepiglottic fold and medial wall of the pyriform sinus above the level of the vocal cord. There must be no fixation of the vocal cord, and pyriform sinus involvement must not extend inferior to the cricoarytenoid joint.

Subtotal Laryngectomy (Subtotal Glottic-Supraglottic Laryngectomy, Three-Quarter Laryngectomy)

Subtotal, or three-quarter, laryngectomy theoretically consists of resection of both a vertical and a horizontal half of the larynx. Beyond this basic definition, however, the procedure and its indications differ as used by various surgeons in different parts of the world. A key element in all such operations is reconstruction, because loss of a vocal cord in addition to loss of the supraglottic structures would otherwise entail profound functional disability.

In 1965, Ogura and Dedo[42] described a procedure for resection of T2 supraglottic cancers involving the arytenoid cartilages and the glottis with minimal subglottic extension. The supraglottic resection continued downward to include the true vocal cord, with the arytenoid if necessary. The cord was reconstructed by infracturing a triangular wedge of thyroid cartilage, which was then covered with a flap of hypopharyngeal mucosa.

In Japan, a more extensive "subtotal laryngectomy" was described by Iwai[43] for T3 transglottic lesions of the larynx. The vertical component of the resection included not only the vocal cord but also the ipsilateral thyroid ala and possibly part of the cricoid cartilage. The glottis was reconstructed by rotating the superior cornu of the thyroid cartilage to replace the resected portion of the laryngeal framework, with resurfacing with a flap of hypopharyngeal mucosa. Sekula[44] reported a variety of procedures performed at his clinic in Cracow, Poland, for the resection of glottic tumors with supraglottic extension and of supraglottic tumors with glottic extension. The procedures, which are categorized as "subtotal laryngectomy," were often performed within "narrow limits of safety" as far as tumor margins were concerned. Early postoperative radiotherapy was frequently used. The author pointed to favorable early results and to the advantages of offering these procedures to patients who would have refused total laryngectomy. Some severe problems with postoperative deglutition were encountered.

In the United States, Biller and Lawson[45] developed a partial laryngectomy for transglottic tumors that was suitable for glottic tumors with superior extension, for supraglottic tumors with inferior extension, or for tumors that originated within the ventricle and spread bidirectionally. Resection combined the supraglottic laryngectomy with hemilaryngectomy (three-quarter laryngectomy), with reconstruction by a large flap of thyroid cartilage pedicled on the inferior constrictor muscle. The procedure was limited to lesions 2 cm or less in diameter without vocal cord fixation, subglottic extension, anterior commissure or cartilage involvement, or prior radiation therapy.

Friedman et al.[46] employed a horizontal subtotal partial laryngectomy with vertical extension for supraglottic carcinomas extending onto the arytenoid cartilage or the vocal cord, as well as for transglottic cancers with minimal subglottic extension and minimal cephalic extension onto the ventricle and the false cord, without invasion of cartilage. The procedure was employed in selected patients with vocal cord fixation as well as previous radiation therapy; the key factor in selection of patients was the unequivocal preoperative demonstration by CT of the absence of cartilage invasion.

While a number of subtotal laryngectomy procedures have been employed by various surgeons, the procedure described by Biller and Lawson[45] is the only one with which I have personal experience and will be described in detail.

Indications

Biller and Lawson have enumerated the following criteria for subtotal laryngectomy: (1) a tumor 2 cm or less in diameter, (2) no evidence of vocal cord fixation, (3) absence of subglottic extension, (4) no involvement of the anterior commissure, (5) no evidence of cartilage invasion on CT scan, and (6) no prior radiation therapy. The procedure was employed by these authors mainly for glottic carcinoma with superior extension, but it is suitable for supraglottic tumors that extend inferiorly. It is more effective in treatment of either glottic or supraglottic tumors that do not invade the paraglottic space deeply, than for true ventricular tumors with significant paraglottic space involvement.

Technique of Subtotal Laryngectomy

Figure 6–3A. Bone and cartilage cuts are shown. Perichondrium is reflected inferiorly from the portion of thyroid cartilage to be resected (not shown) and is preserved by its attachment to the cricothyroid membrane. The position of the anterior commissure is determined in the midline, one third of the distance from the base of the thyroid notch to the inferior border of thyroid cartilage. From this point, an oblique cut is made to the midportion of the contralateral thyroid cartilage, and a vertical cut is made in the midline to the inferior border of the thyroid cartilage. A third vertical cut is placed on the ipsilateral thyroid ala approximately 1.5 cm anterior to its posterior border.

Figure 6–3B. The hypopharynx is entered through the valleculae, and the incisions are extended medially and laterally until the epiglottis can be delivered through the incision with a traction suture. The vertical entry into the larynx is commenced on the contralateral side with an incision through the aryepiglottic fold and ventricle, continuing in the line of the thyrotomy incision to the anterior commissure, where it continues inferiorly in the midline.

Figure 6–3C. The subglottis is now incised, anterior to posterior, along the superior border of the cricoid cartilage. As this incision progresses, the ipsilateral hemilarynx is reflected laterally, providing complete exposure of the tumor and the proposed resection margins.

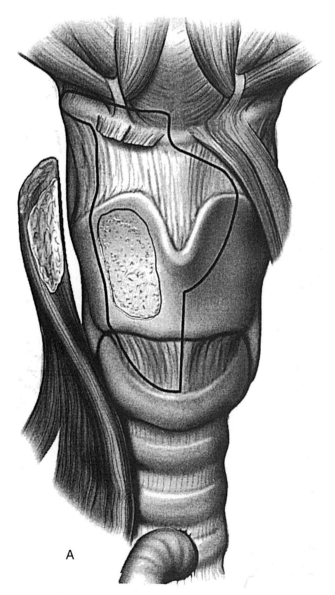

A

Figure 6–3. Subtotal (three-quarter) laryngectomy.

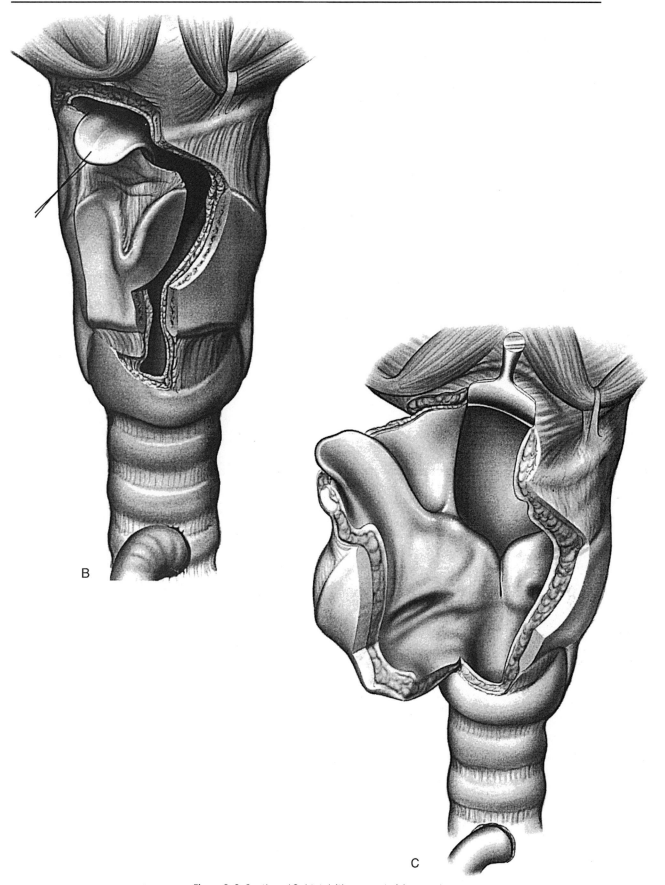

Figure 6–3 *Continued* Subtotal (three-quarter) laryngectomy.

Illustration continued on following page

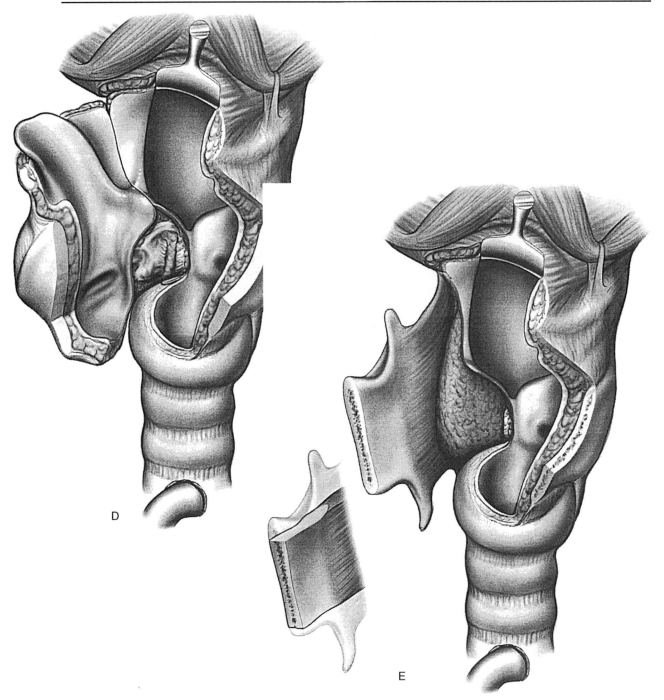

Figure 6–3 *Continued* Subtotal (three-quarter) laryngectomy.

Figure 6–3*D***.** The cricoarytenoid joint is separated along the inferior mucosal incision, and the interarytenoid mucosa and interarytenoid muscle are incised. Superiorly, the ipsilateral glossoepiglottic ligament and superior hypopharyngeal mucosa are incised, commencing the downward posterolateral incision. This is continued through the aryepiglottic fold, until the incision joins the posterior midline incision. The remaining attachments to the pyriform sinus are separated (not shown), and the specimen is removed without injury to the pyriform

sinus mucosa. A cricopharyngeal myotomy is performed (not shown).

Figure 6–3*E***.** The remaining portion of the larynx is shown. The preserved portion of the posterior lamina of the ipsilateral thyroid cartilage is mobilized by freeing the cricothyroid joint and freeing the superior cornu from its superior attachments. The cartilage segment, pedicled on the inferior constrictor muscle, will be used to replace the resected vocal cord and arytenoid cartilage.

Figure 6–3F. The cartilage flap is trimmed and rotated into position over the cricoid cartilage. It is fixed in the anterior and posterior midlines with wire or heavy polyglactin sutures.

Figure 6–3G. The cartilage flap is covered on the superior and the inferior surfaces by a flap of postarytenoid mucosa and pyriform sinus mucosa, as far as can be accomplished. This flap should be mobilized and sutured in place before the cartilage is fixed. Biller and Lawson[45] suggest reducing the depth of anesthesia in order to ensure adequate glottic closure on adduction and adequate respiratory passage on abduction.

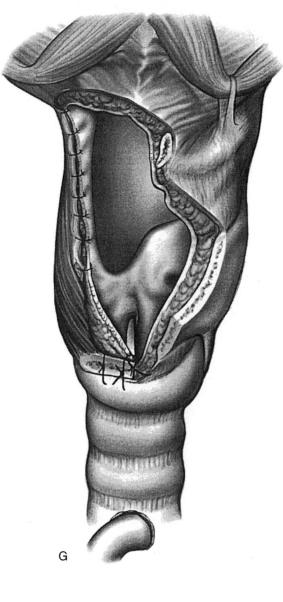

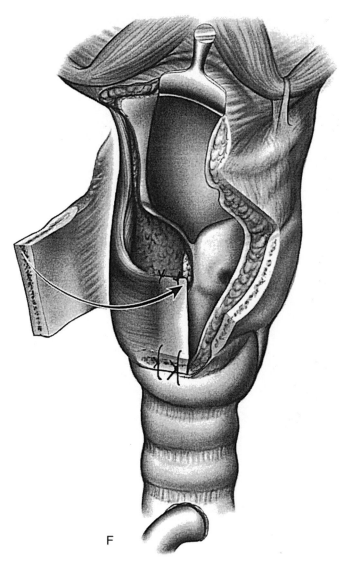

Figure 6–3 *Continued* Subtotal (three-quarter) laryngectomy.

Illustration continued on following page

Figure 6–3*H.* A nasogastric feeding tube is inserted. The larynx is closed by approximation of the base of the tongue and the vertical laryngeal borders to the perichondrium and the transected strap muscles in a single layer.

Figure 6–3*I.* The strap muscles form a complete layer of closure over the larynx. As with all partial laryngectomies, the larynx need not be airtight as long as a patent tracheostomy tube is in place. It is necessary to preserve sufficient mucosa for resurfacing one side of the larynx at the glottic level and to provide enough tissue for nonepithelialized healing of all remaining mucosal defects.

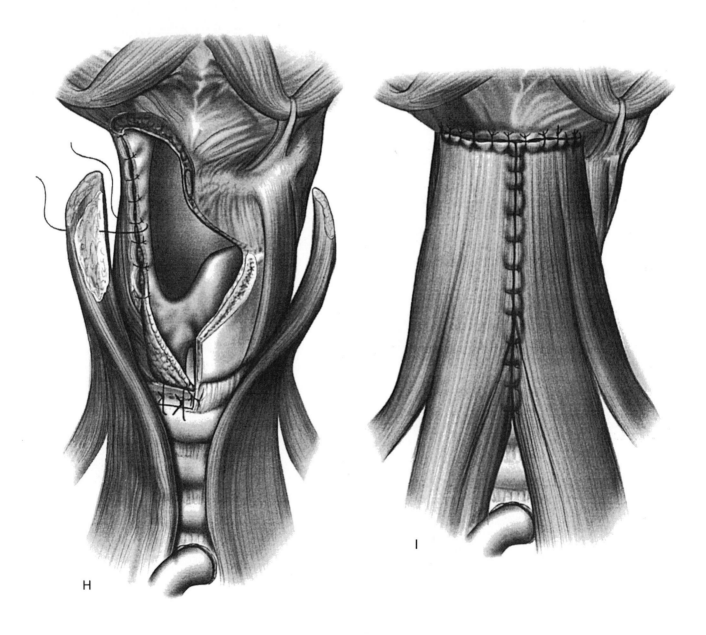

Figure 6–3 *Continued* Subtotal (three-quarter) laryngectomy.

Results

The results of subtotal laryngectomy are difficult to evaluate because of the small numbers of cases reported and the variation in the indication for this procedure. Sekula[44] and Iwai[43] used this procedure for resection of transglottic tumors in their relatively small series of cases and achieved cure rates between 60% and 70%. Ogura and Dedo[42] reported no recurrences and good laryngeal function in four patients followed 9 to 21 months after subtotal laryngectomy, performed for the indications described above.

Five patients operated on by Biller and Lawson[45] were free of tumor for periods greater than 1½ years, at the time of their report. Friedman et al.[47] reported 3-year survival of 70% in a series of 24 patients with similar tumors, some with fixed vocal cords (stage T3).

Surgical Measures to Assist Deglutition

The major problem encountered after SSL is restoration of deglutition without aspiration. Loss of the supraglottic structures not only removes the anatomic protection of the laryngeal introitus, but also interrupts the sequential sensory input of the swallowing mechanism. This sensory derangement is the most important factor in the loss of adequate deglutition after supraglottic resections.[48] This deficiency in sensory reception can be compensated for by the residual structures, provided damage to the external branch of the superior laryngeal nerve and to the recurrent laryngeal nerve is avoided.[49] In extensive resections for larger tumors, which may include arytenoid resection and tongue base excision, injury to these nerves, as well as erratic healing, edema, and scarring, may further reduce sphincteric function.

The loss of ability to close the glottis tightly because of resection or from paralysis of a vocal cord will significantly reduce the patient's ability to regain deglutitory function. If a vocal cord or arytenoid cartilage is to be resected during surgery, it is important to restore glottic competence by reconstruction of the glottic defect and to position the paralyzed cord in the midline. Biller et al.[50] emphasized that partial arytenoid resection with exposure of the residual cartilage is the most common cause, leading frequently to arytenoid fixation in the abducted position. These authors suggested that covering the exposed cartilage with a mucosal flap may avoid chondritis and, ultimately, fixation of the cord. For cases with partial arytenoid resection, they recommended fixation of the arytenoid cartilage in the posterior midline with a nonabsorbable

suture, and for cases in which the entire arytenoid cartilage was to be resected, they advised employing a free or pedicled thyroid cartilage flap to prevent a posterior glottic defect.

Cricopharyngeal myotomy at the time of initial resection, and preservation of the hyoid bone have been employed as means of minimizing postoperative aspiration. Division of the cricopharyngeal muscle ostensibly prevents the failure of relaxation of the sphincter during the second phase of swallowing. A retrospective analysis by Flores et al.[51] of 51 patients operated on at the Cleveland Clinic indicated that preservation of the hyoid bone facilitated closure but improved deglutition only if both superior laryngeal nerves were preserved along with the hyoid, which is not feasible in most resections. Cricopharyngeal myotomy could not be shown to affect ultimate success in swallowing, but it seemed to facilitate a more rapid return of deglutition.

Calcaterra[52] and Goode[53] have advocated suspension of the larynx to minimize postoperative aspiration. The thyroid cartilage is fixed to the mentum of the mandible or digastric muscles with heavy suture material (we prefer slowly absorbed polyglactin for this). The sutures are placed so that the larynx is tilted forward slightly. We have not noticed any significant improvement in postoperative deglutition in patients in whom we have performed this procedure. However, we find laryngeal suspension useful for closure of large supraglottic defects in cases for which resection of a portion of the base of the tongue is required.

Preservation of the internal laryngeal nerve has been discussed as a means of preventing aspiration. However, it is not possible to resect a supraglottic carcinoma adequately without sacrificing this nerve. In cases in which lateral pharyngotomy is used for nonmalignant conditions, the nerve may be preserved by dissection and retraction, but this causes marked restriction of exposure. Because the sensory field of the internal laryngeal nerve is almost completely resected in SSL, preservation of this nerve would serve little purpose.

Postoperative Management

Management of the patient after SSL is essentially the same as that after vertical partial laryngectomy, except that more difficulty can be anticipated in recovery of deglutition. No oral feedings are offered until the wounds are well healed. Then, small amounts of semisolids, such as gelatin dessert or custard, are tried. Occlusion of the tracheostomy tube while eating and leaning to the lesser-involved side while swallowing may assist deglutition without aspiration. In difficult cases, decannulation of the tracheostomy and removal of the nasogastric feeding tube may help. A "three swallow" technique has been described by Tucker.[48] The patient, while holding a deep breath, takes a small bolus of semisolid material, swallows twice, and then coughs and swallows a third time. Liquids should be attempted only after semisolid food can be managed reasonably well. It is necessary for the patient to "practice" swallowing for short periods frequently throughout the day before reflexes are properly reeducated. With patience and persistence, even the poorest candidates for supraglottic laryngectomy will usually learn to swallow. Occasionally, "completion" laryngectomy is necessary because of persistent glottic incompetence.

Complications

The complication rate is not high after supraglottic laryngectomy. Bocca[54] reported 28 complications in a series of 223 patients (12.5%), and Som[17] noted significant complications in 9 of 93 patients (9.6%). Table 6–2 summarizes the frequency with which various complications occurred in several large series of cases.[17, 54, 55]

Aspiration and Pneumonia

Sessions et al.[55] found aspiration of food to be the most common problem after supraglottic laryngectomy, whereas airway obstruction occurred infrequently. The true extent of the aspiration problem may not be appreciated by many surgeons. Flores et al.[51] determined that relatively normal swallowing could be expected in only 85% to 90% of patients after supraglottic laryngectomy. Approximately one half of the remaining patients in the study could swallow and cough well enough to prevent pneumonia but were unable to ingest sufficient food to maintain adequate nutrition and required either gastrostomy or completion laryngectomy. The remaining 5% to 7% developed persistent pulmonary infection and required completion laryngectomy.

Murray,[56] in a retrospective study of patients after SSL, noted that respiratory infections and deaths from pneumonia occurred more often than was generally realized. With the increasing use of SSL in older patients and in patient with tumors involving the hypopharynx, a higher frequency of postoperative aspiration will be noted. Thus, when the indications for this procedure are extended to include these less favorable cases, surgeons must be willing to use corrective surgical measures for the incompetent glottic insufficiency that will develop in some patients, including thyroid cartilage implants, possible laryngeal suspension, and cricopharyngeal myotomy (see Surgical Measures to Assist Deglutition).

Surgical procedures have been developed to treat problems of aspiration arising from glottic incompetence. The use of injectable collagen has been discussed in Chapter 5. Biller et al.[50] have used a cartilage implant to correct posterior glottic incompetence after supraglottic laryngectomy with arytenoid resection. Unlike other techniques, which employ an anterior thyrotomy approach for insertion of the implant and are suitable for anterior glottic defects, a posterior approach similar to a Woodman type of external arytenoidectomy is used. After disarticulation of the inferior cricoarytenoid joint, the posterior cricoid is exposed submucosally, and the implant is inserted and fixed with a wire into the bed of the previously resected arytenoid. Good results were reported in four of six patients followed for a minimum of 18 months.

Airway Obstruction

Airway obstruction may arise from differing causes. The most common type occurs in the early postoperative period and is due to lymphedema of unresected supraglottic mucosa. This problem is prevented by removing the entire false vocal cord at the time of initial resection, even if inclusion of this structure is not necessary to ensure an adequate resection margin. The problem may be treated by excision of the edematous mucosa by suspension laryngoscopy. The carbon dioxide laser is ideal for this purpose.

Table 6–2. COMPLICATIONS OF SUPRAGLOTTIC LARYNGECTOMY				
	Sessions et al.[55]	Bocca[54]	Som[17]	Total	Percent of Total Reported Complications
Aspiration	17	6	2	25	36
Pneumonia	3	3	2	8	12
Airway obstruction	2	11	2	15	22
Infection or fistula	—	8	13	21	30
Total number of complications	22	28	19	69	

A more persistent type of airway obstruction occurs as a result of laryngeal infection and necrosis. Loss of mucosa and cartilage with eventual web or stricture formation is not as frequent after supraglottic laryngectomy as after vertical partial laryngectomy. Management of this problem has been discussed in detail in Chapter 5. Simple glottic webs may be treated with a "keel." More extensive strictures require excision of the scar and all devitalized tissue and laryngeal reconstruction with skin flaps or grafts. The carbon dioxide laser may be helpful in cases in which extensive destruction of the laryngeal framework has not occurred.

Infection, Necrosis, and Fistulae

Infection, necrosis, and fistulae are related, as one causes the other. The incidence of such complications is low in SSL performed in nonirradiated patients for tumor confined to the larynx. Even when postoperative infection and fistula formation do occur, healing takes place readily. Large supraglottic fistulae within open neck wounds will often heal spontaneously, without formal closure by lined flaps or other elaborate procedures. When, however, supraglottic laryngectomy is extended to include resection of various portions of the hypopharynx, fistula formation occurs more readily, and staged surgical procedures are often necessary for closure.

As stated previously, infection, necrosis, and fistulae are more likely to occur in irradiated patients. Many surgeons, therefore, regard previous high-dose radiotherapy as a contraindication to SSL. Although we prefer to operate on nonirradiated patients, we have found that SSL can be performed after high-dose radiotherapy if certain precautions are observed: (1) the lesion must have been suitable for supraglottic laryngectomy prior to radiotherapy; (2) only selective neck dissection should be employed electively; and (3) the perichondrial flap and strap muscles should not be relied on for closure. We have used a large sternomastoid muscle flap to reinforce the closure. Creation of a temporary laryngostoma may be considered, if adequate tissue is not available for closure.

Voice

Voice problems are much less frequent after SSL than after vertical partial laryngectomy. Sessions et al.[55] noted only one "minor" problem with the voice after supraglottic laryngectomy. Som[17] reported postoperative fixation of the ipsilateral vocal cord in 4 of his 93 cases. He felt this resulted from inadvertent incision into the arytenoid cartilage during the resection, with resultant fixation by scar.

SUPRACRICOID LARYNGECTOMY WITH CRICOHYOIDOPEXY

Segmental resection of the larynx from the cricoid cartilage to the hyoid bone has been popular in Europe, but not in the United States, for the past decade. The initial concept of a partial laryngeal resection in which reconstruction was accomplished by suturing the hyoid bone to the cricoid cartilage was described by Majer and Rieder in 1959.[57] The concept was refined and reported in the English language literature by Piquet et al.[58] in 1974, and it has been used extensively in Europe.[59–61] The procedure has been employed for supraglottic carcinomas with preepiglottic space, paraglottic space, and thyroid cartilage involvement that were not amenable to conventional or extended SSL. The operation is similar to the supracricoid laryngectomy with cricohyoidoepiglottopexy employed for glottic carcinomas, described in detail in Chapter 5.

Indications

Based on experience with 68 patients, none of whom had local recurrence, Laccourreye et al.[60] listed the indications for supracricoid laryngectomy with cricohyoidopexy as follows:

1. T1 or T2 supraglottic lesions extending to the ventricle, the infrahyoid epiglottis, and the posterior third of the false vocal cord
2. T1 or T2 supraglottic lesions extending to the glottis and the anterior commissure with or without impaired mobility of the true vocal cord
3. T3 transglottic carcinomas with marked limitation of the true vocal cord
4. Selected cases of T4 transglottic carcinomas invading the thyroid cartilage

The authors consider the following conditions as contraindications to the procedure:

1. Subglottic extent greater than 10 mm anteriorly and 5 mm posteriorly, because these tumors involve the cricoid cartilage
2. Preoperative clinical examination that reveals arytenoid cartilage fixation, because these lesions invade the posterior intrinsic laryngeal muscles, the cricoarytenoid joint, or the arytenoid cartilage
3. Massive invasion of the preepiglottic space observed preoperatively either during the clinical examination or with CT (limited invasion of the preepiglottic space is not considered a contraindication, because this compartment is totally resected during the procedure)
4. Supraglottic and transglottic lesions that involve the pharyngeal wall, the vallecula, the base of the tongue, the postcricoid, and the arytenoid region
5. Cricoid cartilage invasion

Technique of Supracricoid Laryngectomy with Cricohyoidopexy

Figure 6–4A. The initial steps are similar to those described with supracricoid laryngectomy with cricohyoidoepiglottopexy (CHEP) (see Chapter 5):

1. The oral airway is intubated if feasible.
2. Either a transverse or a U-shaped incision is made, depending on the extent of neck dissection to be performed.
3. The skin flap raised to 1 cm above the hyoid bone.
4. The sternohyoid and sternothyroid muscles are transected along the superior border of thyroid cartilage, and after downward reflection of the sternohyoid muscles, the thyrohyoid muscles are transected along the inferior border of thyroid cartilage. The inferior pharyngeal constrictors and thyroid perichondrium are sectioned along the posterior borders of the thyroid alae. The pyriform sinuses are dissected from beneath the thyroid alae.

5. The cricothyroid joints are disarticulated.
6. The thyroid isthmus is ligated.
7. The anterior wall of the trachea is bluntly dissected to the carina, to permit elevation of the trachea for laryngeal closure.
8. A transverse incision is made through the cricothyroid membrane at the upper border of the cricoid cartilage, and an endotracheal tube is inserted to replace the oral endotracheal tube, which is withdrawn.

The periosteum of the hyoid bone is now incised anteriorly and laterally, and the preepiglottic space is separated from the posterior surface of the hyoid bone. The hypopharynx is now entered superiorly, behind the hyoid bone, through the valleculae.

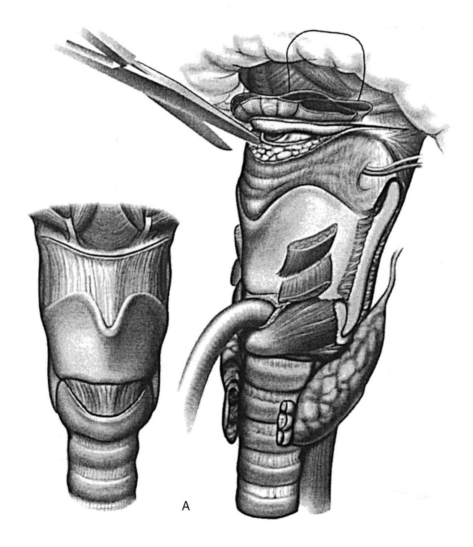

A

Figure 6–4. Supracricoid laryngectomy with cricohyoidopexy.

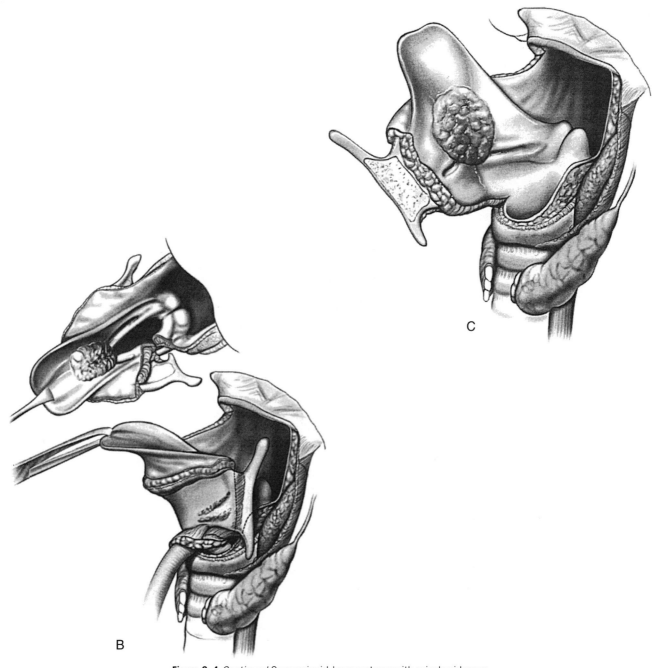

Figure 6–4 *Continued* Supracricoid laryngectomy with cricohyoidopexy.

Illustration continued on following page

Figure 6–4*B*. This superior transverse incision is now enlarged laterally to one side, until the epiglottis can be grasped with a tenaculum or suture and pulled through the incision, permitting visualization of the larynx and the tumor.

On the lesser involved (left) side, a vertical incision is made through the aryepiglottic fold, anterior to the arytenoid, and extended inferiorly to the upper border of the cricoid.

Figure 6–4*C*. The vertical prearytenoid incision and the inferior transverse incision are now connected with an incision along the superior border of

the cricoid cartilage. At this point, as with CHEP, the thyroid cartilage is grasped between the surgeon's hands and fractured in the midline, as if "opening a book." Complete visualization of the endolarynx and the side of greater involvement is now achieved. The tumor may now be excised under direct vision by completing the incision on the ipsilateral (right) side along the superior border of the cricoid cartilage, preserving the arytenoid cartilage if possible, with a vertical prearytenoid incision, or removing it, if necessary, by carrying the incision to the posterior midline.

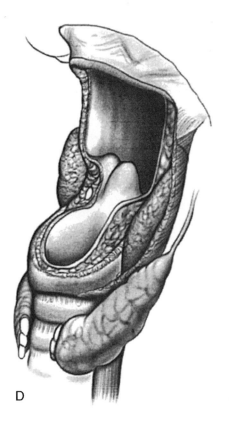

D

Figure 6–4 *Continued* Supracricoid laryngectomy with cricohyoidopexy.

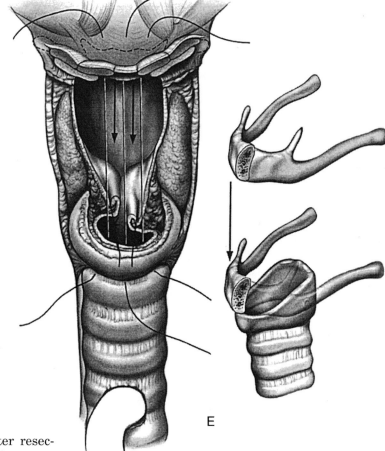

E

Figure 6–4D. The laryngeal remnant after resection is shown. Both arytenoid cartilages, the entire cricoid cartilage, and the hyoid bone (not shown) remain.

Figure 6–4E. The mucosa of the upper part of the arytenoid cartilages is repaired, leaving the inferior aspects bare. If one arytenoid cartilage has been removed, the raw surfaces are not covered. The arytenoid cartilages are fixed to the midline of the cricoid with "air sutures" if necessary, in order to prevent rotation or posterior displacement. Three submucosal heavy polypropylene sutures are now placed around the cricoid cartilage and the hyoid bone. The first suture is placed in the midline, and the lateral sutures are placed about 1 cm on each side.

Figure 6–4F. With upward traction on these sutures, a tracheostomy tube is placed at the level of the skin incision and the hyoid bone is impacted onto the cricoid cartilage. No gap must be left between the cricoid cartilage and the hyoid bone, and the anterior borders of the cricoid cartilage and the hyoid bone must be carefully aligned. Reapproximation of sternohyoid muscles completes the repair.

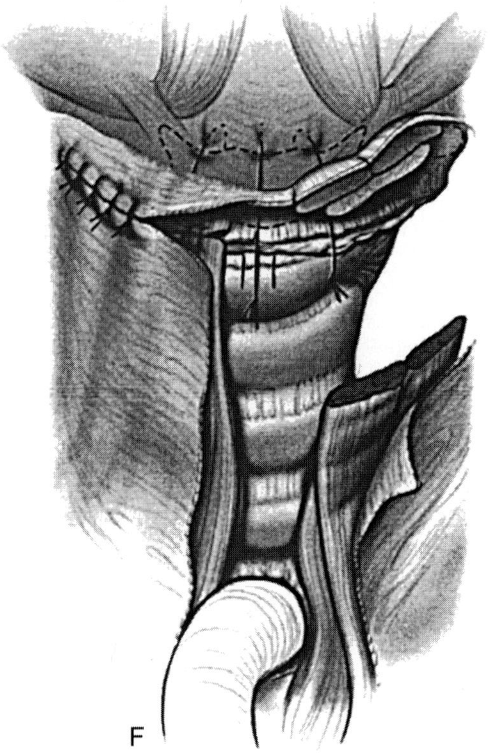

F

Figure 6–4 *Continued* Supracricoid laryngectomy with cricohyoidopexy.

Oncologic Results

Laccourreye et al.[60] reported results of treatment of 68 patients operated on at the Laennec Hospital in Paris between 1974 and 1986. The minimum follow-up time was 18 months, and 39 patients were followed at least 3 years. There were no local recurrences. Four of 68 patients (5.8%) developed tumor recurrence in the neck. All had preoperatively palpable cervical lymph nodes, and all had been treated, at the time of primary resection, with radical neck dissection and postoperative radiation therapy. Eight of the patients (8.8%) developed distant metastases. The 3-year actuarial survival rate was 71.4%. Ten patients died from recurrence of the primary tumor, two from distant metastases, and two from intercurrent disease.

Laccourreye et al.[61] reported results in 19 patients with infrahyoid epiglottic squamous cell carcinoma with gross preepiglottic space invasion, not amenable to SSL for various reasons, including massive invasion of the petiole, invasion of the anterior commissure, invasion of the true vocal cord, involvement of the floor of the ventricle, and marked limitation of true vocal cord mobility. In most of the patients one arytenoid cartilage was either totally or partially removed. The 5-year actuarial survival was 84.2%. There was only one instance of local recurrence and one of nodal recurrence. The 5-year actuarial rate of death from distant metastasis was 5.6% and from second primary tumors, 30%. The second primary tumor was the cause of death in five of six patients who died.

Postoperative Function and Complications

In the series of 68 patients reported by Laccourreye et al.,[60] all patients were decannulated within 8 weeks with the exception of one patient who died of a ruptured aortic aneurism on the third postoperative day. The average time of decannulation was 7 days. Normal postoperative deglutition was achieved by 50 of 67 patients (75%) within the first postoperative month. Physiologic phonation without tracheostomy was achieved in all patients within the same time period. Fifteen patients required temporary gastrostomy, and in two patients, permanent gastrostomy was required—one because of resection of the base of the tongue for a second primary tumor. Laccourreye et al.[61] found, by multivariate analysis, that swallowing problems occurred with significantly greater frequency in patients who underwent partial or complete resection of an arytenoid cartilage.

In the latter study of Laccourreye et al.,[61] various complications were found related to postoperative radiation therapy. These included persistent laryngeal edema in 4 of 19 patients, reduced mobility of the remaining arytenoid cartilage in 3 patients and chondroradionecrosis in 2 patients. There was 1 instance each of glottic stenosis and of cervical fibrosis with phrenic nerve paralysis.[61]

REFERENCES

1. Frazier EJ. The development of the larynx. *J Anat Physiol* 1909; 44:156–191.
2. Hast MH. Applied embryology of the larynx. *In* Alberti PW, Bryce DP (eds): *Workshops from the Centennial Conference on Laryngeal Cancer,* pp 6–10. New York, Appleton-Century-Crofts, 1976.
3. Ogura JH. Supraglottic subtotal laryngectomy and radical neck dissection: one stage operation for carcinoma of the epiglottis. *Laryngoscope* 1958; 68:983–1003.
4. Rouviere H. *Anatomy of the Human Lymphatic System.* Ann Arbor, Mich, Edwards Brothers, 1931.
5. Bocca E, Pignataro O, Mosciaro O. Supraglottic surgery of the larynx. *Ann Otol Rhinol Laryngol* 1968; 77:1005–1026.
6. Kirchner J, Som ML. Clinical and histological observations on supraglottic cancer. *Ann Otol Rhinol Laryngol* 1971; 80:638–644.
7. Vermund H. Role of radiotherapy in cancer of the larynx as related to the TNM system of staging. *Cancer* 1970; 24:485–504.
8. Coates HL, DeSanto LW, Devine KD, et al. Carcinoma of the supraglottic larynx: a review of 221 cases. *Arch Otolaryngol* 1976; 102:686–689.
9. Jankovic I, Merkas, Z. Radiotherapy as the primary approach in the treatment of laryngeal cancer. *In* Alberti PW, Bryce DP (eds): *Workshops from the Centennial Conference on Laryngeal Cancer,* pp 881–888. New York, Appleton-Century-Crofts, 1976.
10. Ogura JH, Sessions DG, Spector GJ. Conservation surgery for epidermoid carcinoma of the supraglottic larynx. *Laryngoscope* 1975; 85:1808–1815.
11. Goepfert H, Jesse RH, Fletcher GH, et al. Optimal treatment for the technically resectable squamous cell carcinoma of the supraglottic larynx. *Laryngoscope* 1975; 85:14–32.
12. Lee NK, Goepfert H, Wendt CD. Supraglottic laryngectomy of intermediate stage cancer: UTMD Anderson Cancer Center experience with combined therapy. *Laryngoscope* 1990; 100:831–836.
13. Mendenhall WM, Parsons JT, Stringer SP, et al. Carcinoma of the supraglottic larynx: a basis for comparing the results of radiotherapy and surgery. *Head Neck* 1990; 12:204–209.
14. Gilbert RW, Birt D, Shulman H, et al. Correlation of tumor volume with local control in laryngeal carcinoma treated by radiotherapy. *Ann Otol Rhinol Laryngol* 1987; 96:514–518.
15. Mancuso AA. Evaluation and staging of laryngeal and hypopharyngeal cancer by computed tomography and magnetic resonance imaging. *In* Silver CE (ed): *Laryngeal Cancer,* pp 46–94. New York, Thieme, 1991.
16. Isaacs J, Mancuso AA, Mendenhall WM, et al. Deep spread patterns in CT staging of T_{2-4} squamous cell laryngeal carcinoma. *Otolaryngol Head Neck Surg* 1988; 99:455–464.
17. Som ML. Conservation surgery for carcinoma of the supraglottis. *J Laryngol Otol* 1970; 84:655–678.
18. DeSanto L, Lillie J, Devine K. Surgical salvage after radiation of laryngeal cancer. Laryngoscope 1976; 86:649–657.
19. Biller H, Ogura J, Davis W, et al. Planned preoperative irradiation for carcinoma of the larynx and laryngopharynx treated by total and partial laryngectomy. *Laryngoscope* 1969; 79:1387–1395.
20. Ogura JH, Biller H. Pre-operative irradiation for laryngeal and laryngopharyngeal cancers. *Laryngoscope* 1970; 80:802–810.
21. Goepfert H, Lee N, Wendt C, Peters L. Treatment of cancer of the supraglottic larynx. *In* Silver CE (ed): *Laryngeal Cancer,* pp 176–182. New York, Thieme, 1991.
22. Trotter W. The Hunterian lectures on the principles and technique of operative treatment of malignant diseases of the mouth and pharynx. Lancet 1913; 1:1075.
23. Trotter W. A method of lateral pharyngotomy for the exposure of large growths in the epilaryngeal region. *J Laryngol Otol* 1920; 35:289–295.
24. Trotter W. Operations for malignant disease of the pharynx. *Br J Surg* 1929; 16:485–495.

25. Colledge L. Repair of pharyngeal defects after operation for removal of malignant tumors. *Proc R Soc Med* 1931; 24:14.
26. Orton HB. Lateral transthyroid pharyngotomy. *Arch Otolaryngol* 1930; 12:320–338.
27. Orton HB. Cancer of the laryngopharynx. *Arch Otolaryngol* 1938; 28:344–354.
28. Alonso JM. Conservative surgery of cancer of the larynx. *Trans Am Acad Opthalmol Otolaryngol* 1947; 51:633–642.
29. Alonso JM, Jackson CL. Conservation of function in surgery of cancer of the larynx: bases, techniques and results. *Trans Am Acad Ophthalmol Otolaryngol* 1952; 56:722.
30. Som ML. Surgical treatment of carcinoma of the epiglottis by lateral pharyngotomy. *Trans Am Acad Ophthalmol Otolaryngol* 1959; 63:28–47.
31. Zeitels SM, Vaughan CW. Preepiglottic space invasion in early epiglottic cancer. *Ann Otol Rhinl Laryngol* 1991; 100:789–792.
32. Bocca E, Pignataro O, Oldini C. Supraglottic laryngectomy: 30 years of experience. *Ann Otol Rhinol Laryngol* 1983; 92:14–18.
33. Burnstein FD, Calcaterra TC. Supraglottic laryngectomy: series report and analysis of results. *Laryngoscope* 1985; 95:833–836.
34. Maceri DR, Lampe HB, Makielski KH, et al. Conservation laryngeal surgery: a critical analysis. *Arch Otolaryngol* 1985; 111:361–365.
35. Robbins KT, Davidson W, Peters LJ, et al. Conservation surgery for T2 and T3 carcinomas of the supraglottic larynx. *Arch Otolaryngol Head Neck Surg* 1988; 114:421–426.
36. Ogura JH, Biller H, Calcaterra TC, et al. Surgical treatment of carcinoma of the larynx, pharynx, base of tongue and cervical esophagus. *Int Surg* 1969; 52:29–40.
37. Ogura JH, Jurema AA, Watson RK. Partial laryngopharyngectomy and neck dissection for pyriform sinus cancer. *Laryngoscope* 1960; 70:1399–1417.
38. Ogura JH, Mallen RW. Partial laryngopharyngectomy for supraglottic and pharyngeal carcinoma. *Trans Am Acad Ophthalmol Otolaryngol* 1965; 69:832–845.
39. Ogura JH, Sessions DG, Ciralsky RH. Supraglottic carcinoma with extension to the arytenoid. *Laryngoscope* 1975; 85:1327–1331.
40. Reference deleted.
41. Bocca E, Pignataro O, Oldini C, et al. Extended supraglottic laryngectomy: review of 84 cases. *Ann Otol Rhinol Laryngol* 1987; 96:384–386.
42. Ogura JH, Dedo HH. Glottic reconstruction following subtotal glottic-supraglottic laryngectomy. *Laryngoscope* 1965; 75:865–878.
43. Iwai H. Limitations of conservation surgery in carcinoma involving the arytenoid. *In* Alberti PW, Bryce DP (eds): *Workshops from the Centennial Conference on Laryngeal Cancer,* pp 426–431. New York, Appleton-Century-Crofts, 1976.
44. Sekula J. The subtotal operation in the treatment of cancer of the larynx. *Laryngoscope* 1967; 77:1996–2006.
45. Biller HF, Lawson W. Partial laryngectomy for transglottic cancers. *Ann Otol Rhinol Laryngol* 1984; 93:297–300.
46. Friedman WH, Katsantonis GP, Siddoway JR, et al. Contralateral laryngoplasty after supraglottic laryngectomy with vertical extension. *Arch Otolaryngol Head Neck Surg* 1989; 107:742–745.
47. Friedman WH, Katsantonis GP. Subtotal laryngectomy with contralateral laryngoplasty. *In* Silver CE (ed): *Laryngeal Cancer,* pp 183–192. New York, Thieme, 1991.
48. Tucker H. Deglutition following partial laryngectomy. *In* Silver CE (ed): *Laryngeal Cancer,* pp 197–200. New York, Thieme, 1991.
49. Ward PH. The second Joseph H. Ogura Memorial Lecture. Compilations of laryngeal surgery: etiology and prevention. *Laryngoscope* 1988; 98:54–57.
50. Biller HF, Lawson W, Sacks S. Correction of posterior glottic incompetence following partial laryngectomy. *Ann Otol Rhinol Laryngol* 1982; 91:448–449.
51. Flores TC, Wood BG, Levine HL, et al. Factors in successful deglutition following supraglottic laryngeal surgery. *Ann Otol Rhinol Laryngol* 1982; 91:579–583.

52. Calcaterra T. Laryngeal suspension after supraglottic laryngectomy. *Arch Otolaryngol* 1971; 94:306–309.
53. Goode R. Laryngeal suspension in head and neck surgery. *Laryngoscope* 1976; 86:349–354.
54. Bocca E. Supraglottic cancer. *Laryngoscope* 1975; 85:1318–1326.
55. Sessions DG, Ogura JH, Ciralsky RH. Late glottic insufficiency. *Laryngoscope* 1975; 85:950–959.
56. Murray GM. Pulmonary complications following supraglottic laryngectomy. *Clin Otolaryngol* 1976; 1:241–247.
57. Majer E-H, Rieder W. Technique de laryngectomie permettant de conserver la perméabilité respiratoire. (La crico-hyöido-pexie). *Ann Otolaryngol* 1959; 76:677–681.
58. Piquet J-J, Desaulty A, Decroix G. La crico-hyöido-epiglotto-pexie: Technique opératoire et résultats Fonctionnels. *Ann Otolaryngol Chir Cervicofac* 1974; 91:681–686.
59. Piquet J-J, Darras JA, Berrier A, et al. Les laryngectomies subtotales fonctionelles avec crico-hyöido-pexie: technique, indications, résultats. *Ann Otolaryngol Chir Cervicofac* 1986; 103:411–415.
60. Laccourreye H, Laccourreye O, Weinstein G, et al. Supracricoid laryngectomy with cricohyoidopexy: a partial laryngeal procedure for selected supraglottic and transglottic carcinomas. *Laryngoscope* 1990; 100:735–741.
61. Laccourreye O, Brasnu D, Merite-Drancy A, et al. Cricohyoidopexy in selected infrahyoid epiglottic carcinomas presenting with pathological preepiglottic space invasion. *Arch Otolaryngol Head Neck Surg* 1993; 119:881–886.

Chapter 7

Total Laryngectomy
Carl E. Silver and Alfio Ferlito

BACKGROUND

The first total laryngectomy was carried out in 1873 by Billroth,[1] and techniques for successful performance of this radical procedure were developed throughout the first quarter of the twentieth century. Nevertheless, widespread acceptance of the procedure did not occur for many decades. During the period between World War I and World War II, many leading institutions placed a major emphasis on radiation therapy for the treatment of head and neck tumors, and of the larynx in particular. According to Martin,[2] no laryngectomies were performed at Memorial Hospital, New York, between 1918 and 1933. The lack of enthusiasm for total laryngectomy, as well as for other radical head and neck operations, was understandable in view of the condition of surgical techniques. In the absence of antibiotics, postoperative pneumonia occurred frequently, often with fatal results, and wound breakdown was almost inevitable after total laryngectomy. The only anesthetic agents available were inhalants, such as chloroform or ether, and administration by open drop or face mask was cumbersome as well as dangerous. Local anesthesia was often used for total laryngectomy, but this was not particularly pleasant, either for the patient or for the surgeon.

With regard to the effect of the new availability of antibiotics on laryngeal surgery, Martin's comments[2] are most impressive: "Only those surgeons whose experience spans this transition period can appreciate the impact of the sudden dramatic changes in the prevention and/or control of surgical sepsis and postoperative pulmonary complications as the result of the sulfas and penicillin. For example, in total laryngectomy, healing by primary intention without salivary fistula now often took place. After partial laryngectomy there had always been a risk of hemorrhage 4–7 days after operation due to septic necrosis of the raw wound surface within the larynx. In such cases, the aspiration of blood and bronchopneumonia were inevitable. With the new facilities, prompt healing was the rule."

Several modifications in technique developed during the 1930s. A subperichondrial laryngectomy was described by Crowe and Broyles.[3] The larynx was resected by stripping off the perichondrium with its attached muscles. Difficulties with closure were minimized by this technique, but the procedure was useful only for early lesions, which today are more suitably treated by partial laryngectomy or radiation. The narrow-field laryngectomy of Jackson and Jackson[4] attempted to minimize the difficulties in pharyngeal closure by preserving tissue while widening the field of resection suffi-

ciently to permit extirpation of more extensive tumors that were still confined to the larynx. The operation was recommended for intrinsic carcinoma without perichondrial involvement or perichondritis and without evidence of lymphatic metastases. In this operation the larynx was skeletonized extraperichondrially.

Wide-field laryngectomy was described by Jackson and Babcock[5] in 1931 for the resection of lesions with perichondrial involvement, palpable lymphatic metastases, or extrinsic involvement. Jackson and Jackson[4] clearly preferred radiation for such lesions, but if surgical resection absolutely had to be done, the wide-field procedure was recommended. This operation involved the elevation of wide skin flaps and excision of the larynx and all lymphatic tissue from one jugular vein to the other. This procedure was closer to the present-day laryngectomy than to its predecessors, yet emphasis was still placed on conserving muscle tissue. No portion of the thyroid gland was resected, and the cricoid cartilage, or at least a portion of it, was often left attached to the trachea. The hyoid bone and the upper part of the epiglottis were not resected.

The laryngectomy currently in use is based on the principle of the wide-field operation, but it differs from the surgical procedure performed in the 1930s. Portions of the hyoid bone, the epiglottis, and the cricoid cartilage may be left unresected, in selected instances, only for the purpose of constructing a phonatory neoglottis. The modern laryngectomy usually involves wide resection of the strap muscles and the perilaryngeal tissue, including the ipsilateral thyroid lobe, particularly when done in continuity with a neck dissection. The bilateral jugular node dissection of the 1930s, considered to be useful only as a staging procedure during the era from the 1950s through the 1980s, has evolved into the bilateral selective lateral neck dissection.*

PATIENT SELECTION

Although in the past the most widely accepted surgical treatment for stage III and stage IV cancer of the larynx was total laryngectomy, it is no longer appropriate to assume that the larynx must be removed when laryngeal cancer is advanced, or that all T3 and T4 cancers of the larynx require combined therapy (laryngectomy and postoperative radiotherapy). The availability of alternative treat-

---

*The subject of neck dissection, in conjunction with laryngectomy and its various techniques and indications, is discussed in detail in Chapter 11.

ments has served to limit the indications for total extirpation of the larynx. These alternatives include surgical procedures for resection of less than the entire larynx with preservation of varying degrees of laryngeal function, as well as nonsurgical "larynx saving" protocols employing chemotherapy and radiation sequentially. It is therefore not possible to state with authority what the indications for total laryngectomy are, because these indications vary from surgeon to surgeon and from institution to institution, depending on individual or institutional philosophy and capabilities, as well as on patient preference.

SURGICAL ALTERNATIVES

The development of procedures that exceed the magnitude of resection achieved with conventional conservation surgery has provided surgical alternatives to total laryngectomy for treatment of locally advanced laryngeal cancer. Thus, the various forms of extended vertical and horizontal partial laryngectomy and the supracricoid laryngectomies, described in Chapters 5 and 6, permit resection of various T3 and a limited number of T4 glottic and supraglottic cancers, with local control and survival rates that match those achieved with total laryngectomy for the same lesions. The procedure of near-total laryngectomy, described in Chapter 8, has provided an alternative to total extirpation of the larynx for even more advanced lesions, including endolaryngeal lesions with significant paraglottic space involvement and extra-laryngeal spread, as well as for hypopharyngeal tumors.

The popularity of these procedures varies among surgeons and even according to geographic area. For example, supracricoid laryngectomy is widely employed in Europe, but it has not achieved general acceptance in the United States.[6] Similarly, there is considerable controversy as to whether extended conservation procedures can or should be employed in patients after failure of radiation therapy.

NONSURGICAL ALTERNATIVES

In 1991, the Department of Veterans Affairs Laryngeal Cancer Study Group[7] published the results of a prospective randomized study in which 332 patients with previously untreated stage III or stage IV squamous cell carcinoma of the larynx were treated either with chemotherapy followed by definitive radiation therapy or with total laryngectomy and postoperative radiation. In the chemotherapy group, 59 patients (36%) who had not re-

sponded even partially were referred for total laryngectomy. Two-year survival rates were statistically identical in the surgery and radiation groups. The larynx was preserved in 64% of patients treated initially with the chemotherapy protocol and in 64% of the patients alive and free of disease. The authors concluded that the positive response to chemotherapy could be used as a way to select radiation therapy rather than surgery for patients with advanced laryngeal tumors; use of radiation would allow preservation of the larynx in a high percentage of patients without compromising overall survival. Similar results for laryngeal cancer were reported by Shirinian et al.[8] and Nikolau et al.,[9] although the same benefits were not obtained in patients with hypopharyngeal and oropharyngeal cancer.[8]

Wolf and Fisher[10] noted that despite preservation of the larynx in 64% of the patients treated according to the same chemoradiation protocol, overall survival was not improved when compared to conventional treatment. The authors studied the response of cervical node disease to chemotherapy and noted that patients whose neck disease failed to respond usually required "salvage" neck dissection after radiation therapy, and that the overall death rate was increased and survival time decreased in this group of patients. They advised that neck disease should be assessed independently of primary tumor response in trials of organ preservation strategies using induction chemotherapy, and that failure to achieve a complete clinical response in the neck should warrant a planned, early salvage neck dissection in order to achieve improved overall survival.

Critics of the Department of Veterans Affairs study note the lack of improvement in overall survival, the higher incidence of local recurrence compared with surgical treatment, and the time and morbidity involved in administering three cycles of chemotherapy followed by irradiation. DeSanto[11] recently pointed out that this important study must be considered with caution; there was no evidence that the chemotherapy contributed to survival because there was no radiotherapy-alone group. The failure of adjuvant and neoadjuvant therapy to improve the survival of patients with head and neck cancer has been well documented. Stell[12] presented an overview of 23 trials of adjuvant chemotherapy in squamous cell carcinoma of the head and neck. Meta-analysis showed an insignificant overall improvement in cancer mortality of 0.5% but indicated that toxicity and mortality rates from chemotherapy were high. Similarly, Tannock and Cummings[13] observed that neoadjuvant chemotherapy has no demonstrated role as yet and should therefore not be considered for the routine management of patients with squamous cell carcinoma of the larynx, stating that "any treatment that adds toxicity without benefit is bad treatment."

CHOICE OF MODALITY

With the above considerations noted, it remains necessary in each individual case to select a modality for treatment of laryngeal cancer at any stage. It is important to consider medical, social, and emotional factors in determining treatment modality. Patients who present unacceptable degrees of medical risk or those with severe emotional instability are not good candidates for laryngectomy and should be offered nonsurgical treatment first. On the other hand, potentially noncompliant patients are not good candidates for radiation therapy, particularly if it is preceded by neoadjuvant chemotherapy. If laryngectomy will cause a previously independent elderly patient to become institutionalized, it should be avoided if possible. Many persons adapt well to laryngectomy; the availability of prosthetic means of voice restoration is of great help in this respect. Usually the surgeon can gain some insight into the patient's probable reaction to surgery, and this should be taken into consideration when treatment is recommended.

INDICATIONS FOR TOTAL LARYNGECTOMY

While the indications for total laryngectomy may depend on factors such as geography, surgical philosophy, and capabilities, there remain certain instances in which, if treatment is to be surgical, total laryngectomy is the only feasible procedure for adequate tumor extirpation. These restricted situations are as follows:

1. Cancer with bilateral cord fixation
2. Cancer with postcricoid involvement
3. Cancer extending across the interarytenoid area
4. Extensive multiregional and nonunilateral cancer
5. Annular subglottic cancer
6. Full-course radiation failure with chondroradionecrosis

AIRWAY MANAGEMENT

Many patients with laryngeal tumors requiring total laryngectomy have some degree of airway ob-

struction. Although this may not be clinically apparent when the patient is fully awake and at rest, a dangerous degree of obstruction may occur when the patient receives sedation, particularly in the course of an endoscopic examination. The combination of sedation, a supine position, extension of the neck, and manipulation of the larynx may precipitate an emergency, requiring a hurried tracheostomy if this possibility has not been anticipated.

Airway Control During Endoscopy

It is difficult to formulate a foolproof method to avoid the problem of having to perform a preliminary tracheostomy on every laryngectomy patient on a routine basis. This is unnecessary, and the presence of a previous tracheostomy makes subsequent laryngectomy slightly more difficult. In addition, there is evidence that the incidence of stomal recurrence is higher in patients who have had a previous tracheostomy.[14, 15] Perhaps the best advice that can be given is to anticipate the possibility of severe airway obstruction in every patient with a sizeable laryngeal neoplasm who is to undergo endoscopy or any other surgical procedure. Preoperative sedation should be avoided and consent for possible tracheostomy should be obtained in every case. The tracheostomy instruments should be opened and ready for immediate use during the endoscopy.

Endoscopy is safest when performed under topical anesthesia. If only a biopsy is needed for a patient who will obviously require a total laryngectomy, the indirect laryngoscopy biopsy technique is the least traumatic and will cause minimal interference with the airway. If complete evaluation of the larynx and hypopharynx under anesthesia is required, a small endotracheal tube can be inserted while the patient is awake, after which anesthesia can be induced and a direct laryngoscopy performed. The endotracheal tube should not be removed until the patient has fully recovered from anesthesia, 12 to 24 hours later. It is usually safe to assume that if a patient is able to breathe comfortably before the endoscopic procedure, he or she will be able to breathe well once he or she has fully recovered from anesthesia. If the preoperative endoscopy has been hampered by the presence of an endotracheal tube, laryngoscopy can be repeated at the time of laryngectomy (either total or partial), after tracheostomy has been performed.

The surgical laser has proved useful for debulking large intralaryngeal tumors in order to minimize airway obstruction and, in many cases, to avoid the need for tracheostomy.

Tracheostomy

Some patients should have an "elective" preliminary tracheostomy. Such patients include those who are clinically dyspneic and stridulous and those with pulmonary sepsis resulting from ineffective cough due to obstruction. When a tracheostomy is required, it is always simpler to perform it after the airway has been controlled by some form of intubation than to operate on a struggling dyspneic patient. It may be difficult for the anesthesiologist to intubate a larynx that has a large neoplasm. A 6-mm ventilating bronchoscope or a specially designed tracheoscope can be used effectively for intubation in these cases. The instrument can be passed with the patient fully awake and can be visually guided through the laryngeal lumen. A large straight-bladed anesthetist's laryngoscope can facilitate passage of the bronchoscope in difficult cases. Once the bronchoscope has been passed, it is connected to the anesthesia apparatus as a closed system. The patient can be sedated or anesthetized, the neck extended, and the tracheostomy performed. The bronchoscope, laryngoscope, and anesthesia connections should be available during any procedure to be performed on a patient with a potentially obstructing laryngeal tumor who does not already have a tracheostomy.

Recently, the technique of "awake" transnasal intubation with the nasotracheal tube passed over a fiberoptic laryngoscope or bronchoscope has proven useful in patients difficult to intubate by conventional means. This technique, useful for intubating patients with cancer at many sites in the upper aerodigestive track, is often useful for laryngeal tumors, but it may prove difficult in patients with extremely bulky laryngeal neoplasms.

In performing tracheostomy in a patient who is to undergo total laryngectomy, both the skin incision and the incision into the trachea should be placed as high as possible, without entering the tumor. Preoperative imaging studies, such as computed tomography or magnetic resonance imaging, will demonstrate the inferior extent of the tumor and should be performed if feasible. If the tumor does not extend below the cricoid cartilage, the tracheostomy should be placed through the first tracheal ring. High placement of the skin and tracheal incisions will facilitate the subsequent laryngectomy, during which the skin around the temporary tracheostomy will be excised and the trachea sectioned inferiorly.

If a separate preliminary tracheostomy has not been performed before the laryngectomy, the surgeon will have to decide whether to perform it at the beginning of the procedure or to perform the neck dissection and most of the laryngectomy with a transoral endotracheal tube, waiting until the trachea is sectioned before cannulating it and removing the transoral tube. In the illustrations presented here, the latter technique is shown, mainly to enhance the clarity and simplicity of the drawings. In actual practice, many patients will either have had a previous tracheostomy or will have a tracheostomy performed at the start of the laryngectomy. Because it is easier to work without a tracheostomy tube in the operative field, and because endotracheal intubation does not appear to be an important factor in causing stomal recurrence,[15] the delayed tracheal section technique is preferred when feasible.

Emergency Laryngectomy

In an effort to avoid having to perform preliminary tracheostomy as a separate procedure, some surgeons have performed "emergency" laryngectomy (laryngectomy performed within 24 hours of detecting a previously untreated and undiagnosed malignancy). However, this practice has obvious drawbacks, and there is little evidence that it reduces either patient mortality or stomal recurrence. McCombe and Stell[16] studied 31 patients who underwent emergency laryngectomy for airway obstruction between 1974 and 1990 and found no significant difference in early postoperative mortality, stomal recurrence rates, or survival between this group and a comparison group undergoing elective laryngectomy. Narula et al.[17] concluded that emergency laryngectomy offers no particular advantage, in terms of survival, on comparison with urgent tracheostomy and delayed laryngectomy. It also presents several disadvantages, such as the need to rely on frozen-section analysis, the difficulty in obtaining expert anesthetic support, the inability to provide thorough and complete nutritional and metabolic work-up before major surgery, and inadequate opportunity to address the psychologic needs of the patient and the family. The authors found stomal recurrence to be connected with the extent of the neoplasm at presentation rather than to preliminary tracheostomy.

TECHNIQUE OF TOTAL LARYNGECTOMY FOR ENDOLARYNGEAL TUMOR

Figure 7–1A. This coronal view is of a massive transglottic tumor that will require total laryngectomy. The lesion crosses the ventricle, fills the paraglottic space, and extends subglottically below the cricothyroid membrane. A lesion of this size and nature will often invade the laryngeal framework (not shown).

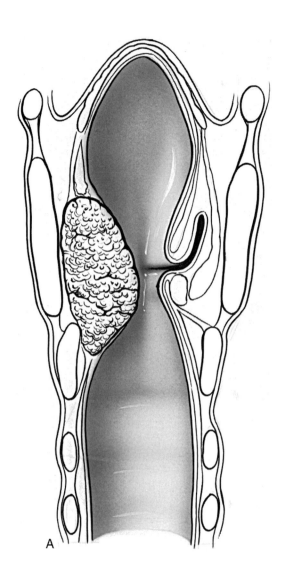

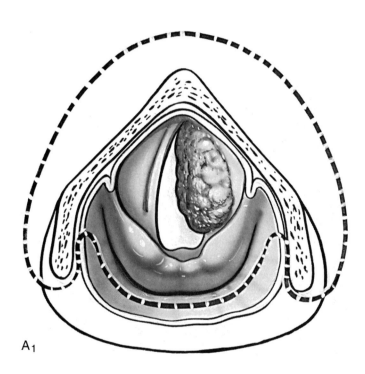

A₁

Figure 7–1. Total laryngectomy.

Illustration continued on following page

Figure 7–1A_1. This transverse view shows the tumor. The mucosa of the uninvolved (left) pyriform sinus will be preserved, whereas the entire pyriform sinus on the ipsilateral (right) side will be resected.

Figure 7–1*B.* This illustration demonstrates the surgical field at the conclusion of right radical neck dissection, before laryngectomy is commenced. The carotid artery is exposed along its length. The jugular vein and the sternocleidomastoid muscle have been included in the neck dissection. The entire neck dissection specimen is tied into a small bag for convenience and is reflected onto the larynx, to which it is left broadly attached.

Figure 7–1*B₁.* If a neck dissection is not performed, the procedure is commenced by mobilizing the ipsilateral sternomastoid muscle and separating the jugular vein and the carotid artery from the midline structures. The omohyoid muscle is divided.

Figure 7–1*C.* The ipsilateral (right) side is mobilized inferiorly. The sternohyoid and sternothyroid muscles are transected low in the neck, revealing the thyroid gland, the trachea, and the esophagus. The ipsilateral thyroid lobe will be resected. The inferior thyroid artery is divided, as are the paratracheal structures inferior to the thyroid lobe, including the recurrent laryngeal nerve. The paratracheal tissue is divided, bringing the trachea into view. The surface of the trachea should be dissected free along the line of resection. If there has been a previous tracheostomy, this dissection is complicated by the presence of fibrosis and adhesions secondary to that procedure. It is necessary to clear and transect the trachea through uninvolved tissue, below the field of tracheostomy, which will be included in the resection.

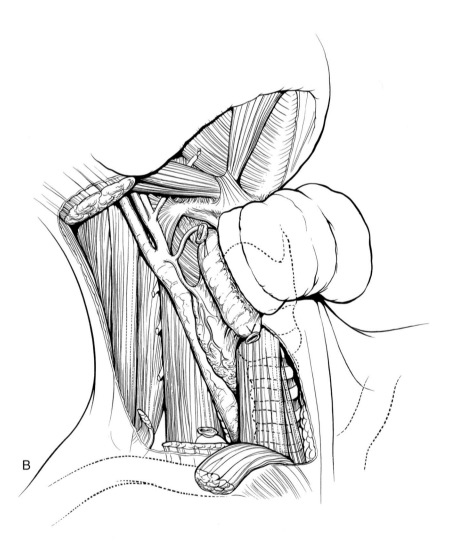

B

Figure 7–1 *Continued* Total laryngectomy.

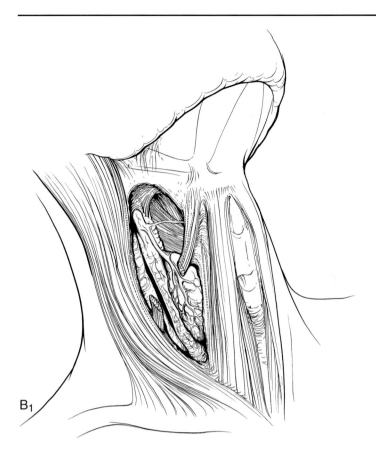

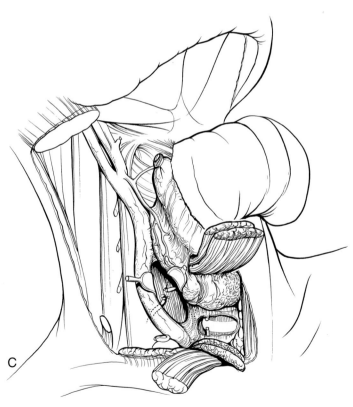

Figure 7–1 *Continued* Total laryngectomy.

Illustration continued on following page

Figure 7–1*D.* The ipsilateral side continues to be mobilized superiorly. The superior thyroid artery is divided. The suprahyoid muscles are severed along the superior border of the body and the greater cornu of the hyoid bone. As the hyoglossus muscle is being separated from its origin on the greater cornu, care must be taken not to injure the hypoglossal nerve, which is on the superficial surface of that muscle, and to avoid the lingual artery, which is just deep to the muscle. The lesser cornu should be left attached to the hyoid bone. The muscles that attach to the body of the hyoid bone are thick and must be transected completely before the external aspect of the hypopharyngeal mucosa is reached. If tumor in the valleculae is suspected, the suprahyoid muscles should be left attached to the body of the hyoid bone.

Figure 7–1*E.* The contralateral side is mobilized. The sternomastoid muscle is retracted laterally, the omohyoid muscle is divided as it crosses the jugular vein, and the internal jugular vein and carotid artery are separated from the midline structures. The sternohyoid and sternothyroid muscles are transected low in the neck. The thyroid isthmus is divided. The thyroid lobe on this side will be preserved. The inferior and superior thyroid arteries are therefore left intact. The paratracheal tissues, including the recurrent laryngeal nerve, are transected at a level corresponding with the trachea already cleared on the opposite side, thereby exposing and clearing the tracheal surface.

Figure 7–1*F.* The contralateral (left) thyroid lobe is separated from the trachea. The superior vascular pedicle is left intact. This procedure is somewhat tedious, usually requiring clamping and ligature of multiple points of attachment. If a previous tracheostomy has been done, the portion of the thyroid lobe outside the field of the tracheostomy is preserved. If involvement of the thyroid gland with tumor is suspected, particularly in pharyngoesophageal or subglottic tumors, total thyroidectomy should be done.

The superior laryngeal artery is divided and ligated, leaving the superior thyroid artery intact. Separation of the suprahyoid musculature continues by severing of the attachment of the hyoglossus muscle and the digastric sling from the left greater and lesser cornua.

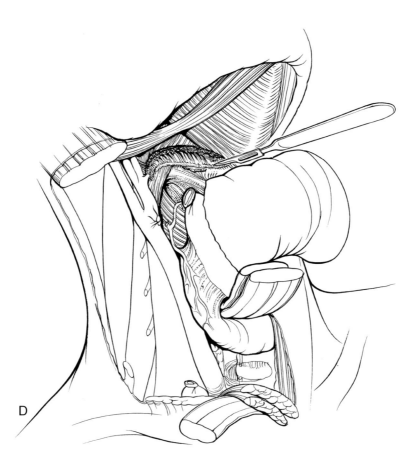

D

Figure 7–1 *Continued* Total laryngectomy.

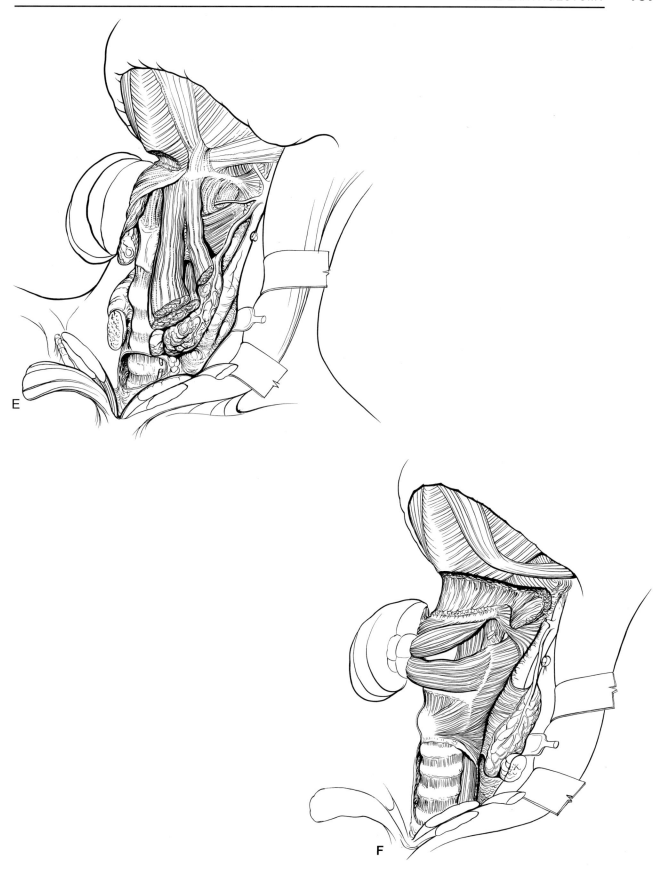

Figure 7–1 *Continued* Total laryngectomy.

Illustration continued on following page

Figure 7–1G. If there is no possibility of involvement of the contralateral pyriform sinus with tumor, the mucosa on this side may be preserved, to simplify closure of the hypopharynx. The inferior constrictor muscle fibers are incised along the posterior edge of the thyroid ala, exposing the pyriform sinus mucosa beneath. The mucosal reflection is dissected from the inner aspect of the thyroid cartilage to liberate as much tissue as possible. (The neck specimen and the perilaryngeal soft tissue have been removed from the illustration for clarity.)

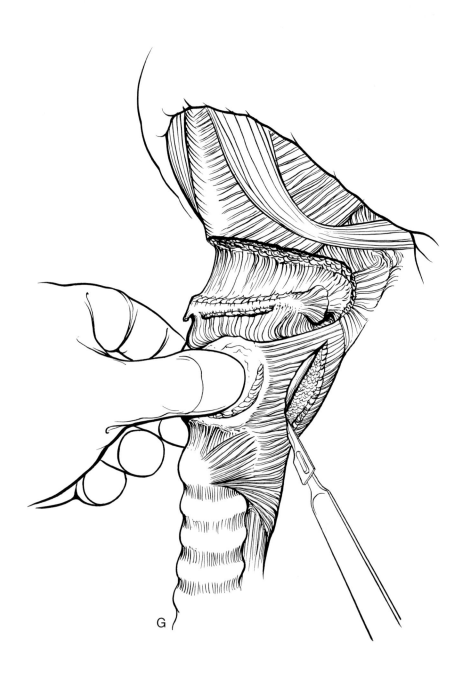

Figure 7–1 *Continued* Total laryngectomy.

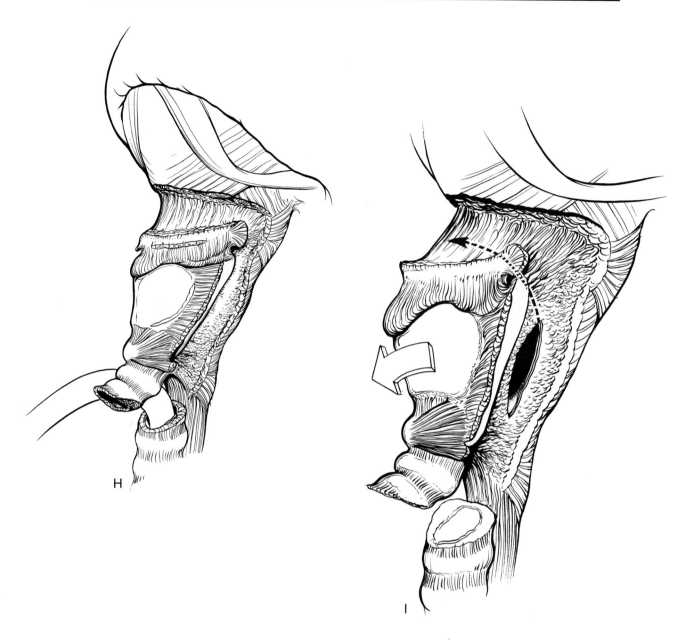

Figure 7–1 *Continued* Total laryngectomy.

Illustration continued on following page

Figure 7–1*H*. The larynx is now completely mobilized. The trachea is transected and a cuffed endotracheal tube is inserted into the distal segment for control of the airway by the anesthesiologist. The trachea is divided at an appropriate level, depending on the inferior extent of the tumor and the presence of a previous tracheostomy. In this example, the trachea is divided between the second and third rings. If possible, the trachea should be divided at least 2 cm below the inferior limit of the tumor or 1 cm inferior to the tracheostomy site. If the resection margin permits, the tracheal incision should be beveled upward posteriorly to maximize the size of the tracheostoma. The proximal posterior tracheal wall and the cricoid cartilage are separated from the esophagus.

Figure 7–1*I*. The hypopharynx is entered through the contralateral pyriform sinus. It is also possible to enter the pharynx through the valleculae or through the posterior mucosa. The site of entry should be as far from the tumor as possible. The mucosal incision is enlarged superiorly, and the mucosal surface is carefully inspected before cutting, to maintain an adequate resection margin.

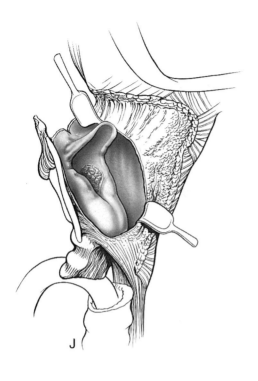

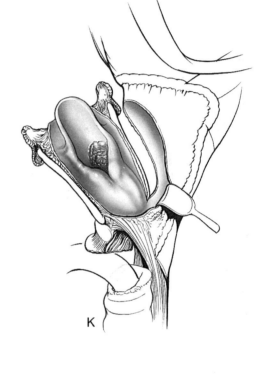

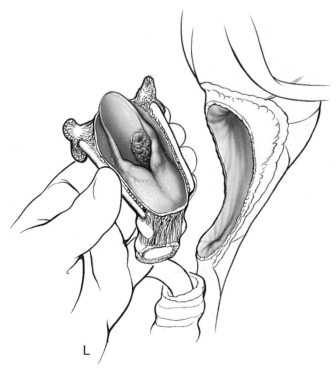

Figure 7–1 *Continued* Total laryngectomy.

Figure 7–1J. As the incision is extended through the valleculae, the entire hypopharynx can be visualized and the line of resection can be planned. The ipsilateral pyriform sinus will be resected fairly widely around the tumor. It should be kept in mind that the pyriform sinus forms the posterior wall of the paraglottic space, which, in the case demonstrated, is involved with tumor.

Figure 7–1K. The mucosal incision is completed through the posterior region, and the remaining attachments of the larynx are severed.

Figure 7–1L. This is a continuation of the procedure described in Figure 7–1K.

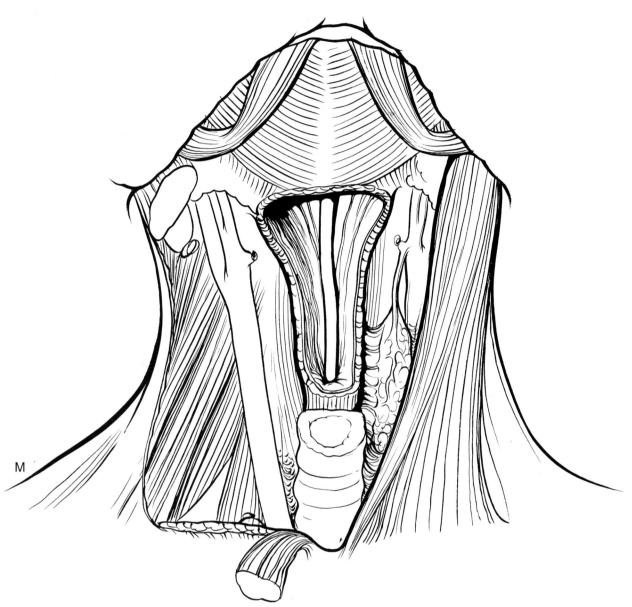

M

Figure 7–1 *Continued* Total laryngectomy.

Illustration continued on following page

Figure 7–1 *M*. Before closure, the hypopharyngeal defect is large and triangular. A nasogastric tube is passed and secured to the nasal columella with a suture. Flexion of the neck will minimize the hypopharyngeal defect and relieve tension on the suture line.

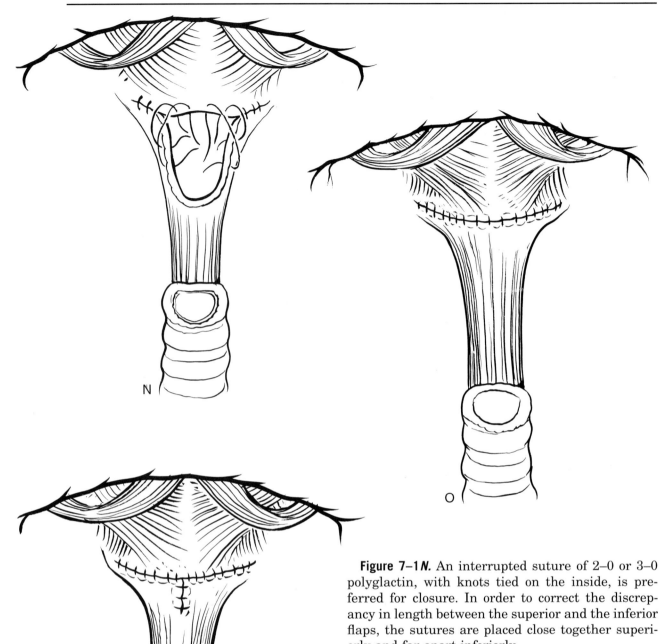

Figure 7–1 *Continued* Total laryngectomy.

Figure 7–1*N*. An interrupted suture of 2–0 or 3–0 polyglactin, with knots tied on the inside, is preferred for closure. In order to correct the discrepancy in length between the superior and the inferior flaps, the sutures are placed close together superiorly and far apart inferiorly.

Figure 7–1*O*. In most cases it will be possible to achieve a transverse linear closure after resection for endolaryngeal tumors. This is preferable to a T or Y closure because of a lower incidence of postoperative fistula.

Figure 7–1*O$_1$*. If a transverse linear closure cannot be achieved, the inferior flap is closed vertically, forming a T or a Y. The closure is reinforced by approximating the cut edges of the inferior constrictor muscle to the suprahyoid muscles. A tightly constricting muscular ring should be avoided. In many instances where the muscles cannot be approximated, the preserved thyroid lobe is used to reinforce the closure.

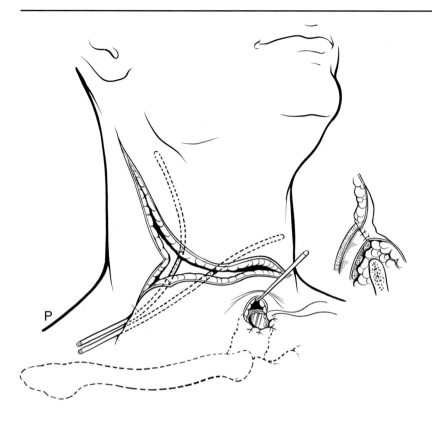

Figure 7–1 *Continued* Total laryngectomy.

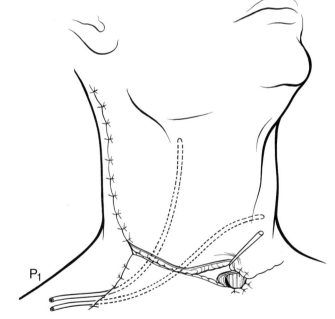

Figures 7–1P and P₁. The tracheostoma is constructed by suturing the skin edges with interrupted 3–0 or 4–0 nylon. The endotracheal tube is intermittently removed to permit placement of sutures when necessary. The tracheostoma is placed either in the main incision or through a separate small incision in the inferior flap. The latter is preferable, because there is less likelihood of postoperative stricture, but it is usually not feasible if there has been a previous tracheostomy.

COMPLICATIONS

Hemorrhage

Hemorrhage occurring in the immediate postoperative period (first 12 hours) often manifests as a continuous flow of blood through the wound catheters and is usually associated with swelling of the skin flaps because of accumulated blood and clots. Blood may also issue from the tracheostoma or appear in the pharynx. This type of bleeding is usually the result of an unligated vessel or dislodgment of a ligature and requires prompt exploration of the wound, removal of the clot, irrigation, and ligation of the bleeding vessel. Occasionally, immediate postoperative bleeding occurs because of loss of clotting factors, particularly in patients with severe liver disease or patients who have received multiple transfusions during surgery. This possibility should be considered in all cases, and it is wise to perform an immediate work-up of coagulation factors whenever postoperative hemorrhage occurs. As it may often be difficult to detect a clotting factor deficiency precisely and immediately, the rapid administration of several units of fresh frozen plasma may stop the bleeding very effectively.

Hemorrhage occurring from 4 days to several weeks (or longer) after surgery is invariably due to rupture of one of the carotid arteries as a result of infection, necrosis, or exposure to air and salivary contents. As blood may dissect beneath the skin flaps and appear at apparently remote locations, including the oral cavity or the trachea, bright red hemorrhage occurring any time after the immediate postoperative period should lead to the working diagnosis of carotid artery rupture. The wound should be immediately explored. The initial bleeding is often intermittent, and the temporary cessation of bleeding should not cause complacency but should be viewed as an opportunity to move the patient to the operating room where an orderly exploration can be conducted.

Airway Obstruction

The laryngectomized patient is extremely susceptible to airway obstruction because there is no alternative airway around the matured tracheostoma. In the immediate postoperative period, obstruction of the trachea or laryngectomy tube with clotted blood is the greatest danger. Under no circumstances should a patient leave the operating room with a single-cannula anesthesia endotracheal tube in the airway. This should be removed and replaced with a short, double-cannula No. 10 or No. 12 laryngectomy tube. It is preferable to suture these tubes

to the skin rather than to tie tapes around the cervical skin flaps, particularly if a chest flap has been used for reconstruction. If ventilatory assistance is required postoperatively, a double-cannula No. 8 or No. 10 cuffed plastic tracheostomy tube is used. Care must be taken to prevent the tracheostomy tube from passing beyond the carina. If it is inconvenient to place a laryngectomy tube in the tracheostoma, the patient is better off without any than with a tube that may be easily dislodged or obstructed or that will cause pressure necrosis of a skin flap. The sutures are removed from the tracheostoma on the 10th to the 12th postoperative day in uncomplicated cases. After the sutures have been removed, the patient usually does not require a laryngectomy tube. Once decannulated, however, the patient must be observed closely for several days to prevent tracheal obstruction from crusted secretions and other solid material. Application of a petrolatum-based antibiotic ointment to the mucocutaneous junction and periodic instillation of 1 to 2 ml of sterile saline or sodium bicarbonate solution into the trachea will help prevent the accumulation of obstructing material in patients who are so prone. The breathing of a laryngectomy patient should be completely silent. Personnel who attend to these patients should be taught that noisy breathing is a sign of tracheal obstruction.

Detachment of the trachea from the skin can occur in the early-to-intermediate postoperative period (3 days to 3 weeks after surgery). This complication, in addition to usually causing an immediate airway problem, will also lead to severe stricture of the tracheostoma when healing occurs. According to Young and Maran,[18] the causes of this complication are poor surgical technique, poor tissue quality, poor condition of the patient in general, and excessive tension on the trachea. For reconstruction, it is necessary to control local infection, to débride all necrotic tissue, and to re-create the tracheostoma without tension by elevating adequate skin flaps for this purpose.

Stricturing of the tracheostoma with the formation of a microstoma can occur in the late postoperative period (3 weeks to 1 year after surgery). The etiology, prevention, and management of this problem is discussed in detail in Chapter 13.

Infection, Fistula, and Necrosis

Part of a skin flap may become necrotic because of inadequate circulation, in the absence of either a fistula or infection. Débridement and skin grafting, if necessary, will usually suffice to correct this situation. Simple wound infections, unassociated with necrosis, skin loss, or fistula, also occur occasionally. Opening the wound to provide adequate drainage constitutes adequate treatment.

Salivary fistulae, manifested by drainage beneath the intact skin flaps and escape of usually purulent saliva through the suture lines or the drainage site, occur with some frequency. The extent and severity of a fistula depend on the amount of associated tissue necrosis. Thus, fistulae may range from narrow tracts surrounded by relatively healthy tissue, to massive open wounds with wide exposure of the hypopharynx and often of the carotid artery. All fistulae will delay the onset of oral feeding and increase the length of hospitalization, and the more severe varieties can set the stage for carotid artery rupture. Pharyngocutaneous fistulae are often responsible for significant metabolic depletion, and by delaying the administration of postoperative radiotherapy they may contribute to recurrence of cancer.

Factors Predisposing to Fistula Formation

Previous radiation therapy has long been considered a predisposing factor to fistula formation, although there are differences of opinion as to whether radiation increases the rate of fistula formation[19–21] or increases the severity and duration of the fistulae.[22, 23] Other factors that have been implicated are positive resection margins,[24, 25] anemia,[26, 27] wound tension, tumor burden, and preoperative weight loss. Before the availability of myocutaneous flaps for the closure of large pharyngeal defects, the extent of mucosal resection was an important predisposing factor for postoperative fistula formation.[23, 25]

Management of Pharyngocutaneous Fistula

Most fistulae occurring beneath intact skin flaps may be treated by establishing continuous drainage, with frequently changed sump catheters and irrigation, and will heal without further surgical treatment. As the fistula drains freely through the catheters, the surrounding tissue granulates and the fistulous tract eventually becomes narrower. The catheters are removed when the tract contains healthy granulation tissue.

Larger fistulae require surgical closure. Such closure requires two epithelial surfaces: one to line the pharynx and one to resurface the cervical skin. In many instances, one or both of these surfaces may be developed from local tissue. More complicated problems occur when disruption of the pharyngeal closure and leakage of pharyngeal contents beneath the skin flaps is associated with necrosis of the overlying skin and loss of coverage of the neck wound. In these cases, fistula, necrosis, and infection are combined. Such wounds require débridement and control of infection, as well as surgical closure, which can be accomplished only by moving a large flap of healthy tissue to provide both internal and external surfaces for repair of the defect.

The timing of surgery will often depend on whether the carotid artery is exposed in the wound, and hence, on whether there is danger of its rupturing. If the carotid artery has been successfully covered with a muscle flap or dermal graft and thus does not become exposed, rupture will probably not occur, and immediate resurfacing of the neck is not mandatory. The surgeon may opt for a period of wound débridement, antibiotic therapy, and hyperalimentation before surgically closing the wound. If the carotid artery is exposed, however, it must be immediately covered with healthy skin, muscle, or a myocutaneous flap. We have reported successful results with a "sandwich" pectoral muscle myocutaneous flap for coverage of large necrotic cervical defects associated with pharyngeal fistula, infection, and carotid exposure.[28] Departing from the previously standard procedure, we do not wait for clean granulation tissue to develop at the recipient site, but débride the wound in the operating room and immediately apply the myocutaneous flap to the freshly débrided cervical tissue. The skin paddle is turned inward to close the defect in the pharyngeal mucosa, while a meshed skin graft is applied to the external aspect of the pectoral muscle in order to resurface the skin defect. Using the skin graft avoids sacrificing unnecessarily large amounts of pectoral skin for repair of the complex wound.

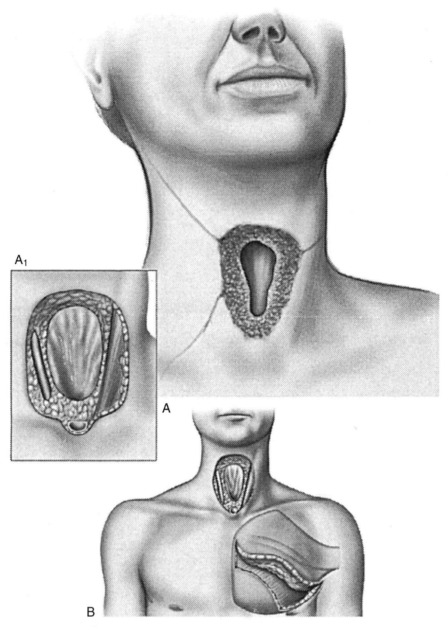

Figure 7–2. Transfer of greater pectoral muscle "sandwich" flap.

Transfer of Greater Pectoral Muscle "Sandwich" Flap

Figure 7–2A. The procedure reported by Goldstein et al.[28] from our service is shown. A large necrotic cervical defect is shown, typical of that resulting from dehiscence of the pharyngeal closure after laryngectomy, with loss of the overlying skin from necrosis.

Figure 7–2A₁. The hypopharynx is widely exposed within the wound, and the carotid artery is partly exposed in the base of the defect, adjacent to the pharynx. The patient is taken to the operating room, and the wound is débrided immediately.

Figure 7–2B. A myocutaneous flap from the greater pectoral muscle is developed on the left side of the chest. This will be transferred to the neck beneath the intervening upper thoracic and remaining intact cervical skin.

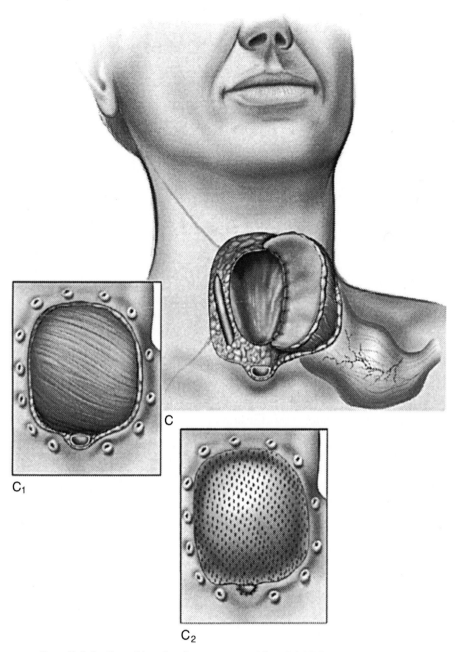

C

C₁

C₂

Figure 7–2 *Continued* Transfer of greater pectoral "sandwich" flap.

Figure 7–2C. The skin paddle is turned inward and sutured to the mucosal edge of the pharyngeal defect. This closure continues circumferentially, until the defect has been closed completely.

Figure 7–2C₁. The cervical skin edges have been undermined, and the pectoral muscle, wider than the skin paddle, is tucked under the skin edges, covering the carotid artery and providing a base of healthy tissue for skin grafting. The muscle is se-

cured beneath the skin edges with sutures tied over bolsters.

Figure 7–2C₂. A meshed split-thickness skin graft is applied over the exposed portion of the pectoral muscle, resurfacing the neck. It is not necessary to make a bilobed paddle of thoracic skin in order to provide external coverage for the neck over the intact pectoral muscle.

Swallowing Difficulties

Esophageal Motility Disorders

Postlaryngectomy patients may experience varying degrees of dysphagia because of alterations in esophageal motility. Duranceau et al.[29] performed esophageal motility studies in 10 patients after total laryngectomy and noted marked derangements in the function of the upper esophageal sphincter and the body of the esophagus in all 10 of the patients. The function of the lower esophageal sphincter did not differ from controls. Five of the 10 patients complained of dysphagia.

Dysmotility and loss of sphincteric motor function may result from interruption of the upper digestive tube, interruption of the pharyngeal branches of the vagus nerve, bilateral division of the superior laryngeal nerves, anterior fixation of tracheal structures because of surgically induced cicatrix, loss of the negative pressure generated by the pharyngoesophageal segment, and inefficient peristalsis of the pharyngoesophageal musculature.[29–32]

Hypopharyngeal Stenosis

Postlaryngectomy dysphagia may be caused by hypopharyngeal stenosis. Although it is uncommon after conventional total laryngectomy for endolaryngeal cancer, postoperative stenosis occurs frequently when mucosal resection is extended to include portions of the hypopharynx, particularly when primary closure has been attempted.[33, 34] At least 3 cm of hypopharyngeal mucosa are required for tension-free primary closure without compromising the lumen.[35] In cases in which insufficient mucosa remains for adequate primary closure, the hypopharynx should be repaired by transfer of myocutaneous flaps or by free transfer of revascularized jejunal or fasciocutaneous flaps. These techniques are discussed in detail in Chapter 9.

Relatively mild hypopharyngeal stenosis may be managed in the early postoperative period by progressive dilatation. Once mature cicatrical narrowing has occurred, surgical correction is required. Short stenotic segments may be repaired by release of scar tissue, cricopharyngeal myotomy, or Z-plasty. Patients with long segments of stenosis may require replacement or bypass of the stenotic segment. We have employed the tubed major pectoral myocutaneous flap for this purpose.[36, 37] If preferred, any of the methods of esophageal replacement, such as visceral interposition or transfer of revascularized jejunal or fasciocutaneous flaps, may be used to correct benign postlaryngectomy pharyngo-

esophageal stenosis. These techniques are discussed in detail in Chapter 10.

Hypothyroidism and Hypoparathyroidism

In most total laryngectomies, one lobe of the thyroid gland and its related parathyroid tissue are preserved, thus preserving normal thyroid and parathyroid function. Occasionally, however, infarction or resection of thyroid, parathyroid, or both tissues may result in endocrine deficiencies. The reported incidence of hypothyroidism has ranged from 3.5%[38] to 29.1%.[39] Symptoms and signs may be minimal, and unrecognized hypothyroidism may exert a profoundly detrimental effect on wound healing and postoperative recovery. Several authors have reported dramatic improvement in general condition and in healing of pharyngocutaneous fistulae after initiation of thyroid hormone therapy for hypothyroid patients.[40, 41]

For subglottic, hypopharyngeal, and postcricoid carcinomas, intentional resection of the thyroid gland may be required. In these cases hypoparathyroidism is prone to occur, particularly when the cervical esophagus has been resected along with the larynx and the hypopharynx (pharyngolaryngectomy-esophagectomy) for postcricoid and cervical esophageal carcinomas[42, 43]. Krespi et al.[44] reviewed three groups of laryngectomized patients to assess the incidence of hypoparathyroidism. The incidence of hypoparathyroidism was 12% after conventional total laryngectomy with thyroid preservation, 50% after total laryngectomy with mediastinal dissection, and 75% after total pharygolaryngectomy-esophagectomy with gastric transposition. Intravenous calcium and oral vitamin D are employed in the early postoperative period to manage hypocalcemia. If oncologically feasible, intraoperative parathyroid autotransplantation may prevent permanent hypoparathyroidism. Bypass of the duodenum and the proximal jejunum by jejunostomy feeding after the gastric transposition procedure can exacerbate hypocalcemia, which is often relieved by commencing oral feeding.[45]

Medical Complications of Total Laryngectomy

Patients undergoing major extirpative procedures in the head and neck are often spared the fluid compartment shifts, pain, and disturbance of basic physiologic functions associated with intraabdominal and intrathoracic procedures, particularly with regard to ambulation and genitourinary and gastrointestinal function.[46] Dramatic improvement of airway obstruction, pulmonary toilet, and life-threatening aspiration may be achieved by total laryngectomy in patients with advanced tumors. The nonsurgical complications after total laryngectomy involve primarily the cardiovascular, neurologic, and pulmonary systems.

Arriaga et al.[47] evaluated 414 patients after total laryngectomy. The mortality was 1.2%. Major, nonfatal medical complications occurred in 6.3% of the patients. There were 7 instances of stroke, 3 cases of myocardial infarctions, and 2 cases of pulmonary embolus. Twelve patients developed respiratory failure requiring mechanical ventilation. Although patients over 65 years of age experienced a greater number of postoperative medical problems than did younger patients, major complications such as respiratory failure, myocardial infarction, pulmonary embolus, and stroke did not occur with significantly greater frequency in the elderly. Rather, postoperative mortality was associated with specific risk factors—myocardial infarction, with preexistant heart disease; stroke, with diabetes mellitus; and respiratory failure, with chronic obstructive pulmonary disease. Advanced age, in itself, should not be considered a contraindication to total laryngectomy.

RESULTS OF TOTAL LARYNGECTOMY

It is meaningless to discuss the "cure rate" of total laryngectomy because this procedure is employed for a variety of tumors involving different origins, different sites, and different stage groupings. Total laryngectomy is the last resort in the management of laryngeal cancer, not in the sense that is should be employed only after other modalities or operative procedures have failed, but rather in the sense that it should be employed only when it is the procedure that will produce the best chance of cure for a specific situation. Other sections of this chapter and of this book discuss the efficacy of alternative procedures and modalities by comparing the results of those procedures with the results that would be obtained by total laryngectomy.

A review of the literature indicates that for endolaryngeal cancers, total laryngectomy produces cure rates of 65% to 70% for T3, N0 laryngeal cancers and cure rates of 45% to 50% for T4, N0 cancers.[48] Lower cure rates are usually achieved in patients who have failed to respond to radiation therapy or in those with cervical lymph node metastases.[49]

With the armamentarium of rehabilitative and supportive measures available for restoration of voice, as well as for restoration of an acceptable quality of life, total laryngectomy remains an effective and often the optimal procedure for management of advanced laryngeal cancer

LARYNGECTOMY FOR SUBGLOTTIC CARCINOMA

Primary subglottic carcinomas arising independently in the subglottic region, rather than by downward extension of glottic tumors, are rare. Such tumors compose 4% to 6% of all laryngeal carcinomas.[50, 51] Extension through the conus elasticus into the subglottic area may occur in more than 20% of glottic cancers.[52] Pathologic and clinical behavior and problems in management are similar for the primary subglottic tumors and for the so-called extension or glottic-subglottic tumors. Although histologic evaluation of larynges with as little as 3 mm of subglottic extension of glottic tumors has revealed findings similar to those described for primary subglottic cancers,[51] true clinical similarity and indications for mediastinal extension of total laryngectomy apply only to lesions with extensions greater than 1 cm below the true cord. These tumors traverse the cricothyroid membrane and extend into the cricoid ring. Sessions et al.[53] found that the recurrence rate of subglottic extension tumors more than doubled when the tumor extended 15 mm or more below the vocal cord.

Primary subglottic tumors are almost always seen initially in a relatively advanced state because absence of vocal cord involvement at an early stage causes the lesion to be asymptomatic. Most patients present with airway obstruction, often necessitating tracheostomy, which further complicates surgical management. In some cases it may be difficult to insert the tracheostomy tube without violating the tumor. Endoscopic debulking by lasers may be feasible in some instances.

Causes of Treatment Failure

Harrison[51] has listed the causes of failure in treatment of subglottic tumors as follows:

1. Inadequate resection of the trachea below the tumor, particularly if there has been a previous tracheostomy.

2. Extension of tumor over the superior rim of the cricoid, which can lead to recurrence in the margins of the pharyngeal repair.

3. Extension of tumor posteriorly below the cricoid cartilage to involve the cervical esophagus.

4. Involvement of the thyroid gland. Although this was found in only 5 of 25 specimens,[52] it is

impossible to detect clinically and will inevitably lead to recurrence if the involved thyroid gland is left behind.

5. Metastases to paratracheal lymph nodes. This occurrence of metastases is also clinically undetectable, but microscopic metastases have been found in 50% of all larynges with primary subglottic carcinoma examined by serial section. Welsh[54] injected radioactive gold into the subglottic area of human subjects and found that 96% of the material concentrated in the ipsilateral paratracheal nodes.

Treatment of Subglottic Carcinoma

Harrison[51] concluded that total thyroidectomy, low sectioning of the trachea, and resection of lymph nodes from the paratracheal gutters are required for adequate treatment of subglottic carcinoma. This is accomplished by removing the manubrium as far as the first interspace, which permits resection of at least three additional centimeters of trachea and removal of the paratracheal adipose tissue, the lymphatics, and the nodes above the left innominate vein. The tracheostoma is placed directly into the bed of the resected manubrium as far inferiorly as is convenient. No functional problems are created by resection of the manubrium. In 1975, Harrison[52] reported 3-year survival in 5 of 8 patients with primary subglottic tumors and in 10 of 17 patients with glottic-subglottic lesions. Examination of the paratracheal nodes was of prognostic significance. Every patient who had involved nodes at the lower end of the chain died of cancer. The patients whose lower nodes were uninvolved survived.

Postoperative radiation therapy is of value in preventing stomal recurrence in subglottic carcinoma. Tong et al.[55] administered elective postoperative irradiation to 26 patients at high risk for stomal recurrence. In 22 of these patients, the stomas were included in the field and no stomal recurrences developed. In 4 patients, the stomas were shielded, and stomal recurrences developed in 2 of the 4. More recently, Weber et al.[56] evaluated results of paratracheal lymph node dissections in 141 patients with laryngeal and hypopharyngeal cancer. Eight of 30 patients (26.7%) with subglottic extension had paratracheal lymph node metastases. Peristomal recurrences developed in 6 of 141 patients (4%), and metastasis to the peritracheal lymph nodes was identified in one third of these patients. No peristomal recurrence developed in any of the patients who received postoperative radiotherapy to the stoma.

Choice of Surgical Procedure

Although there is general agreement that low resection of the trachea and resection of the paratracheal nodes is necessary to reduce the incidence of tracheal or stomal recurrence in subglottic carcinoma, most surgeons do not perform routine manubrial resection and mediastinal dissection. Nevertheless, there are instances in which the size and location of the tumor and the habitus of the patient render adequate resection impossible without partial manubriectomy. This situation is most likely to arise in instances of primary subglottic carcinoma situated well below the vocal cords. If it is felt that at least a 2-cm margin of normal trachea can be obtained, the paratracheal nodes adequately removed, and the tracheostoma created without tension, then manubrial resection is not necessary. Postoperative radiation should be administered, and it should include the stoma in all cases of laryngectomy for subglottic tumors.

REFERENCES

1. Gussenbauer C. Über die erste durch Th. Billroth am Menschen ausgeführte Kehlkopf-Extirpation und die Anwendung eines künstlichen Kehlkopfes. *Arch Klin Chir* 1874; 17:343–356.
2. Martin H. *Surgery of Head and Neck Tumors.* New York, Hoeber-Harper & Row, 1957.
3. Crowe SJ, Broyles EN. Carcinoma of the larynx and total laryngectomy. *Trans Am Laryngol Assoc* 1938; 60:47.
4. Jackson C, Jackson CL. *Cancer of the Larynx.* Philadelphia, Saunders, 1939.
5. Jackson C, Babcock W. Laryngectomy for carcinoma of the larynx. *Surg Clin North Am* 1931; 11:1207.
6. Laccourreye H, Laccourreye O, Weinstein G, et al. Supracricoid laryngectomy with cricohyoidopexy: a partial laryngeal procedure for selected supraglottic and transglottic carcinomas. *Laryngoscope* 1990; 100:735–741.
7. Department of Veterans Affairs Laryngeal Cancer Study Group. Induction chemotherapy plus radiation compared with surgery plus radiation in patients with advanced laryngeal cancer. *N Engl J Med* 1991; 324:1685–1690.
8. Shirinian MH, Weber RS, Lippman SM, et al. Laryngeal preservation by induction chemotherapy plus radiotherapy in locally advanced head and neck cancer: the M.D. Anderson Cancer Center experience. *Head Neck* 1994;16:39–44.
9. Nikolau A, Fountzilas G, Kosmidis P, et al. Laryngeal preservation in cases of advanced laryngeal cancer treated with platinum based induction chemotherapy before local treatment. *J Laryngol Otol* 1991; 105:930–933.
10. Wolf GT, Fisher SG. Effectiveness of salvage neck dissection for advanced regional metastases when induction chemotherapy and radiation are used for organ preservation. *Laryngoscope* 1992; 102:934–939.
11. DeSanto, LW. Cancer of the larynx. *Curr Opin Otolaryngol Head Neck Surg* 1993; 1:133–136.
12. Stell PM, Rawson NS. Adjuvant chemotherapy in head and neck cancer. *Br J Cancer* 1990; 61:779–787.
13. Tannock IF, Cummings BJ. Neoadjuvant chemotherapy in head and neck cancer: no way to preserve a larynx. *J Clin Oncol* 1992; 10:343–346.
14. Keim WF, Shapiro MJ, Rosen HO. Study of postlaryngectomy stomal recurrences. *Arch Otolaryngol* 1965; 81:183.

15. Stell PM, Van Den Broek P. Stomal recurrence after laryngectomy: aetiology and management. *J Laryngol Otol* 1971; 85:131–140.

16. McCombe A, Stell PM. Emergency laryngectomy. *J Laryngol Otol* 1991; 105:463–465.

17. Narula AA, Sheppard IJ, West K, et al. Is emergency laryngectomy a waste of time? *Am J Otolaryngol* 1993; 14:21–23.

18. Young HA, Maran AG. Detachment of the trachea following total laryngectomy. *J Laryngol Otol* 1977; 91:111–117.

19. Stell PM, Cooney TC. Management of fistulae of the head and neck after radical surgery. *J Laryngol Otol* 1974; 88:819–834.

20. Lundgren J, Olofsson J. Pharyngocutaneous fistulae following total laryngectomy. *Arch Otolaryngol* 1979; 4:13–23.

21. Johansen LV, Overgaard J, Elbrond O. Pharyngo-cutaneous fistulae after laryngectomy: influence of previous radiotherapy and prophylactic metronidazole. *Cancer* 1988; 61:673–678.

22. Cummings CW, Johnson JT, Chung CK, et al. Complications of laryngectomy and neck dissection following planned preoperative radiotherapy. *Ann Otol* 1977; 86:745–750.

23. Weingrad DN, Spiro RH. Complications after laryngectomy. *Am J Surg* 1983; 146:517–520.

24. Gall AM, Sessions DG, Ogura JH: Complications following surgery for cancer of the larynx and hypopharynx. *Cancer* 1977; 39:624–631.

25. Shemen LJ, Spiro RH. Complications following laryngectomy. *Head Neck Surg* 1986; 8:185–191.

26. Lavelle RJ, Maw AR. The aetiology of post-laryngectomy pharyngo-cutaneous fistulae. *J Laryngol Otol* 1972; 86:785–793.

27. Mendelsohn MS, Bridger GP. Pharyngocutaneous fistulae following laryngectomy. *Aust N Z J Surg* 1985; 55:177–179.

28. Goldstein RD, Komisar A, Silver CE, Strauch B. Management of necrotic neck wounds with a "sandwich" pectoralis myocutaneous flap. *Head Neck Surg* 1988; 10:246–251.

29. Duranceau A, Jamieson G, Hurwitz AL, et al. Alteration in esophageal motility after laryngectomy. *Am J Surg* 1976; 131:30–35.

30. Silver CE, Henick D. Complications of laryngeal surgery. *In* Weissler MC, Pillsbury HC: *Complications in Head and Neck Surgery,* pp 107–121. New York, Thieme, 1995.

31. McConnel FM, Cerenko D, Mendelsohn MS. Dysphagia after total laryngectomy. *Otolaryngol Clin N Am* 1988; 21:721–726.

32. Lund WS. A study of the cricopharyngeal sphincter in man and in the dog. *Ann R Coll Surg Engl* 1965; 37:225–246.

33. Kaplan JN, Dobie RA, Cummings CW. The incidence of hypopharyngeal stenosis after surgery for laryngeal cancer. *Otolaryngol Head Neck Surg* 1981; 89:956–959.

34. Gates GA, Hearne EM III. Predicting esophageal speech. *Ann Otol Rhinol Laryngol* 1982; 91:454–457.

35. Stell PM. Total laryngectomy: *In* Silver CE (ed): *Laryngeal Cancer,* pp 212–223. Thieme, New York, 1991.

36. Cusumano RJ, Silver CE, Brauer RJ, et al. Pectoralis myocutaneous flap for replacement of cervical esophagus. *Head Neck* 1989; 11:450–456.

37. Silver CE, Cusumano RJ, Fell SC, et al. Replacement of upper esophagus: results with myocutaneous flap and with gastric transposition. *Laryngoscope* 1989; 99:819–821.

38. Zohar Y, Ben Tovim R, Laurian N, et al. Thyroid function following radiation and surgical therapy in head and neck malignancy. *Head Neck Surg* 1984; 6:948–952.

39. Vrabec DP, Heffron TJ. Hypothyroidism following treatment for head and neck cancer. *Ann Otol Rhinol Laryngol* 1981; 90:449–453.

40. Talmi YP, Finkelstein Y, Zohar Y. Pharyngeal fistulas in postoperative hypothyroid patients. *Ann Otol Rhinol Laryngol* 1989; 98:267–268.

41. Alexander MV, Zajtchuk JT, Henderson RL. Hypothyroidism and wound healing. *Arch Otolaryngol* 1982; 108:289–291.

42. Isaacson SR, Lowry LD, Snow JB Jr. Hypoparathyroidism secondary to surgery for carcinoma of the pharynx and larynx. *Trans Am Acad Opthalmol Otolaryngol* 1977; 84:584–591.

43. Buchanan G, West TE, Woodhead JS, et al. Hypoparathyroidism following pharyngolaryngo-esophagectomy. *Clin Oncol* 1975; 1:89–96.

44. Krespi YP, Wurster CF, Wang TD, et al. Hypoparathyroidism following total laryngopharyngectomy and gastric pull-up. *Laryngoscope* 1985; 95:1184–1187.

45. Price JC, Ridley MB. Hypocalcemia following pharyngoesophageal ablation and gastric pull-up reconstruction: pathophysiology and management. *Ann Otol Rhinol Laryngol* 1988; 97:521–526.

46. Jun M, Strong E, Salzman E, Gerold F. Head and neck cancer in the elderly. *Head Neck Surg* 1983; 4:376–382.

47. Arriaga MA, Kanel KT, Johnson JT, et al. Medical complications in total laryngectomy: incidence and risk factors. *Ann Otol Rhinol Laryngol* 1990; 91:611–615.

48. Silver CE. *Surgery for Cancer of the Larynx and Related Structures.* New York, Churchill Livingstone, 1981.

49. Silver CE, Moisa II. The role of surgery in the treatment of laryngeal cancer. *CA Cancer J Clin* 1990; 40:134–149.

50. Batsakis JG. *Tumors of the Head and Neck.* Baltimore, Williams and Wilkins, 1974.

51. Harrison DFN. The pathology and management of subglottic cancer. *Ann Otol Rhinol Laryngol* 1971; 80:6–12.

52. Harrison DFN. Laryngectomy for subglottic lesions. *Laryngoscope* 1975; 85:1208–1210.

53. Sessions DG, Ogura JH, Fried MP. Carcinoma of the subglottic area. *Laryngoscope* 1975; 85:1417–1423.

54. Welsh LW. The normal human laryngeal lymphatics. *Ann Otol Rhinol Laryngol* 1964; 73:569–582.

55. Tong D, Moss WT, Stevens KR. Elective irradiation of the lower cervical region in patients at high risk for recurrent cancer at the tracheal stoma. *Radiology* 1977; 124:809–811.

56. Weber RS, Marvel J, Smith P, et al. Paratracheal lymph node dissection for carcinoma of the larynx, hypopharynx and cervical esophagus. *Otolaryngol Head Neck Surg* 1993; 108:11–17.

Chapter 8

Near-Total Laryngectomy

Carl E. Silver and Idel I. Moisa

Near-total laryngectomy (NTL) is a voice-preserving operation designed for the oncologic resection of selected advanced unilateral carcinomas involving the larynx.[1-4] Conventionally, these lesions are treated with total laryngectomy. Nevertheless, an oncologically sound resection with a "true" hemilaryngectomy that includes the cricoid cartilage and the superior tracheal rings and yet preserves a portion of the uninvolved contralateral larynx may be feasible for lesions sufficiently localized to one side. The tumors for which this procedure is indicated are too extensive for conventional conservation surgery. They are often transglottic tumors with invasion of the paraglottic space and fixation of the vocal cord. The procedure is useful for glottic, subglottic, supraglottic, and pyriform sinus carcinomas.

The operation ablates one hemilarynx entirely and usually the anterior portion of the contralateral vocal cord. The entire contralateral vocal cord may be preserved in cases of pyriform sinus carcinoma with minimal endolaryngeal involvement. The resection extends posteriorly to the midline, and inferiorly it includes the ipsilateral cricoid cartilage, the thyroid lobe, and portions of the upper tracheal rings, if necessary. Superiorly, the entire preepiglottic space, the epiglottis, the hyoid bone, and the valleculae may be excised. A segment of the larynx is preserved on the uninvolved contralateral side, which includes the recurrent laryngeal nerve, the posterior thyroid cartilage, the arytenoid cartilage, and a portion of the thyroarytenoid muscle.

The remaining laryngeal tissue is insufficient for reconstruction of an adequate airway, but preservation of a myomucosal segment of intrinsic larynx along with its recurrent laryngeal nerve and arytenoid cartilage permits the creation of a "dynamic" tracheoesophageal shunt for preservation of the voice. This mucosa-lined tube connects the trachea with the pharynx and can function as a neoglottis during expiration, allowing lung-powered voice production. The shunt is composed of endolaryngeal muscle innervated by the vagus nerve and thus is closed by sphincteric action during swallowing, thereby preventing aspiration. Breathing is maintained by a permanent tracheostomy that must be manually occluded to produce voice. In suitable patients, a valved prosthesis may be employed to eliminate the need for manual occlusion.[5, 6]

TERMINOLOGY

This operation was originally termed "extended hemilaryngectomy,"[1] and subsequently, "subtotal laryngectomy."[2] Eventually, because of confusion with other surgical procedures bearing the same names, this procedure became known as "near-total laryngectomy" (NTL),[7-9] or as "near-total laryngopharyngectomy" (NTLP), when applied to resection of hypopharyngeal (pyriform sinus) lesions.[10, 11] For larger resections requiring complex reconstruction of the pharynx, the name "extended near-total laryngopharyngectomy" has been suggested.[7] The term "near-total laryngectomy" continues to be applied occasionally to different extended conservation operations in which the laryngeal airway is preserved, thereby creating some confusion in terminology. Perhaps the description "Pearson near-total laryngectomy" would be most specific in reference to the procedure discussed in this chapter.

INDICATIONS AND CONTRAINDICATIONS
(Table 8–1)

The NTL procedure is most suitable for resection of unilateral T3 and T4 laryngeal carcinomas, transglottic cancer, and cancer of the pyriform sinus. This procedure has been employed instead of total laryngectomy in resections of tongue base and pharyngeal cancers in which the larynx must be sacrificed because of inability to preserve its function.[4, 11, 12]

The preservation of laryngeal function is an important consideration in the management of lesions that may be anatomically suitable for partial laryngectomy or for extended conservation surgery, but which occur in patients in whom such procedures may be physiologically unworkable because of age, chronic lung disease, or the necessity of extending the resection into the tongue or the pharynx. In such patients, NTL may represent an alternative to total laryngectomy. While larynx preservation with combined chemotherapy and irradiation has supplanted laryngectomy for some patients, there are many individuals in whom direct surgical management is preferable, because of anticipated noncompliance, the inability to tolerate chemotherapy, or the presence of lesions that are unlikely to respond to nonsurgical treatment.

Extensive pyriform sinus carcinoma that involves the aryepiglottic fold, the tongue base, or the tonsil and that requires pharyngectomy and flap reconstruction of the pharynx may be resected adequately with NTL if the lesion is sufficiently localized to one side and if one normal pyriform fossa can be preserved.[11, 13]

With the need to preserve one arytenoid cartilage and at least two thirds of the uninvolved cord in order to create the vocal shunt, tumor involvement of the postcricoid area or the interarytenoid region is the principal contraindication to this operation.

Table 8–1. INDICATIONS FOR NEAR-TOTAL LARYNGECTOMY, NEAR-TOTAL LARYNGOPHARYNGECTOMY, AND EXTENDED NEAR-TOTAL LARYNGOPHARYNGECTOMY

Site	Pearson and Keith[11]	DeSanto et al.[12]	Chandrachud et al.[18]	Singh and Hardcastle[19]	Su and Hwang[24]	Tang et al.[28]	Levine et al.[15]	Silver and Moisa[27]	Total Number of Sites
Glottic	24	0	3	1	2	0	3	3	34
Transglottic	14	0	5	2	0	0	0	4	25
Supraglottic	32	28	3	0	5	0	5	0	73
A-E fold	6	0	0	0	0	0	0	0	6
Subglottic	1	0	0	0	0	0	0	0	1
Laryngeal	0	0	0	0	0	10	0	0	10
Pyriform fossa	24	0	0	1	13	3	2	1	44
Posterior hypopharyngeal wall	0	0	0	0	0	0	1	0	1
Tongue base	5	1	0	0	0	0	0	0	6
Pharynx	0	8	0	0	0	0	0	0	8
Oral tongue	1	0	0	0	0	0	0	0	1
Tongue base and pharynx	0	0	0	0	1	0	0	1	2
Thyroid	0	1	0	0	0	0	0	0	1
Cervical esophagus	0	0	0	0	0	0	0	0	1
Total number of tumors	107	38	11	4	21	13	11	9	214

Involvement of the anterior portion of the opposite cord is not a contraindication, provided the cord moves normally and the arytenoid cartilage is free of tumor.

In studies of whole organ sections, Dumich et al.[10] determined that involvement of the apex and the paraglottic space with pyriform sinus carcinoma, immobilization or involvement of the ipsilateral vocal cord, and invasion of the cricoid and thyroid cartilages, do not necessarily represent oncologic reasons for removing the contralateral uninvolved laryngeal tissues. By contrast, bilateral vocal cord fixation, postcricoid involvement, and extension of the tumor across the interarytenoid area represent clear contraindications to NTL. The value of preoperative assessment and frozen-section monitoring in the proper selection of patients for this procedure was emphasized. Comparable results were noted by Robbins and Michaels[14] in a similar study. These authors concluded that NTL is a technically viable alternative for many patients who would otherwise undergo total laryngectomy.

Opinion is divided regarding the place of NTL after radiation therapy. Total laryngectomy may be preferable in such cases because the tumor margins may be obscure and the safety of preserving the contralateral arytenoid cartilage is uncertain.[9, 11] NTL, after radiation failure, may be considered for tumors that were treated with radiation at the T1 stage but that have progressed to the T3 stage at the time that the recurrence is recognized.[11] The operation has been used successfully, after radiation failure, for treatment of supraglottic carcinoma.[1, 8]

Cervical metastases and extralaryngeal spread of the tumor are not contraindications to NTL. A neck dissection may be performed before laryngeal surgery begins.

Postoperative radiation therapy after NTL does not seem to have a deleterious effect on the subsequent development of speech or deglutition.[12, 15]

ADVANTAGES AND DISADVANTAGES OF NEAR-TOTAL LARYNGECTOMY COMPARED TO TOTAL LARYNGECTOMY

The alternative to NTL, and a far more widely employed procedure, is total laryngectomy, with immediate or delayed insertion of a voice prosthesis. There is little doubt that the ease and quality of speech obtained through the biologic shunt that is created by NTL surpass those forms of fistula voice in which the upper esophageal sphincter is the vibrating source. Also, because there is no prosthesis to be taken care of, the NTL shunt is reliable and maintenance free. In the authors' experience, patients with successful NTL have a better quality of life and a more natural voice than do patients who have had total laryngectomy.

Nevertheless, NTL has not achieved widespread acceptance among surgeons. Although the procedure was originally described in 1980,[1] by 1991 we had published the results of only 160 cases reported in the literature,[16] and in this book we summarize 213 reported cases, including our own series of 7 cases. Several factors have discouraged the use of this procedure, among them being the greater complexity of NTL, as well as the longer operating time (usually 30 to 60 minutes), compared to total laryngectomy. An important disadvantage of NTL is that correction of an improperly functioning shunt is difficult. Although a stenotic shunt may respond to dilatation, this is not successful in some instances, and the subsequent insertion of a voice prosthesis may be onerous. The problem of aspiration can be even more difficult to correct, particularly if the shunt is adynamic; the surgeon and the patient may have to choose between closing the shunt permanently or tolerating the sometimes disabling aspiration. Perhaps the greatest deterrent to the use of NTL is the lack of confidence that the occasionally close margins obtained after resection of large tumors will produce results equivalent to those obtained with the simple, reliable standard total laryngectomy. For the treatment of large tumors, the ability to place a voice prosthesis in almost every patient immediately after total laryngectomy, and thus provide the patient with satisfactory voice rehabilitation, strongly favors total laryngectomy over the more technically complicated and possibly oncologically questionable NTL.

TECHNIQUE

The complex surgical procedure has been described in detail in previous publications.[1, 2, 7, 11] In the accompanying illustrations, the resection of a right-sided transglottic carcinoma with extension inferiorly is demonstrated.

Figure 8–1A. A tracheostomy is created through the third tracheal ring. The tracheostomy may be placed lower, if required by subglottic extension, but higher placement may interfere with proper construction of the shunt. The ipsilateral (right) larynx is mobilized in the same manner as for total laryngectomy, with the thyroid lobe, the prelaryngeal muscles, and the adjacent lymphoareolar structures included in the resected specimen. On the contralateral (left) side, the larynx is skeletonized as for vertical hemilaryngectomy. The central portion of the thyroid cartilage is outlined as shown and removed.

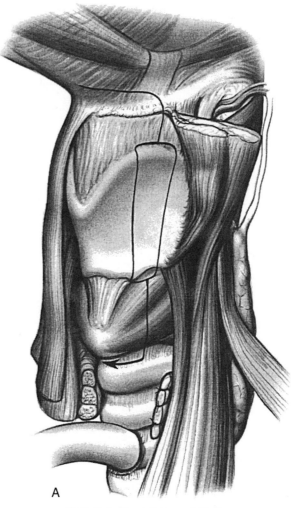

A

Figure 8–1. Near-total laryngectomy.
Illustration continued on following page

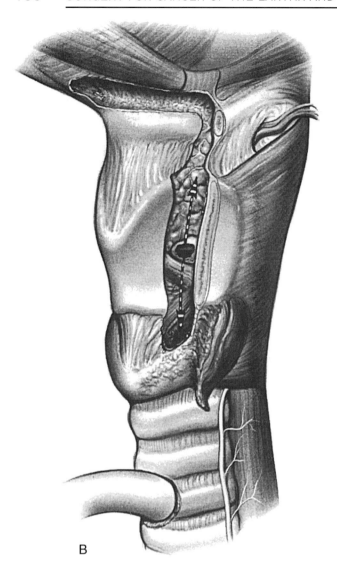

B

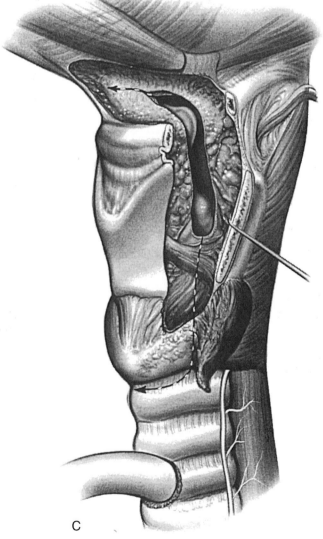

Figure 8–1B. Removal of the cartilage exposes the ventricular mucosal defect through which the larynx will be entered, at about the midportion of the contralateral vocal cord. Subsequent superior and inferior incisions into the endolarynx are indicated by the dotted line. For resection of hypopharyngeal tumors that do not involve the endolarynx, the laryngotomy may be performed closer to the midline to preserve more mucosa for the shunt.

Figure 8–1C. The mucosal incision is extended superiorly, exposing the epiglottis, and then carried medially through the valleculae. The inferior incision, to be made through the vocal cord and then medially, inferior to the cricoid, is outlined. For resection of lesions confined to the glottis, the epiglottis need not be resected, and the transverse medial incision may be made through the petiole. This procedure results in a smaller pharyngeal defect that will require closure.

C

Figure 8–1 *Continued* Near-total laryngectomy.

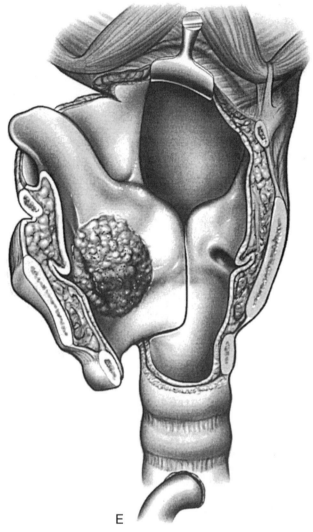

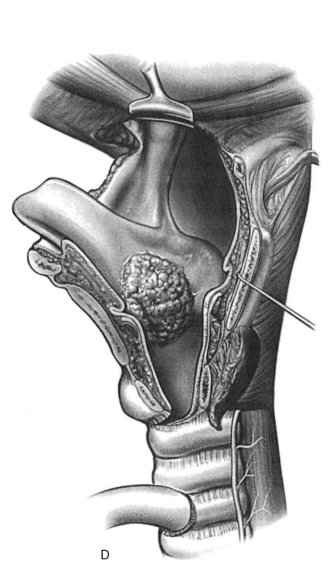

Figure 8–1 *Continued* Near-total laryngectomy.
Illustration continued on following page

Figure 8–1*D.* Completion of the inferior incision permits inspection of the laryngeal interior, which reveals the tumor. The left (contralateral) and the inferior resection margins have been determined by the incisions made earlier for entry into the larynx.

Figure 8–1*E.* The inferior incision continues beneath the cricoid cartilage as far as the midline, where it will course vertically between the arytenoid cartilages. As this incision is continued, the portion of the larynx to be resected is rotated outward, providing a better exposure of the tumor and the resection margins.

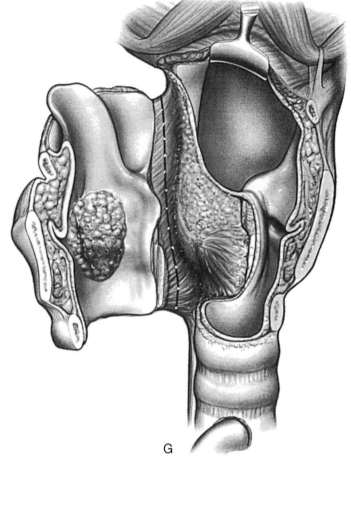

G

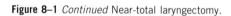

Figure 8–1 *Continued* Near-total laryngectomy.

Figure 8–1F. The mucosa of the posterior midline is incised, the anterior perichondrium of the cricoid lamina is scored, and the cricoid cartilage is fractured manually, by placing a finger in the hypopharynx for control, as shown. The remaining deep structures in the posterior midline, namely the posterior perichondrium and the interarytenoid muscle, are divided, with care being taken not to injure the anterior hypopharyngeal mucosa. Because the pyriform sinus is not to be resected in this case, the mucosal incision continues along the right aryepiglottic fold, completing the resection margin.

Figure 8–1G. The specimen is freed from the hypopharyngeal and pyriform sinus mucosa, and the remaining attachments, consisting mostly of the right inferior constrictor muscle, are divided, completing the resection.

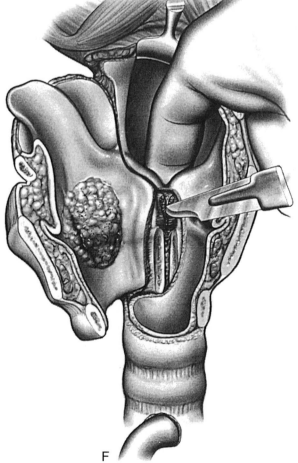

F

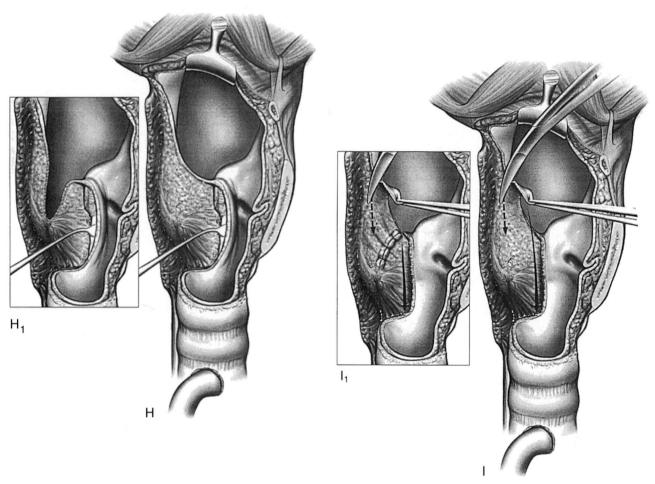

H₁

H

I₁

I

Figure 8–1 *Continued* Near-total laryngectomy.

Illustration continued on following page

Figures 8–1*H* **and 8–1***H₁*. The reconstructive phase of the procedure commences with submucosal dissection and piecemeal removal of a sufficient amount of residual (left) cricoid cartilage to permit tubing of the subglottic mucosa. Figure 8–1*H₁* shows a defect in the pyriform sinus when that portion of the mucosa has been resected. This defect will be closed by direct suture, as far as the reflection of the postcricoid mucosa (see Fig. 8–1*I₁*).

Figures 8–1*I* **and 8–1***I₁*. The remaining laryngeal structures now include a strip of mucosa from the trachea to the posterior half of the contralateral (left) hemilarynx, the left arytenoid cartilage, the vocal muscle, the recurrent laryngeal nerve, and the posterior portion of the thyroid cartilage. The phonatory shunt will be created from the myomucosal tissue of the left hemilarynx, the subglottis, and the upper trachea. In most cases of endolaryngeal tumor, there will be insufficient laryngeal mucosa remaining to form a shunt of adequate diameter. The mucosa available for tubing may be augmented by rotating a flap of the pyriform sinus mucosa inferiorly and suturing it to the remaining laryngeal mucosa. This flap is developed from the pyriform sinus mucosa, as shown. The flap is developed similarly, whether the pyriform sinus mucosa has been saved (Fig. 8–1*I*) or resected and repaired (Fig. 8–1*I₁*).

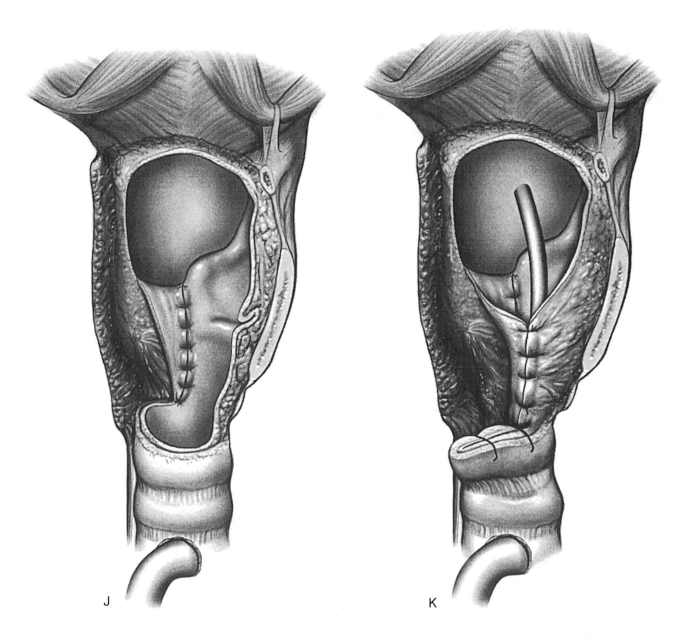

J

K

Figure 8–1 *Continued* Near-total laryngectomy.

Figure 8–1*J.* The augmentation flap is rotated downward and sutured vertically to the cut posterior midline margin of the laryngeal mucosa, thus increasing the amount of tissue available for tubing. If the laryngotracheal remnant can be tubed without an augmentation flap, then the flap need not be created.

Figure 8–1*K.* Commencing at the anterior superior border of the cut edge of the trachea, the myomucosal segment is now tubed, using a small catheter as a template. Pearson originally recommended a No. 14 Fr catheter for the purpose of producing a shunt of adequate caliber, and this was originally employed on our service. More recently, we have used a 14-gauge polyethylene catheter to construct a shunt of narrower diameter, as suggested by Gavilan et al.[17] In our experience, this has worked satisfactorily for voice production, and the narrower shunt is less likely to permit aspiration.

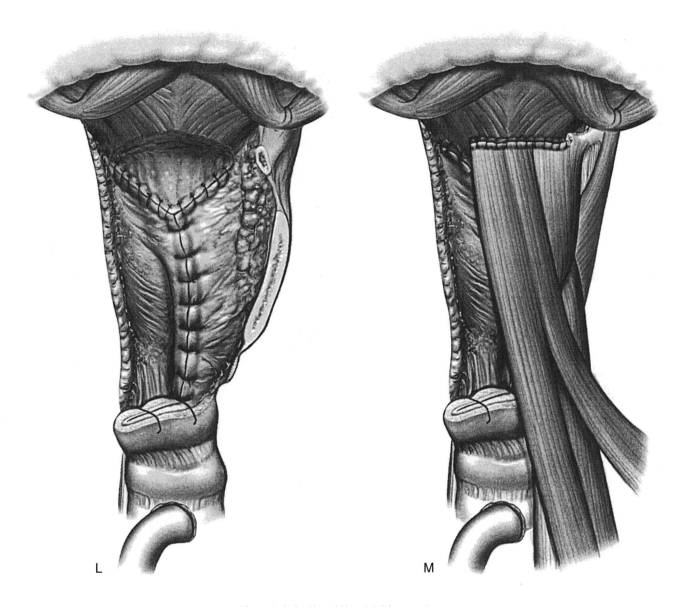

L

M

Figure 8–1 *Continued* Near-total laryngectomy.

Illustration continued on following page

Figure 8–1*L.* After construction of the shunt, the hypopharyngeal mucosa is closed.

Figure 8–1*M.* The infrahyoid muscles are sutured to the suprahyoid muscles, covering the shunt and the pharyngeal closure. The tracheostomy opening will be sutured to a corresponding incision in the skin, creating a permanent tracheostoma.

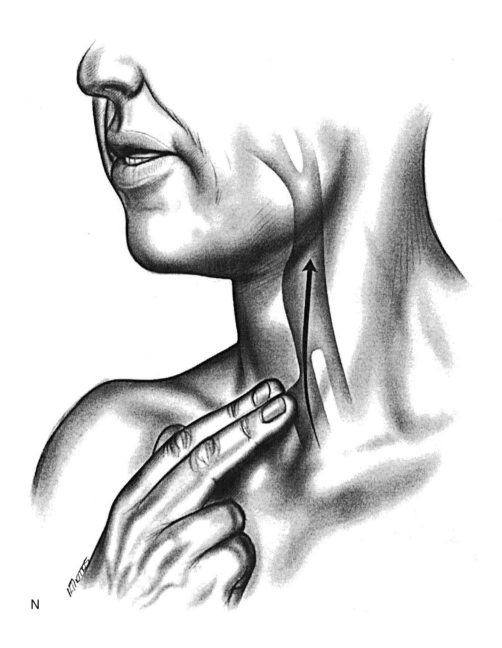

Figure 8–1 *Continued* Near-total laryngectomy.

Figure 8–1N. In order to speak, the patient must occlude the stoma with a finger, forcing air through the shunt into the pharynx. During swallowing, the shunt contracts from the action of the preserved vocal muscle and arytenoid cartilage. Respiration occurs through the unoccluded tracheostoma.

RESULTS

Cure Rates

NTL appears to be as effective as total laryngectomy for the local control of suitable lesions. Pearson and Keith[11] reported an overall 3-year cure in 35 of 66 patients (53%). Nine patients died of causes unrelated to their laryngeal cancer, producing a determinate cure rate of 61%.

Tables 8–2 and 8–3 summarize the cure and recurrence rates for individual sites reported in various studies. Local recurrence was the cause of death in only two of the patients reported by Pearson and Keith; both had failed radiation therapy for supraglottic carcinoma. Distant metastases accounted for the highest number of deaths (8 out of 20 deaths) in patients with hypopharyngeal tumors.

DeSanto et al.[12] reported the results of 39 patients operated upon between 1980 and 1985 at the Mayo Clinic. Twenty-six of the patients (67%) demonstrated no recurrences, while 13 (33%) died of their disease.

Chaudrachud et al.[18] reported no deaths and no local recurrences among 11 patients who underwent NTL between 1983 and 1987, although 1 patient developed cervical metastasis, which required neck dissection. Four patients in this series (2 patients with stage T3N0 supraglottic tumors and 2 with stage T3N0 transglottic tumors) were radiation fail-

ures. Singh and Hardcastle[19] reported good short-term oncologic results in their series of 4 patients.

Levine et al.[15] reported their experience with 11 patients who underwent NTL between 1989 and 1992. Two of these patients subsequently required completion laryngectomy because of wound complications. Eight (89%) of the remaining 9 patients have had a mean disease-free survival period of 25.5 months.

Voice Production

In order to produce voice following NTL, the shunt walls must be healed sufficiently so that postoperative edema does not prevent air from entering the pharynx when the stoma is occluded.[11] Most of our patients have acquired the ability to phonate by the second postoperative week, although a longer period of healing and education is required for establishment of good fistula speech. A dedicated speech pathologist is invaluable during this phase. As previously mentioned, voice production usually requires finger occlusion of the stoma. Many of our patients have found it difficult to occlude the uncannulated stoma during the months after surgery but have functioned well with tracheostomy or laryngectomy tubes, which are easier to occlude. When completely healed, some patients may be fitted with adhesive expiratory stomal valves, designed originally for tracheoesophageal puncture prostheses.

Table 8–2. CURE RATES WITH NEAR-TOTAL LARYNGECTOMY

Study	No. of Patients	Period	Cure Rate by Site No. Tumor-Free/Total No.		Overall Cure Rate No. Tumor-Free/Total No. (%)
Pearson and Keith[11]	66	3 years	Transglottic, glottic, and subglottic	20/29	35/66 (53%)
			Supraglottic	8/17	
			Hypopharynx	7/20	
DeSanto et al.[12]	39	1980–1985	Supraglottic		26/39 (67%)
Chandrachud et al.[18]	11	1983–1987	Transglottic	5/5	11/11 (100%)
			Glottic	3/3	
			Supraglottic	3/3	
Singh and Hardcastle[19]	4	0.3–1.3 years	Transglottic	2/2	4/4 (100%)
			Pyriform fossa	1/1	
			T3 glottic	1/1	
Su and Hwang[24]	21	1–5 years	Supraglottic	2/5	16/21 (76%)
			Glottic	2/2	
			Pyriform fossa	11/13	
			Tongue base, pharynx	1/1	
Tang et al.[28]	14	2 years	Laryngeal, pyriform fossa, cervical esophagus	—	78.6%
Levine et al.[15]	9	>2 years	Laryngeal, pyriform fossa, posterior pharyngeal wall	—	8/9 (89%)
Silver and Moisa[29]	9	1986–1995	Transglottic	3/4	5/7 (71%)
			Glottic	1/1	
			Pyriform sinus	1/1	
			Hypopharynx	0/1	

Table 8–3. SITE OF TUMOR RECURRENCE AFTER NEAR-TOTAL LARYNGECTOMY

Study	No. of Patients	Site of Original Tumor	Site of Recurrence				New Cancer
			None	*Local*	*Neck*	*Distant*	
Pearson and Keith[11]	29	Glottic, transglottic, subglottic	20	0	4	2	3
	17	Supraglottic	8	2	3	1	3
	20	Hypopharynx	0	0	2	8	3
DeSanto et al.[12]	28	Supraglottic	19	3	3	3	0
	8	Pharynx	5	1	0	2	0
	2	Tongue	0	0	0	0	2
	1	Thyroid	1	0	0	0	0
Chandrachud et al.[18]	11	Various sites	10	0	1	0	0
Singh and Hardcastle[19]	4	Various sites	4	0	0	0	0
Su and Hwang[24]	5	Supraglottic	2	1	1		
	2	Glottic	2	0	0	0	0
	11	Hypopharynx	11	0	0	0	0
	1	Tongue base	1	0	0	0	0
Levine et al.[15]	9	Larynx, pyriform-hypopharynx	8	0	0	1	0
Silver and Moisa[27]	4	Transglottic	3	1	0	0	0
	1	Glottic	1	0	0	0	0
	1	Pyriform-	1	0	0	0	0
	1	Hypopharynx	0	0	1	0	0

The satisfactory results of NTL with regard to the quality of voice, as well the number of patients who have been able to achieve fistula speech, are summarized in Table 8–4.

Objective studies have been performed to evaluate shunt function. Several authors, using laryngoscopy, have described the appearance of the shunt after NTL.[11, 18] The upper end of the shunt flutters and vibrates during phonation; it closes on swallowing, thereby preventing aspiration. Singh[20] used electrolaryngography to study the site and mechanism of phonatory function of the neoglottis in eight patients who had undergone NTL. Substantial similarities were demonstrated in the functional nature of the neoglottis as compared to the normal glottis. The resultant wave patterns revealed that the neoglottis not only controls airflow through it, but also acts as a source of vibration, similar to the normal

vocal cords. In a subsequent report, Singh[21] discussed the utility of this modality for speech rehabilitation in patients after NTL.

Trudeau[22] studied the acoustic characteristics of speech in a single patient who had undergone NTL 4 years previously. Great similarities were noted in the frequency, intensity, and timing of this patient's speech when compared to that of a patient judged to have acquired excellent tracheoesophageal speech using a Blom-Singer prosthesis for the same length of time. The study also suggested that the reconstructed valve offered little resistance to expiratory air but still prevented aspiration.

Videofluoroscopic studies by Chandrachud et al.[18] demonstrated a distinct narrowing of the pharyngoesophageal segment above the myomucosal shunt. Based on this observation, these authors regard the pharyngoesophageal segment, rather than

Table 8–4. VOICE PRODUCTION AFTER NEAR-TOTAL LARYNGECTOMY

Study	Good Fistula Voice	Onset of Voice
	No. of Patients/Total No. (%)	*Length of Time After NTL*
Pearson and Keith[11]	54/66 (82%)	—
DeSanto et al.[12]	29/39 (74%)	—
Chandrachud et al.[18]	10/11 (91%)	—
Singh and Hardcastle[19]	8/8 (100%)	8–10 days
Hoasjoe et al.[25]	11/11 (100%)	—
Su and Hwang[24]	18/21 (86%)	—
Tang et al.[28]	12/14 (86%)	2–5 weeks
Levine et al.[15]	9/11 (82%)	average of 5.3 months
Silver and Moisa[27]	6/7 (86%)	2–3 weeks

the neoglottis, to be the site of voice production following NTL.

Stomal pressures measured in NTL patients who have achieved successful speech average 25 ± 6 cm H_2O at the threshold level and 32 ± 20 cm H_2O during phonation. In comparison, normal subjects with intact larynges generate subglottic pressures of approximately 10 ± 5 cm H_2O. For speech to occur at physiologic airway pressures, the shunt diameter would have to be greater than 6 mm,[23] which is rarely feasible.

Su and Hwang[24] emphasized the value of NTL with major pectoral muscle myocutaneous flap reconstruction for extensive hypopharyngeal carcinoma, noting that, in their series, all four patients who underwent this procedure regained intelligible shunt speech.

Based on high-quality audio recordings that were computer analyzed, Hoasjoe et al.[25] measured quantifiable acoustic characteristics from 11 subjects who had undergone NTL, and compared these with the acoustic characteristics from 11 age-matched laryngeal speakers. Subjects performed vocal tasks that provided acoustic measurements for frequency, intensity, and duration. Substantial intersubject and intrasubject variability was demonstrated in the acoustic measures for NTL patients. These patients demonstrated a general restriction in fundamental frequency, reduced intensity, and a limitation in duration of phonation when compared with laryngeal speakers. Although restricted in their ability to achieve excessive loudness, NTL speakers were, nevertheless, able to produce acceptable intensity levels for general conversational purposes. All 11 NTL patients were able to phonate intelligibly and independently using the speaking shunt, and all, except for one patient who had some cognitive deficits, used the speaking shunt as the primary mode of communication.

The fundamental frequency values during sustained vowel phonation were significantly greater for the NTL than for the normal laryngeal speakers.[25] This was thought possibly to be due to the relatively small area in the speaking shunt through which air passes for phonatory purposes. This means that increased airway constriction in the postsurgical conduit is likely to result in increased air volume velocity and increased fundamental frequency. Further, NTL may reduce the overall effective length of the vocal tract, thereby providing enhanced resonance for higher frequencies.

Significant intersubject variability with regard to fundamental frequency may be expected for patients who undergo NTL because of the differences in the extent of the surgical resection and reconstruction.[25]

Singh and Ainsworth[26] used electrolaryngography to investigate the fundamental frequency in 43 speakers who were matched for age and use of Scottish dialect. The group consisted of 15 neoglottal speakers who had undergone NTL, 17 esophageal speakers who had undergone total laryngectomy, and 11 normal speakers. The average fundamental frequencies of the neoglottal and the male esophageal speakers were higher than those in the normal group, although many fell into the normal range. The average fundamental frequency of the single female neoglottal speaker was higher than the average in the normal group, but the fundamental frequencies of all the female esophageal speakers were lower than those of the normal female speakers.

COMPLICATIONS

The major complications of NTL are aspiration and shunt stenosis (Table 8–5). Aspiration, al-

Table 8–5. COMPLICATIONS AFTER NEAR-TOTAL LARYNGECTOMY		
	Aspiration (Severe or Transient)	Stenosis
Study	No. of Patients with Aspiration/Total No.	No. of Patients with Stenosis/Total No.
Pearson and Keith[11]	8/66	6/66
DeSanto et al.[12]	6/39	—
Chandrachud et al.[18]	1/11	1/11
Singh and Hardcastle[19]	0/4	0/4
Levine et al.[15]	5/9*	0/9
Silver and Moisa[27]	2/6†	1/6

*Mild problem with aspiration. Two patients had a transient problem, three had a permanent problem.
†One patient had a transient problem.

though infrequent, is the more common complication, occurring in 20 of 123 cases (16%) reported in the literature. Pearson and Keith[11] performed dye studies that indicated that the NTL shunt is dynamic and functions to prevent aspiration. Nevertheless, these authors reported serious aspiration problems in 8 of 66 patients, with most of the problems being subsequently corrected without sacrificing speech. Singh et al.[19] did not encounter any problem with aspiration in four patients. Chandrachud et al.[18] described one instance of aspiration and one of stenosis among a series of 11 patients.

Correction of aspiration problems involves the determination, by fiberoptic examination, of whether the shunt is dynamic; that is, whether contraction or "fluttering" of the orifice can be demonstrated. In such cases, the shunt can be dissected and the adynamic (non-muscular) portion of the shunt wall can be excised. If correction is not successful and aspiration is severe, the shunt may be closed or excised. In one of our cases (see next section), aspiration was corrected by means of a prosthesis.

Stenosis occurred in 7 of 90 cases (8%) reported in the literature, in which the occurrence or absence of this complication was noted. Stenosis may be amenable to dilatation, although most authors have not distinguished between patients in whom a single dilatation has been sufficient and those patients in whom repeated dilatations are necessary. To dilate the shunt, a thin, malleable probe is inserted retrograde into the tracheostoma and through the shunt, where it is recovered by endoscopy. A heavy string, followed by a chain of graduated Tucker dilators, is then led through the shunt. Once the dilatation has progressed, it is possible to pass size 30 Fr or larger dilators. The shunt will restore itself to a functional size within a few hours. General anesthesia is required for effective dilatation. Dilatation may not be possible in every case because a completely obliterated lumen will not admit a probe.

THE AUTHORS' EXPERIENCE

Our experience with NTL[16, 27] has been divided into two phases. During the first phase, from 1986 to 1989, seven operations were attempted but only four were completed as NTL. The other three operations were converted to total laryngectomies because of unsatisfactory margins. Of the four patients with NTL, one, with transglottic carcinoma, had an excellent result with good voice, no aspiration, and long-term cure. Another patient with pyriform sinus carcinoma survived but had no vocal function from his shunt, despite attempted dilata-

tion. The other two patients died from recurrence of the tumor. Of these two patients, one had a transglottic carcinoma that was resected with narrow margins; the other had a large hypopharyngeal cancer that required flap reconstruction. The latter patient could not swallow without aspiration. This problem was corrected by insertion of a Shapiro-type periscope prosthesis, which fit well into the shunt.

This unimpressive initial experience (only one of the four patients in whom the operation was completed was cured with good function of the neoglottis) led us to discontinue NTL for several years. The authors' interest in the operation revived after a trip to India in 1992, where NTL was found useful for patients who received little follow-up or rehabilitation therapy. The procedure has since been performed in five additional patients: two patients with transglottic carcinoma with framework invasion, one patient whose surgery was converted from a hemilaryngectomy to NTL when subglottic extension was found at the margin, one elderly patient with glottic subglottic carcinoma, and one patient with pyriform sinus carcinoma. Three of the five patients are alive and free of disease 1 to 4 years after surgery, one is alive with unresectable regional recurrence, and one died of intercurrent disease at 3 years. Shortly after surgery, all patients acquired good shunt speech, which has persisted. Three of the eight patients underwent postoperative irradiation and retained good speech and swallowing function. Two patients had minor difficulty with aspiration after surgery; one has no aspiration problem 1 year after surgery, and the other has a minimal problem with aspiration if liquids are not taken carefully. Aspiration occurred only in patients whose shunts were made wide and with generous augmentation flaps. Narrower shunts produced no aspiration and functioned well for speech.

Thus, in a total of nine patients, four remain free of disease after an interval of 1 to 9 years. Excellent shunt speech was obtained in seven of the nine patients, and satisfactory deglutition in eight of the nine patients. Postoperative irradiation did not affect shunt function.

CONCLUSIONS

NTL is a useful procedure for resection of large unilateral laryngeal and hypopharyngeal tumors, with preservation of a natural phonatory neoglottis. Results of NTL, reported by groups with the greatest experience, are comparable to those achieved by total laryngectomy for the same disease, and the voice that is achieved is easier to produce and superior in quality to esophageal voice or that generated with a prosthesis. Despite these facts, the operation has not gained widespread popularity, as evidenced by the relatively small experience with this procedure reported in the literature. This may be due partly to the technical difficulty of the procedure, but it also results from a preference for extended conservation surgery or for nonsurgical treatment or, perhaps most often, for the proven benefits of total laryngectomy with simultaneous or subsequent tracheoesophageal puncture and prosthesis. The authors' experience has shown how to optimize the results of the procedure by appropriate selection of patients and intraoperative technical considerations.

REFERENCES

1. Pearson BW, Woods RD, Hartman DE. Extended hemilaryngectomy for T3 glottic carcinoma with preservation of speech and swallowing. *Laryngoscope* 1980; 90:1950–1961.
2. Pearson BW. Subtotal laryngectomy. *Laryngoscope* 1981; 91:1904–1912.
3. Pearson BW. The surgical treatment of locoregionally advanced larygeal cancer. *In* Johnson JT, Didolkar MS (eds): *Head and Neck Cancer,* Vol 3, pp 279–288. Amsterdam, Elsevier, 1993.
4. Pearson BW, DeSanto LW. Near-total laryngectomy. *Op Tech Otolaryngol Head Neck Surg* 1990; 1:28–41.
5. Barton B, DeSanto L, Pearson BW, et al. An endostomal tracheostomy tube for leakproof retention of the Blom-Singer stomal valve. *Otolaryngol Head Neck Surg* 1988; 99:38–41.
6. Singh W. Tracheostoma valve for speech rehabilitation in laryngectomees. *J Laryngol Otol* 1987; 101:809–814.
7. Pearson BW. Near total laryngectomy. *In* Silver CE (ed): *Atlas of Head and Neck Surgery,* pp 235–251. New York, Churchill Livingstone, 1986.
8. Pearson BW. The theory and techniques of near-total laryngectomy. *In* Bailey BJ, Biller, HF (eds): *Surgery of the Larynx,* pp 336–346. Philadelphia, Saunders, 1985.
9. Donald PJ, Pearson BW. The larynx. *In* Donald, PJ (ed): *Head and Neck Cancer: Management of the Difficult Case.* Philadelphia, Saunders, 1984.
10. Dumich PS, Pearson, BW, Weiland LH. Suitability of near-total laryngopharyngectomy in pyriform carcinoma. *Arch Otolaryngol* 1984; 110:664–669.
11. Pearson BW, Keith RL. Near-total laryngectomy. *In* Johnson JJ, Blitzer A, Ossoff RH (eds): *American Academy of Otolaryngology-Head and Neck Surgery Instructional Courses, Vol 2,* pp. 309–330. St. Louis, Mosby, 1989.
12. DeSanto LW, Pearson BP, Olsen KD. Utility of near-total laryngectomy for supraglottic, pharyngeal, base-of-tongue, and other cancers. *Ann Otol Rhinol Laryngol* 1989; 98:2–7.
13. Su CY, Hwang CF. Near-total laryngopharyngectomy with pectoralis major myocutaneous flap in advanced pyriform carcinoma. *J Laryngol Otol* 1993; 107:817–820.
14. Robbins KT, Michaels L. Feasibility of subtotal laryngectomy based on whole-organ examination. *Arch Otolaryngol* 1985; 111:356–360.
15. Levine PA, Debo RF, Reibel JF. Pearson near-total laryngectomy: a reproducible speaking shunt. *Head Neck* 1994; 16:323–325.
16. Silver CE, Moisa II. Near-total laryngectomy. *In* Silver CE (ed): *Laryngeal Cancer,* pp. 232–239. New York, Thieme, 1991.
17. Gavilan J, Gavilan C, Herranz J, et al. Near-total laryngectomy: surgical technique. Abstract No. V253. Second World Congress on Laryngeal Cancer, Sydney Australia, February 20–24, 1994.
18. Chandrachud HR, Chaurasia MK, Sinha KP. Subtotal laryngectomy with myomucosal shunt. *J Laryngol Otol* 1989; 103:504–507.
19. Singh W, Hardcastle P. Near-total laryngectomy with myomucosal valved neoglottis. *J Laryngol Otol* 1985; 99:581–588.
20. Singh W. Electrolaryngography in near-total laryngectomy with myo-mucosal valved neoglottis. *J Laryngol Otol* 1987; 101:815–818.
21. Singh W. Clinical application of electrolaryngograph for speech rehabilitation in near-total laryngectomy with myo-mucosal valved neoglottis. *J Laryngol Otol* 1988; 102:335–336.
22. Trudeau, MD. Acoustical characteristics of speech following Pearson's subtotal laryngectomy: a case study. *Folia Phoniatr Logop* 1987; 39:178–182.
23. Woods RW, Pearson BW. Alaryngeal speech and the development of an internal tracheopharyngeal fistula. *Otolaryngol Head Neck Surg* 1980; 88:64–73.
24. Su CY, Hwang CF. Near-total laryngopharyngectomy with pectoralis major myocutaneous flap in advanced pyriform carcinoma. *J Laryngol Otol* 1993; 107:817–820.
25. Hoasjoe DK, Martin GF, Doyle PC, et al. A comparative acoustic analysis of voice production by near-total laryngectomy and normal laryngeal speakers. *J Otolaryngol* 1992; 21:39–43.
26. Singh W, Ainsworth WA. Computerized measurement of fundamental frequency in Scottish neoglottal patients. *Folia Phoniatr Logop* 1992; 44:231–237.
27. Silver CE, Moisa II. Near total laryngectomy. *In* Smee R, Bridger GP (eds): *Laryngeal Cancer. Proceedings of the Second World Congress on Laryngeal Cancer,* pp. 513–517. Amsterdam, Elsevier, 1994.
28. Tang P, Qi Y, Tu G. Near-total laryngectomy in the treatment of advanced laryngeal and hypopharyngeal carcinoma. *Chin J Otorhinolaryngol* 1994; 29:10–12.
29. Silver CE, Deshpande V, Moisa II. Unpublished data.

Chapter 9

The Hypopharynx
Carl E. Silver and Roger J. Levin

More than a century has passed since Isambert[1] and Krishaber[2] began to classify laryngeal tumors as extrinsic or intrinsic. Intrinsic carcinomas, confined to the interior of the larynx, were characterized by slow growth and late development of lymph node metastases. On the other hand, extrinsic tumors, which originated around the laryngeal orifice or the pharyngeal surfaces of the larynx, were found to be rapidly progressive, with early appearance of lymphatic metastases. Extrinsic carcinomas included supraglottic and hypopharyngeal lesions. Subsequent classifications have also separated the two groups. Supraglottic tumors are considered to be laryngeal carcinomas, whereas hypopharyngeal tumors are grouped separately. This is a rational scheme of classification because supraglottic carcinoma behaves like other endolaryngeal lesions do, whereas hypopharyngeal tumors usually follow the more aggressive course previously attributed to extrinsic carcinoma.

BOUNDARIES OF THE HYPOPHARYNX

The hypopharynx is a roughly triangular area extending from a plane through the tip of the epiglottis to a plane through the cricopharyngeal muscle. It consists of three distinct regions: the pyriform sinus, the posterior hypopharyngeal wall, and the postcricoid mucosa. Previously, the superior extent of the hypopharynx was not consistently described. Some authors considered it to extend to 1 cm from the circumvallate line, including the lingual surface of the epiglottis, the vallecula, and the base of the tongue[3]; others considered the anterior superior boundary to be at the level of the tip of the epiglottis.[4, 5] Most authors now classify lesions of the vallecula and the base of the tongue as oropharyngeal tumors, and lesions of the lingual epiglottis and the lateral aryepiglottic fold as supraglottic tumors.

REGIONS OF THE HYPOPHARYNX

Pyriform Sinus

The pyriform sinus forms an inverted pyramid bounded by the lateral glossoepiglottic folds superiorly, the apex of the pyriform sinus inferiorly, the thyroid cartilage laterally, and the aryepiglottic fold and arytenoid cartilage medially. The lateral wall of the pyriform sinus becomes contiguous with the posterior pharyngeal wall at the level of the posterior surface of the arytenoid cartilage. The transition between the supraglottic larynx and the pyriform sinus occurs at the lateral aryepiglottic fold.

Previously, this region had been considered by Ogura et al.[6–8] to comprise a "marginal" area between the supraglottic larynx and the hypopharynx. Marginal lesions, however, behave like pyriform sinus tumors and are therefore included within the same category.

Posterior Hypopharynx

The posterior hypopharynx consists of the expanse of posterior pharyngeal wall from the tip of the epiglottis to the cricopharyngeal muscle. The lateral boundaries, which are rather vaguely defined, are considered to be the junctions with the lateral pharyngeal wall on both sides. Because there is little lateral pharyngeal wall posterior to the pyriform sinus, the precise anatomic junction may be considered to be at the posterior border of the lateral wall of the pyriform sinus (at the level of the posterior border of the arytenoid cartilage). As a practical matter, both posterior and posterolateral pharyngeal wall tumors are treated similarly.

Postcricoid Region

Lesions classified as postcricoid carcinomas arise either on the mucosa covering the posterior surface of the cricoid cartilage anteriorly or within the circumference of the cricopharyngeal muscle. The mucosa between the arytenoid cartilages is rarely the site of origin of a tumor. Lesions of the true esophagus may be distinguished from postcricoid carcinomas by the presence, usually, of a discernible margin of normal mucosa between the lesion and the cricopharyngeal muscle. These tumors usually do not extend upward to involve the hypopharynx.

PATHOLOGY OF HYPOPHARYNGEAL TUMORS

Distribution and Frequency

Cancer of the hypopharynx is not common. It represents less than 10% of cancers of the upper aerodigestive tract and about 0.5% of all malignancies.[9] About 24% of cancers in the laryngeal-hypopharyngeal region occur in the hypopharynx.[3, 10] In the United States, pyriform sinus tumors are considerably more common than any other type of tumor.[3, 4, 11] In northern Europe, however, postcricoid carcinoma occurs with greater frequency than does malignancy of the pyriform sinus.[5, 12]

In the United States, hypopharyngeal tumors occur predominantly in men, although the incidence in women has increased.[4, 11] Postcricoid carcinomas have been noted to occur with greater frequency in women, particularly those of Irish and Scandinavian descent who have Plummer-Vinson syndrome.[12, 13] However, in Kirchner's series of eight cases reported from New Haven, Connecticut, six of the eight patients were men.[11]

The general profile of patients with hypopharyngeal cancer is similar to that of other patients with head and neck cancer. Predisposing factors include smoking tobacco and drinking alcohol. In the series reported by Carpenter et al.[4, 14], 96% of the patients were smokers and 93% were alcohol abusers. The relationship between gastroesophageal reflux and cancer has been explored recently.[15] Chronic inflammation of the hypopharynx, which is associated with reflux, combined with local and systemic insults from tobacco and alcohol, may contribute to the development of cancer in susceptible patients.

Histology

More than 95% of hypopharyngeal malignancies are epidermoid carcinomas. The remaining 5% are mostly adenocarcinomas arising from glandular structures or from islands of ectopic gastric mucosa found in the posterior hypopharyngeal wall and postcricoid region.[16] Although most hypopharyngeal tumors are squamous cell carcinomas, there is a definite tendency for hypopharyngeal tumors to be less differentiated than are laryngeal tumors. Olofsson and van Nostrand[17] reported 55% of the hypopharyngeal lesions in their series to be poorly differentiated, whereas only 13% of the laryngeal tumors in the same series were so classified. Wiernik et al.[18] reported a statistically significant difference in survival when comparing well-differentiated squamous cell carcinomas to anaplastic carcinomas. Nonetheless, Rapoport and Franco[19] reported no difference in prognosis in their series of 126 patients with hypopharyngeal tumors when histopathologic grade alone was evaluated.

Staging

The American Joint Committee[20] staging system for hypopharyngeal tumors, published in 1992, is presented in Table 9–1. Various other staging systems have been devised and used for hypopharyngeal lesions. One of the most useful systems is that devised by Sessions.[3] Regardless of the staging system used, it has been noted repeatedly that hypopharyngeal tumors tend to be large and rather advanced when first diagnosed.[5, 21] Kirchner and Owen[10] classified the tumors from only 11 of 120 patients with pyriform sinus carcinoma as stage T1 or stage T2, whereas the remaining 109 tumors

were staged as T3 tumors. Laccourreye et al.[22] reported 34 lesions staged as T2 tumors in a series of 167 patients with pyriform sinus carcinoma. Florant et al.[23] found a total of 46 cases of stage T1 or stage T2 pyriform carcinomas within a large series. In their series of patients, Carpenter et al.[4] noted the distribution, by stages, for hypopharyngeal tumors to be as follows: stage I, 12 tumors (7%); stage II, 42 tumors (26%); stage III, 82 tumors (51%); and stage IV, 26 tumors (16%).

The late diagnosis of these tumors is probably related to the late appearance of symptoms from the primary tumor, as well as to the rich lymphatic supply of the hypopharynx. Even lesions that appear to be relatively small may prove to be more extensive. Harrison[5] noted that TNM staging is often inaccurate for hypopharyngeal tumors, because extension or fixation of the tumors to surrounding structures may be impossible to detect. In more than 40% of the cases in Harrison's series, the true extent of the lesions was underestimated preoperatively. The tendency for hypopharyngeal tumors to spread submucosally, considerably beyond their apparent mucosal margins, was noted by Hiroto.[17] Harrison[5] found an average of 10 mm of submucosal extension in pyriform sinus tumors and 5 mm of extension for postcricoid lesions.

Behavior and Spread of Hypopharyngeal Carcinoma

Tumors of the Pyriform Sinus

Pyriform sinus tumors extend laterally through the thyroid cartilage to extralaryngeal structures and medially to the larynx. Olofsson and van Nostrand[17] noted lateral spread either through the thyroid cartilage (in 4 patients) or through the cricothyroid space (in 1 patient) in 5 out of 19 patients with pyriform sinus carcinomas. Eleven of the 19 had invasion of one or more laryngeal cartilages. The thyroid ala was the most frequently involved site. Invasion of the cricoid and the arytenoid cartilages occurred less frequently. In 20 out of 51 tissue specimens, Kirchner[11] found invasion of the thyroid cartilage, usually along the posterior edge.

Lesions involving the lateral wall are the ones that most often invade the thyroid cartilage and do so in a high percentage of cases. The apex of the pyriform sinus is usually involved in these instances. Large tumors extend onto the posterior wall of the hypopharynx, across the postcricoid region to involve the opposite side, or superiorly into the base of the tongue. The latter finding portends an ominous prognosis. Pyriform sinus tumors rarely involve the cervical esophagus.[11]

Table 9–1. STAGING SYSTEM FOR CANCER OF THE HYPOPHARYNX*

Primary Tumor (T)

Tx   Primary tumor cannot be assessed
T0   No evidence of primary tumor
Tis Carcinoma in situ
T1   Tumor limited to one subsite of the hypopharynx
T2   Tumor invades more than one subsite of the hypopharynx or an adjacent site, without fixation of the hemilarynx
T3   Tumor invades more than one subsite of the hypopharynx or an adjacent site, with fixation of the hemilarynx
T4   Tumor invades adjacent structures (e.g., cartilage or soft tisues of the neck)

Lymph Nodes (N)

Nx   Regional lymph nodes cannot be assessed
N0   No regional lymph node metastasis
N1   Metastasis in a single lymph node 3 cm or less in greatest dimension
N2   Metastasis in a single ipsilateral lymph node, more than 3 cm but less than 6 cm in greatest dimension, or in bilateral or contralateral lymph nodes, none more than 6 cm in greatest dimension
　　　N2A Metastasis in a single ipsilateral lymph node, more than 3 cm but less than 6 cm in greatest dimension
　　　N2B Metastasis in multiple ipsilateral lymph nodes, none more than 6 cm in greatest dimension
　　　N2C Metastasis in bilateral or contralateral lymph nodes, none more than 6 cm in greatest dimension
N3   Metastasis in a lymph node more than 6 cm in greatest dimension

Distant Metastasis (M)

Mx   Presence of distant metastasis cannot be assessed
M0   No distant metastasis
M1   Distant metastasis

Stage Grouping

Stage O:	Tis	N0	M0
Stage I:	T1	N0	M0
Stage II:	T2	N0	M0
Stage III:	T3	N0	M0
	T1	N1	M0
	T2	N1	M0
	T3	N1	M0
Stage IV:	T4	N0, N1	M0
	Any T	N2, N3	M0
	Any T	Any N	M1

*From Beahr OH, et al. *Manual for Staging of Cancer*, 4th ed, pp. 33–38. Philadelphia, Lippincott, 1992.

Tumors confined to the anterior and the medial walls of the pyriform sinus do not extend laterally into the thyroid cartilage but often extend medially into the larynx, causing impairment of laryngeal function. By histologic assessment of operative specimens, Tani and Amatsu[25] determined that such tumors extend medially and produce vocal cord fixation, usually by invasion of the intrinsic musculature rather than by involvement of the cricoarytenoid joint or the arytenoid cartilage. In 8 of 19 cases of pyriform sinus carcinoma, Olofsson and van Nostrand[17] found invasion of intrinsic laryngeal muscle. Intralaryngeal spread of pyriform sinus carcinoma occurs through the paraglottic space.[11, 12] Thus, once the larynx is involved, pyriform sinus carcinoma behaves similarly to transglottic carcinoma. Because the anterior wall of the pyriform sinus forms the posterior wall of the paraglottic space,[26] tumor spreads easily from one region to the other. Willatt et al.[27] demonstrated that vocal cord paralysis in postcricoid carcinoma was an important prediction of a poor prognosis.

Most pyriform sinus carcinomas have infiltrating rather than "pushing" margins. Kirchner[11] found pushing margins in only 5 of 51 tissue specimens. However, even in these few cases, pushing margins did not ensure a good prognosis, because 2 of the 5 patients died of recurrent cancer. Carbone et al.[28] recently reported on a variant of squamous cell carcinoma that they labeled "superficial extending carcinoma." This entity is a poorly or a moderately differentiated carcinoma that is predominantly mucosal. They identified 6 out of 26 primary hypopharyngeal tumors with this pathologic feature.

Pyriform sinus tumors metastasize mainly into the chain of jugular nodes.[3, 29] Olofsson and van

Nostrand[17] found positive jugular nodes in 12 of 19 specimens for which cervical node dissections were performed. Other node groups are less frequently involved. Wenig and Applebaum[30] determined that the submandibular triangle (level I) is rarely involved in hypopharyngeal carcinomas. Davidson et al.[31] found positive nodes in the posterior triangle (level V) in only 7% of 1,277 neck dissections performed for hypopharyngeal carcinoma; only 1% of necks that were clinically negative (stage N0) had positive nodes at this level. Candela and colleagues[32] reported similar results in a retrospective review of 344 radical neck dissections performed for oropharyngeal or hypopharyngeal carcinoma.

Node groups that are not removed by conventional neck dissection may be at risk for developing metastases. Extension of the tumor to the posterior hypopharynx places the retropharyngeal node of Rouvière at risk.[33, 34] Weber et al.[35] performed paratracheal lymph node dissections in 36 cases of hypopharyngeal tumor resections and found positive nodes in 8.3% of the cases. This correlated with decreased survival.

Sessions[3] found a 50% incidence of positive nodes with primary tumors 5 cm or less in diameter and an 85% incidence of positive nodes with primary tumors greater than 4 cm in diameter. Invasion of thyroid cartilage, muscle, nerve, and extralaryngeal soft tissues were found to be associated with an increased incidence of node metastases. McGavran et al.[29] found metastases in the contralateral node in approximately 10% of patients with pyriform sinus carcinoma and, at necropsy, distant metastases in about 10% to 20% of the patients.

Cure rates for pyriform sinus carcinoma vary according to the modality of therapy and the stage of the lesion being treated. Rapoport and Franco[19] performed a multivariate analysis on 16 parameters and found that only 5 of these parameters affected the prognosis significantly. These significant factors included age, odynophagia, number of clinically positive lymph nodes, number of histologically positive lymph nodes, and treatment with radiation therapy. Sessions[3] found decreased survival to be correlated with involvement of resection margins, presence of poorly differentiated tumors, invasion of thyroid cartilage, and occurrence of more than one positive lymph node.

Tumors of the Posterior Hypopharynx

Posterior pharyngeal wall carcinomas occur most frequently in elderly males and are usually large when first seen. A palpable cervical node is often the first indication of these frequently asymptomatic lesions. Widespread submucosal extension into the oropharynx and cervical esophagus is common. Deep invasion into the underlying prevertebral fascia, the muscles, or the vertebral bodies is difficult to detect. This is probably responsible for the 50% incidence of local recurrence reported by Farr and Arthur[36] for lesions treated by surgery alone. McNeill[37] reported 13 cases of posterior pharyngeal wall lesions, with local control being achieved in only 1 patient.

A characteristic feature of posterior pharyngeal wall carcinoma is its tendency to metastasize to the retropharyngeal nodes,[5, 38] as well as to the jugular chain of nodes. Another characteristic is its frequent association with a second primary tumor seen in 28 out of 164 patients.[5] These various factors combine to produce poor cure rates, ranging from 10% to 20%, for posterior pharyngeal wall carcinoma.[4, 5, 39]

Postcricoid Carcinoma

Postcricoid carcinoma constitutes a unique entity among head and neck cancers. The propensity of this tumor to occur in women has already been mentioned, although this tendency may be more pronounced in the series of cases reported from northern European clinics than in those from the United States. The increased frequency of the disease in northern Europe has also been noted. Postcricoid carcinoma has been associated with the Plummer-Vinson syndrome in female patients.[12, 40]

Postcricoid carcinomas are usually diagnosed at an advanced stage.[5, 41] Olofsson and van Nostrand[17] found invasion of the cricoid cartilage and of the posterior cricoarytenoid muscle in three of seven cases studied by whole-organ serial sectioning. Two of their patients had involvement of the recurrent laryngeal nerves. Harrison[5] has emphasized the tendency of these lesions to metastasize to the paratracheal lymph nodes, as well as to the lower deep cervical nodes. As in the case of subglottic laryngeal carcinoma, he feels that resection of the paratracheal and upper mediastinal nodes through the exposure provided by removal of the upper half of the manubrium is essential for adequate surgical treatment of these lesions. Som and Nussbaum[41] have noted that the apparent recurrence of tumor at the inferior margin of resection is actually often caused by extension of lymphatic metastatic disease. Harrison[5] has attributed treatment failure, which occurs in the majority of cases treated by total pharyngolaryngectomy, to tumor present in the esophageal stump, the paratracheal nodes, or the party wall.

Tumors of the Superior Hypopharynx

As mentioned previously, tumors of the superior hypopharynx are not included by many authors in their definition of hypopharyngeal tumors. The base of the tongue, the pharyngoepiglottic folds, and the valleculae are often considered to be parts of the oropharynx, whereas tumors of the lingual surface of the epiglottis are often considered to be supraglottic laryngeal tumors. These tumors will nonetheless be discussed in this chapter because the surgical procedures used for their treatment are variations of the procedures used to treat other hypopharyngeal tumors.

Sessions[3] found superior hypopharyngeal tumors to constitute 2.8% of all epidermoid carcinomas of the larynx and hypopharynx and approximately 9% of all hypopharyngeal tumors. Three of 12 patients followed for 3 years or more survived, free of tumor. Superior hypopharyngeal tumors are similar to oropharyngeal tumors in their tendency to be poorly differentiated and to metastasize frequently to the chain of jugular lymph nodes.

TREATMENT OF HYPOPHARYNGEAL CARCINOMA

Radiotherapy Versus Surgery

It is generally felt that surgery, either alone or in combination with preoperative or postoperative irradiation, is superior to radiotherapy alone for the treatment of hypopharyngeal tumors.[4, 5, 10, 11, 42–44] Van den Bogaert et al.[45] did not find any significant differences in the survival rates of 90 patients with hypopharyngeal carcinoma, 66 of whom received only radiotherapy. They suggested that the combined surgery-radiotherapy approach allowed for increased local control. Tandon et al.[46] reported survival rates of 62% for stage III hypopharyngeal cancer and 32.4% for stage IV hypopharyngeal cancer after combined treatment with surgery and radiotherapy. Nevertheless, some authors recommend treatment with radical radiotherapy alone, even for stage III and stage IV carcinomas, and reserve surgical resection for salvage or for completion neck dissection.[47–49]

The problem inherent to studies comparing the efficacy of radiotherapy alone to that of combined surgery and radiotherapy is that combined treatment tends to be selected only for potentially curable patients, while the radiotherapy-alone modality is employed for palliation, as well as for cure.

There are suggestions in the literature that postoperative radiotherapy may be more effective than preoperative radiotherapy for the treatment of hypopharyngeal tumors. Vandenbrouck et al.[50] conducted a randomized prospective study comparing the results of preoperative versus postoperative radiotherapy. Their results showed a statistically significant difference in favor of postoperative radiotherapy with regard to survival rates (56% 5-year survival with postoperative radiotherapy versus 20% 5-year survival after preoperative radiotherapy), complications, and quality of life for survivers. Donald et al.[51] found a greater than twofold improvement in survival when postoperative radiotherapy was compared to preoperative radiotherapy. Eisbach and Krause[42] reported a slightly lower cure rate with preoperative radiotherapy, compared with surgery alone. This was ascribed to the impairment of the surgeon's ability to determine the margins of the tumor after the radiotherapy. These authors noted a decrease in the appearance of late contralateral neck metastases in patients who had undergone the combined treatment when compared to treatment with surgery alone; this decrease was attributed to the proved effectiveness of radiotherapy in controlling subclinical neck metastases. Eisbach concluded that surgical excision of the primary tumor with adequate margins and an ipsilateral neck dissection, followed by radiotherapy to both sides of the neck, was the preferred treatment for pyriform sinus carcinoma. Further support for aggressive combined therapy has been documented in more recent studies, one of which demonstrated an almost twofold improvement in survival.[52, 53]

Table 9–2 shows the results of treatment of pyriform sinus carcinoma by the various modalities, as reported for several series of patients in the recent literature. The results of these studies indicate that, whereas surgery appears to be superior to radiotherapy alone, it remains unclear whether combined therapy improves the results achieved by surgery alone.

Chemotherapy

Although systemic chemotherapy has been used for more than two decades, there is no conclusive evidence that single or multidrug chemotherapy regimens either improve survival or decrease distant metastases. Older studies revealed discouraging results with chemotherapy for the treatment of hypopharyngeal carcinomas.[61] One report actually demonstrated a significant decrease in survival in patients treated with radiotherapy combined with multiagent chemotherapy versus survival in patients treated with radiotherapy alone.[62] A more recent study reported the results of treatment with

Table 9–2. SURVIVAL AFTER TREATMENT OF PYRIFORM SINUS CARCINOMA

Authors	Years Posttreatment	Survival: No. of Survivors/Total No. (%)		
		Radiation Therapy Alone	Surgery Alone	Combined Treatment
Kirchner[11]	3	2/55 (4%)	9/28 (32%)	12/33 (36%)
Eisbach and Krause[42]	5	3/23 (13%)	11/16 (69%)	9/16 (56%)
Harrison[5]	3	0/9 (0%)	2/14 (14%)	
Harwick[54]	5		15/59 (25%)	
Lord et al.[43]	5	5/31 (16%)		9/25 (36%)
Routh and Hickman[34]	3	3/12 (25%)		4/9 (44%)
Sasaki et al.[53]	2			13/50 (26%)
Ahmad and Fayos[48]	2.5	19/61 (31%)		3/19 (16%)
Jesse and Lindberg[55]	5		15/67 (22%)	16/49 (33%)
Donald et al.[51]	3	0/6 (0%)		14/25 (56%)
Persky and Daly[56]	5	1/18 (6%)	4/8 (50%)	6/18 (33%)
El Badawi et al.[52]	2	4/9 (44%)	81/203 (40%)	71/142 (50%)
	5		51/203 (25%)	57/142 (40%)
Yates and Crumley[57]	3		13/20 (65%)	18/36 (50%)
	5		10/18 (56%)	10/30 (33%)
Driscoll et al.[58]	3	5/26 (19%)	7/18 (39%)	16/31 (52%)
Vandenbrouck et al.[59]	3	38/152 (25%)		96/199 (48%)
	5	17/127 (13%)		66/199 (33%)
Ogura et al.[60]	3	4/33 (12%)		70/142 (49%)

combined surgery and irradiation, followed by either single-agent (bleomycin) or multiagent chemotherapy. A statistically significant increase in survival was found in the multiagent-treated group.[63]

Conservation Surgery Versus Total Laryngectomy

Hypopharyngeal tumors, known to be more aggressive, extensive, and clinically malignant than laryngeal tumors, were not generally considered suitable for conservation surgery in the past. By 1960, however, Ogura et al.[64] had concluded that in many cases of hypopharyngeal cancer little was gained by sacrificing the entire larynx. Examination of specimens obtained after total laryngectomy had revealed that in many cases of hypopharyngeal malignancy, the arytenoid cartilages and vocal cords were completely free of tumor. Because the cure rates for these lesions treated by total laryngectomy and neck dissection ranged from 32% to 37% only, it was felt that the patients' chances for survival would not be jeopardized by using conservation procedures that resect the lesion adequately while preserving the voice. In 1965, Ogura and Mallen[65] reported 5-year survival in three out of seven patients with pyriform sinus carcinoma and in three out of seven patients with superior hypopharyngeal carcinoma treated by conservation surgery. The contention that conservation surgery would not jeopardize the chances of a cure obtainable by total laryngectomy appeared true enough. In 1969,

Ogura et al.[66] reported 3-year survival in 20 out of 60 patients with pyriform sinus carcinoma treated by total laryngectomy and in 16 out of 29 patients treated by partial laryngectomy. Another report from the same institution[67] noted a 59% 5-year survival rate in 80 patients with pyriform sinus carcinoma treated by preoperative radiotherapy followed by partial pharyngolaryngectomy and a 21% 5-year survival rate in 57 patients treated by preoperative radiotherapy and total laryngectomy. The cure rates, naturally, are lower in the total laryngectomy groups, because it is the more advanced lesions that are treated with this modality.

When results for partial or total laryngectomy for similar lesions are compared, they are seen to be similar. Iwai et al.[68] achieved an overall 30% cure rate in 37 patients treated for hypopharyngeal carcinoma by total laryngectomy and radical neck dissection. Of these, the cure rates were 57% for stage T1 and 47% for stage T2 tumors. In 14 patients with stage T1 or stage T2 lesions that were treated by pharyngolaryngectomy, the cure rate was 53%. The authors concluded that conservation surgery was the preferred treatment for stage T1 and stage T2 hypopharyngeal lesions. Other authors[48, 63] would favor radiotherapy for these earlier lesions (see discussion of radiotherapy vs. surgery).

Although it appears well established that selected hypopharyngeal lesions can be adequately managed by conservation surgery, it is less certain what percentage of hypopharyngeal tumors are actually suitable for conservation surgery. The number of relatively early lesions encountered seems to vary widely. Although certain groups seem to encounter a fairly large percentage of early tumors, others consider such occurrences to be rare. Shah et al.,[44] at the Memorial Sloan-Kettering Cancer Center in New York, felt that only 46 of 301 cases of pyriform sinus carcinoma were appropriate for conservation surgery. Kirchner,[11] in his study of serial sections from 51 specimens of pyriform sinus carcinoma obtained after total laryngectomy, found only 1 lesion that might have been adequately resected by conservation surgery. The advent of newer techniques has extended the ability to resect hypopharyngeal cancers adequately without sacrificing the entire larynx.

Florant et al.[23] performed conservation surgery on 48 patients with pyriform sinus carcinoma, the majority of tumors being stage T1 or T2. These authors extended Ogura's criteria for conservative surgery to include disease on the ipsilateral arytenoid cartilage, providing vocal cord motion was not impaired. Laccourreye and colleagues[22] were able to perform supracricoid hemilaryngopharyngectomy in 34 patients with stage T2 pyriform sinus carcinoma, achieving a 5-year, cause-specific survival rate of 55.8%. Advocates of "near-total laryngectomy" recommend that procedure for tumors not suitable for conservation surgery.[69, 70] Contraindications include bilateral vocal cord fixation, postcricoid involvement, or extension to the posterior commissure (see chapter 8).

SURGICAL PROCEDURES FOR HYPOPHARYNGEAL CARCINOMA

The surgical procedures performed for hypopharyngeal carcinoma are outlined in Table 9–3. The proximity of hypopharyngeal mucosa to the larynx and the tendency, previously discussed, for many hypopharyngeal tumors to invade the larynx make resection of at least that portion of the larynx that is in continuity with adjacent hypopharyngeal structures mandatory for the management of most tumors. In certain instances, particularly with tumors confined to the posterior or posterolateral pharyngeal wall, the resection may be confined to the hypopharyngeal wall without involving the larynx.

The hypopharynx is entirely surrounded by bone and cartilage (as are the mesopharynx and nasopharynx). Thus, all approaches for conservation surgery involve division or removal of portions of the laryngeal skeleton or of the mandible.

Reconstruction after resection of hypopharyngeal tumors, whether by partial or by total laryngectomy, is more complicated than for laryngeal tumors. The defects in hypopharyngeal mucosa often

---

Table 9–3. SURGICAL PROCEDURES FOR HYPOPHARYNGEAL CARCINOMA

Conservation Surgery
  Lateral pharyngotomy approach
    Resection of benign tumors
    Partial pharyngolaryngectomy for superior hypopharyngeal tumors
    Partial pharyngolaryngectomy for pyriform sinus tumors
    Partial pharyngectomy for posterolateral hypopharyngeal wall tumors
  Anterior pharyngotomy approach
    Limited excision of superior hypopharyngeal tumors
    Limited excision of posterior wall tumors
  "Mandibular swing" or median labiomandibular glossotomy approach
    Limited excision of superior hypopharyngeal tumors
    Limited excision of posterior pharyngeal wall tumors
Procedures Requiring Total Laryngectomy
  Extended total laryngectomy
  Total pharyngolaryngectomy
    —with partial esophagectomy
    —with total esophagectomy

---

cannot be closed primarily, and temporary fistulae, skin grafts, or skin and mucosal flaps may be required. The frequent use of pedicled myocutaneous flaps and, more recently, of microvascular free flaps has obviated many of the previously encountered reconstruction problems. For resections involving the entire larynx, the hypopharynx, and various portions of the esophagus, or in the case of a total pharyngolaryngectomy-esophagectomy (TPL-E), elaborate procedures are required to restore alimentary continuity by constructing a new pharyngoesophageal segment. The various methods used to accomplish this are discussed in detail in Chapter 10.

Conservation Surgery for Hypopharyngeal Tumors

The Lateral Pharyngotomy Approach

The lateral approach to the hypopharynx is by far the most useful and versatile for treatment of malignant lesions. This is the approach originally described by Trotter[71] from which the supraglottic subtotal laryngectomy (SSL) and other related procedures evolved. The history of this surgery and its use for treatment of supraglottic laryngeal tumors have been described in detail in Chapters 1 and 6. The lateral pharyngotomy approach, in which the hypopharynx is entered either through the bed of the mobilized hyoid bone or through the upper half of the thyroid cartilage, provides excellent access to lesions of the superior hypopharynx, the pyriform sinus, or the posterolateral pharyngeal wall. It is also useful for the resection of various benign tumors.

Resection of Benign Lesions

Exposure of the hypopharynx for resection of various benign lesions in the superior hypopharynx, the supraglottic region, the arytenoid cartilage, or the ventricle may be obtained by mobilizing and resecting the greater cornu of the hyoid bone and the upper half of the thyroid cartilage. Because there is no need to maintain continuity of the specimen, the bone and the cartilage may be removed separately from the operative field, thereby providing easy access to the structures to be resected. Submucosal masses, such as laryngoceles or ventricular cysts, may often be resected without incising the pharyngeal mucosa. Other lesions, particularly of the vallecula and the epiglottis, require mucosal incision and closure by direct suture or by a perichondrial flap, if the mucosa is deficient anteriorly.

In 1966 we reported the results of treatment of a variety of benign lesions by this approach, including fibrolipoma of the arytenoid, ventricular cyst, desmoid tumor, and laryngocele.[72] More recently, we further detailed our experience in cases of paraganglioma, hemangiopericytoma, and saccular cysts.[73, 74] Other authors have used lateral pharyngotomy for the management of a variety of benign lesions.[75–78]

Figure 9–1A. The surgical approach to a supraglottic paraganglioma of the larynx is shown. The patient presented with an extramucosal supraglottic mass, completely obstructing the larynx, and required a tracheostomy. The endoscopic view is shown in this figure. A biopsy attempted at another institution was non-diagnostic. A second attempt at biopsy, during endoscopic examination on our service, led to considerable bleeding, which required packing through the laryngoscope, while we proceeded with the resection.

Figure 9–1A₁. The relationship of the tumor to the mucosa and the cartilage are demonstrated in this transverse section. The tumor was situated between the supraglottic mucosa and the upper half of the thyroid cartilage. The relationships of this tumor were similar to those of a ventricular cyst or a laryngocele.

Figure 9–1B. The operation commenced with the ligation of the superior laryngeal vessels (not shown), which controlled bleeding from the biopsy site. Following this, the superior half of the thyroid ala was skeletonized, and a perichondrial flap was reflected inferiorly, as for supraglottic subtotal laryngectomy. The greater cornu of the hyoid bone was resected and discarded, providing access to the hypopharyngeal mucosa, which was incised, exposing the epiglottis, and permitting inspection of the laryngeal mucosal aspect of the tumor.

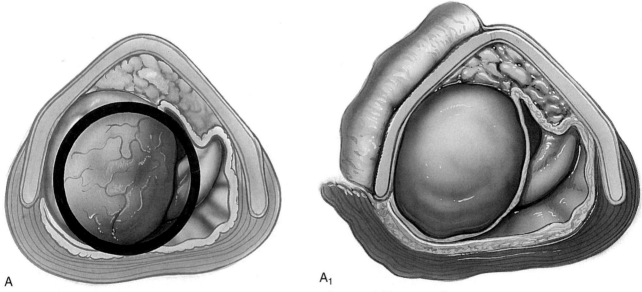

A   A₁

Figure 9–1. Lateral pharyngotomy for supraglottic paraganglioma.

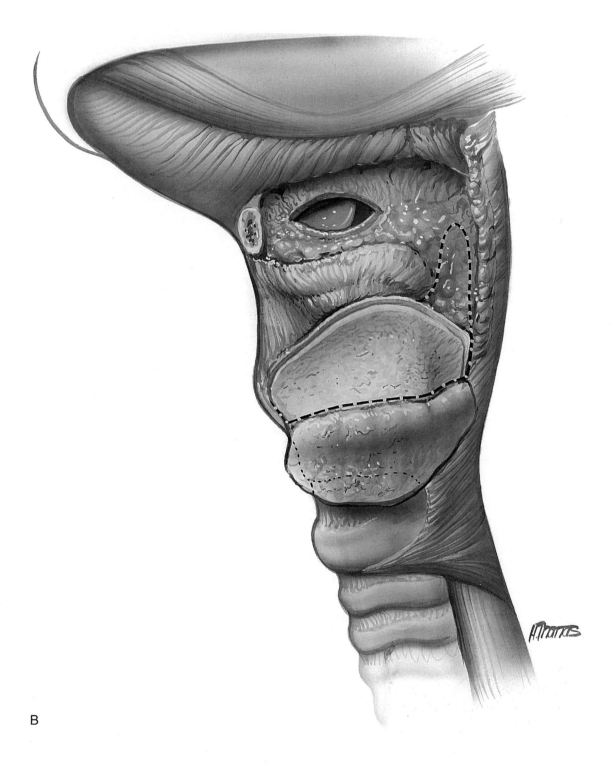

Figure 9–1 *Continued* Lateral pharyngotomy for supraglottic paraganglioma.

Illustration continued on following page

B

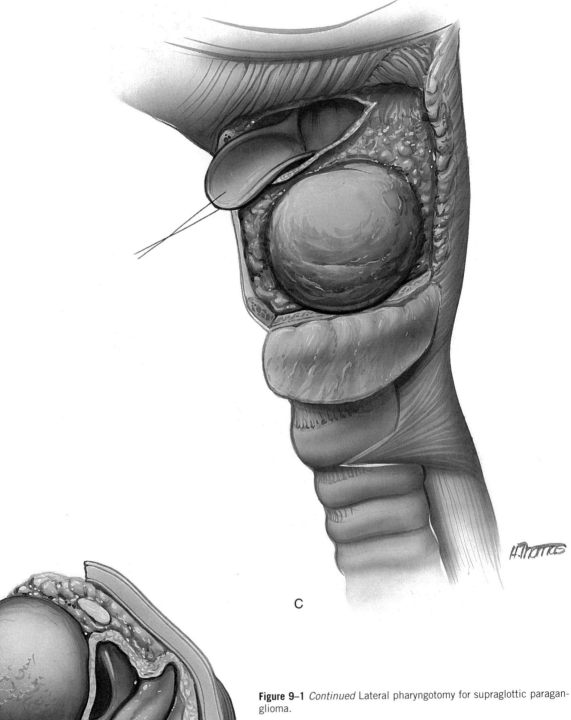

C

C₁

Figure 9–1 *Continued* Lateral pharyngotomy for supraglottic paraganglioma.

Figures 9–1*C* and 9–1*C₁*. The removal of the upper half of the thyroid cartilage exposed the tumor. Complete extramucosal removal was now accomplished. The tumor could have been removed without pharyngotomy, but the ability to visualize both the intra- and the extramucosal aspects of the region facilitated safe resection.

Figures 9–1*D* and 9–1*D₁*. The pharyngotomy was closed with interrupted sutures, after which the perichondrial flap was sutured to the tongue base, providing a second layer of closure. The infrahyoid muscles were approximated to the suprahyoid muscles, in the bed of the resected hyoid cornu, adding a third layer. Following the procedure, airway obstruction was completely relieved, and laryngeal function returned to normal. The patient has been disease-free for 10 years.

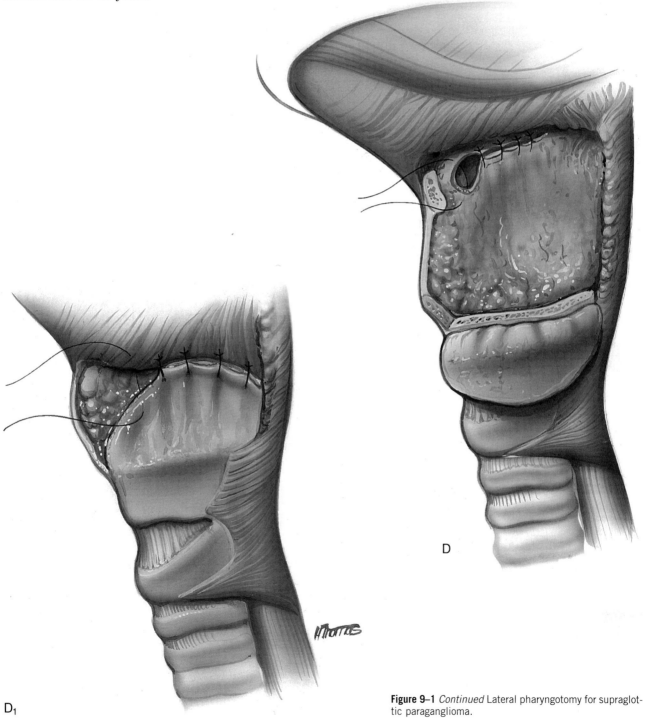

D₁

D

Figure 9–1 *Continued* Lateral pharyngotomy for supraglottic paraganglioma.

Partial Pharyngolaryngectomy for Superior Hypopharyngeal Tumors

In 1965 Ogura and Mallen[65] reported the results of treatment of 15 superior hypopharyngeal cancers by extended supraglottic subtotal laryngectomy. The procedure was used mainly for lesions confined to the valleculae, usually involving the lingual surface of the epiglottis, without extensive infiltration into the base of the tongue. Lesions of 3 cm or less in diameter were felt to be the most appropriate ones for resection by this approach. Massive lesions involving both sides of the valleculae and extending to the circumvallate papillae were considered unsuitable. The authors reported 5-year survival in three out of the seven patients.

We have used partial pharyngolaryngectomy (PPL) on our service for treatment of superior hypopharyngeal tumors and agree with Ogura and Mallen's guidelines for surgery. As with all forms of conservation surgery, caution should be exercised when dealing with radiotherapy failures because of the difficulty of determining tumor margins in the irradiated base of the tongue and difficulties in closing the large anterior-superior defect.

Figure 9–2A. These are transverse and sagittal views showing a lesion in the superior hypopharynx and the line of resection. The specimen will include the base of the tongue, the epiglottis, and the upper half of the thyroid cartilage.

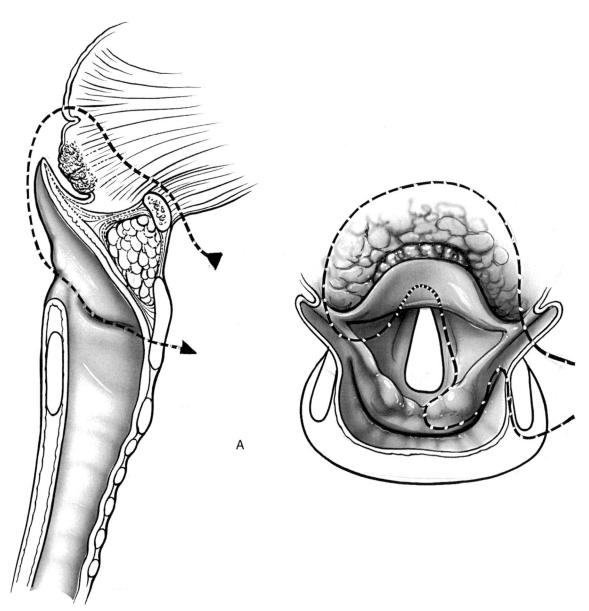

A

Figure 9–2. Partial pharyngolaryngectomy for tumor of the superior hypopharynx.

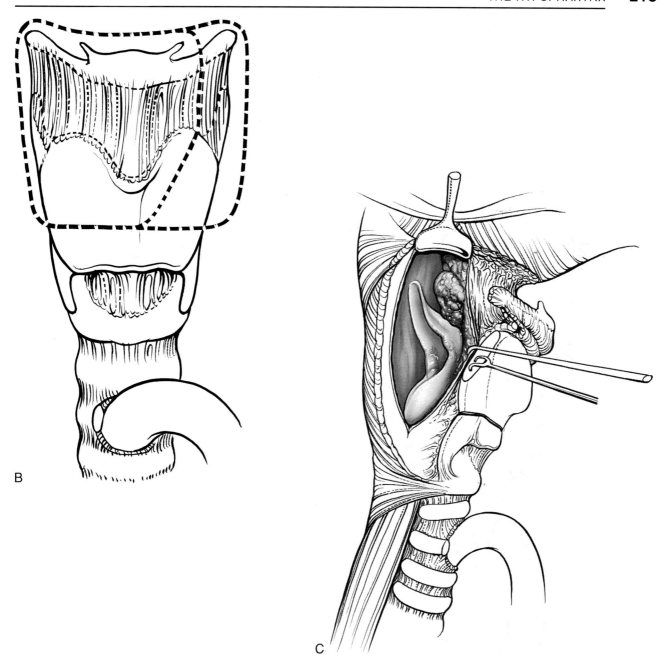

B

C

Figure 9–2 *Continued* Partial pharyngolaryngectomy for tumor of the superior hypopharynx.

Illustration continued on following page

Figure 9–2B. Bone and cartilage cuts are shown. For a lesion localized to one side, these cuts are the same as for SSL. For more extensive lesions involving both valleculae, the entire hyoid complex and the upper halves of both thyroid alae may be resected.

Figure 9–2C. The initial steps in the operation are basically the same as for SSL (see Figs. 6–1A through 6–1H). The hypopharynx is entered posteriorly through the pyriform sinus mucosa, exposing the supraglottic structures and the tumor in the valleculae.

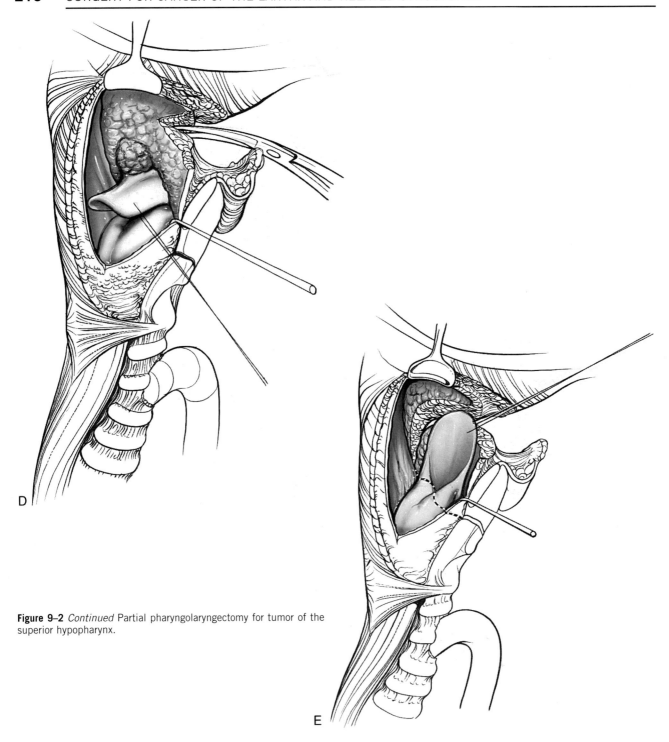

Figure 9–2 *Continued* Partial pharyngolaryngectomy for tumor of the superior hypopharynx.

Figure 9–2D. The epiglottis is retracted downward with a suture. The incision through the base of the tongue is outlined with electrocautery and deepened by cautery or with scissors.

Figure 9–2E. With the tongue incision completed, the remainder of the resection is similar to SSL. Incisions are made through the ipsilateral and then through the contralateral aryepiglottic fold, the false cord, and the ventricle.

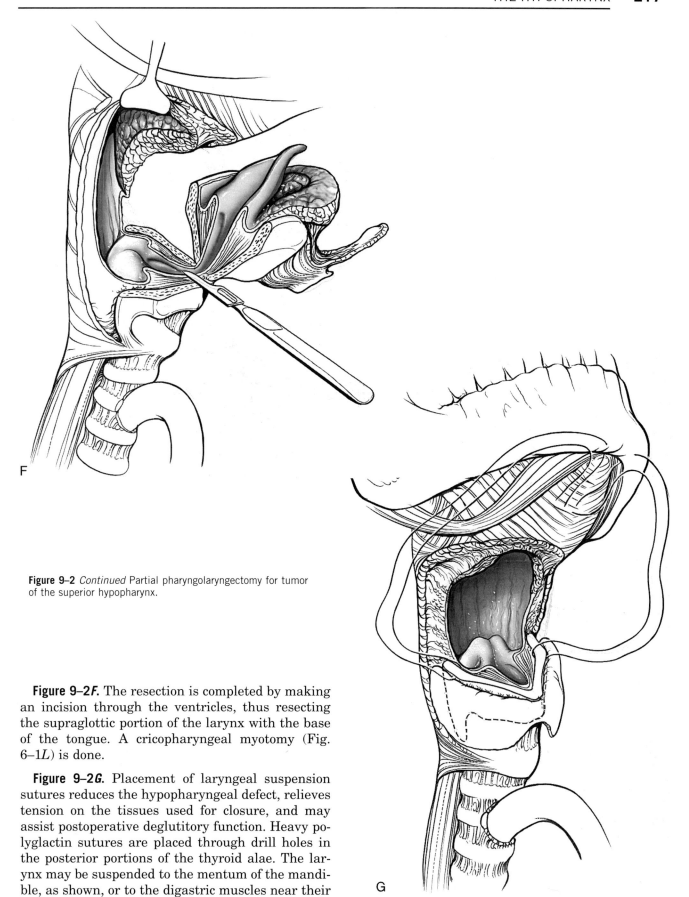

Figure 9–2 *Continued* Partial pharyngolaryngectomy for tumor of the superior hypopharynx.

Figure 9–2F. The resection is completed by making an incision through the ventricles, thus resecting the supraglottic portion of the larynx with the base of the tongue. A cricopharyngeal myotomy (Fig. 6–1*L*) is done.

Figure 9–2G. Placement of laryngeal suspension sutures reduces the hypopharyngeal defect, relieves tension on the tissues used for closure, and may assist postoperative deglutitory function. Heavy polyglactin sutures are placed through drill holes in the posterior portions of the thyroid alae. The larynx may be suspended to the mentum of the mandible, as shown, or to the digastric muscles near their insertion into the mentum.

Illustration continued on following page

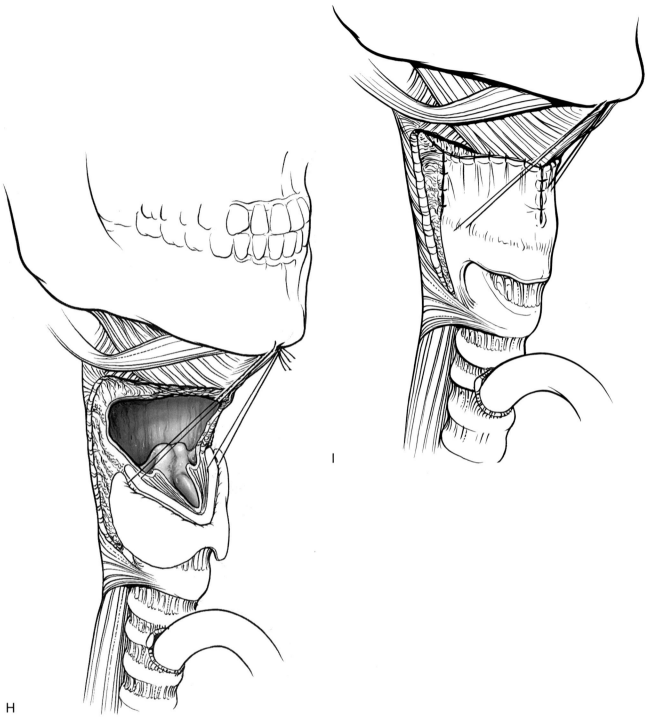

Figure 9–2 *Continued* Partial pharyngolaryngectomy for tumor of the superior hypopharynx.

Figure 9–2H. The suspension sutures are tied, elevating the larynx and tilting it slightly forward.

Figure 9–2I. The hypopharynx is closed by approximation of the mucosae and suture of the perichondrial flap as for SSL. The infrahyoid muscles are sutured to the suprahyoid muscles, as with SSL.

Partial Pharyngolaryngectomy for Pyriform Sinus Tumors of the Medial Wall

Resection of selected pyriform sinus tumors by PPL was reported in 1960 by Ogura et al.[64] in a series of 13 patients. Seven of these lesions were on the medial wall and were resected by an extended SSL that included resection of the arytenoid cartilage. Lesions confined to the lateral wall of the pyriform sinus were managed by the same partial pharyngectomy technique as was used for posterior wall tumors. In 1986, Florant et al.[23] reported the results of 48 pyriform carcinomas treated by PPL.

The technique used for medial wall tumors is useful for lesions of the aryepiglottic fold and lesions involving the anterior wall. It is not useful for lesions involving the lateral or the posterior aspect of the cricoid. The true cords and the arytenoid cartilages must be freely mobile and free of gross tumor involvement, the apex of the pyriform sinus must be uninvolved by tumor, and the thyroid cartilage must be uninvolved. Edema of the arytenoid cartilage is not a contraindication to this procedure.[64]

The results of PPL for the treatment of pyriform sinus tumors have been discussed earlier in this section.

Figure 9–3A. These are views showing the lesion on the medial wall of the right pyriform sinus and the line of resection. The specimen will include the upper half of the right thyroid ala, the epiglottis, the right false cord, the aryepiglottic fold, the arytenoid cartilage, and the mucosa of the upper half of the right pyriform sinus.

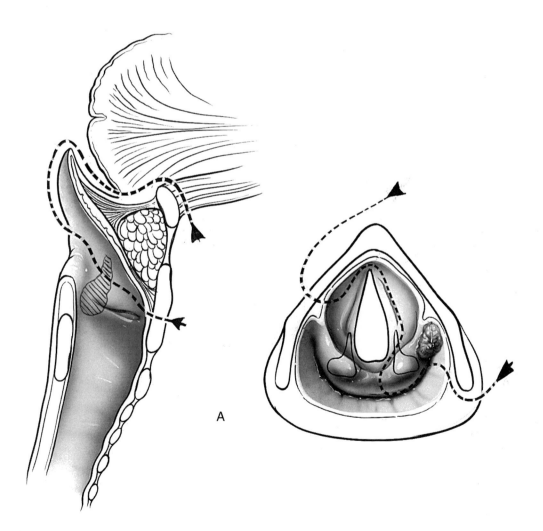

A

Figure 9–3. Partial pharyngolaryngectomy for tumor of the pyriform sinus.

Illustration continued on following page

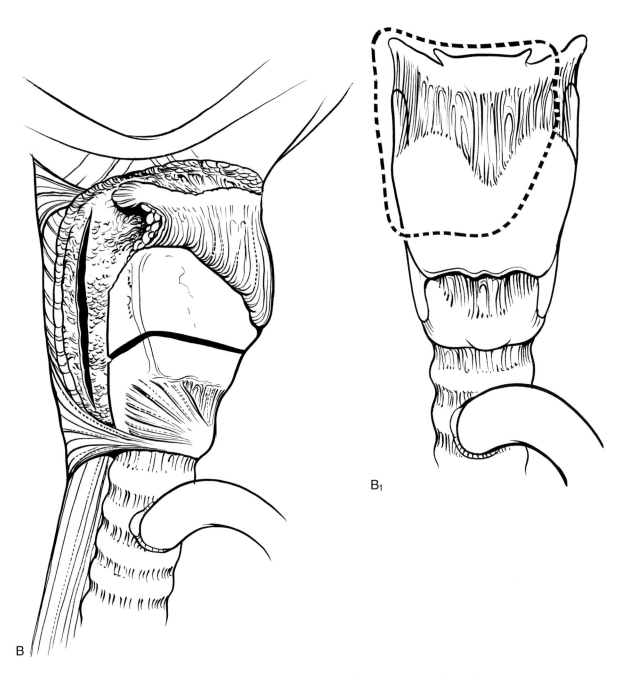

Figure 9–3 *Continued* Partial pharyngolaryngectomy for tumor of the pyriform sinus.

Figures 9–3*B* and Figure 9–3*B₁*. The bone and cartilage cuts are shown. The incision in the right thyroid ala is angled posteriorly in order to remove more of the cartilage over the pyriform sinus. The hypopharynx is entered through the lateral wall of the pyriform sinus.

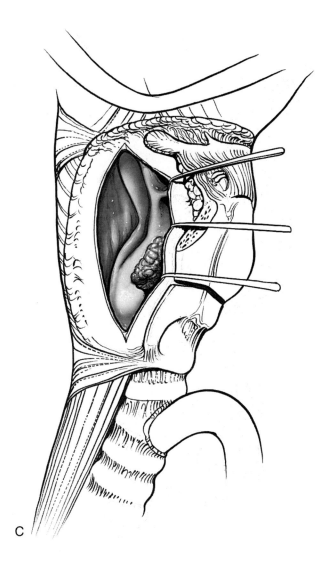

C

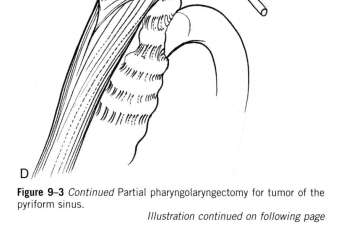

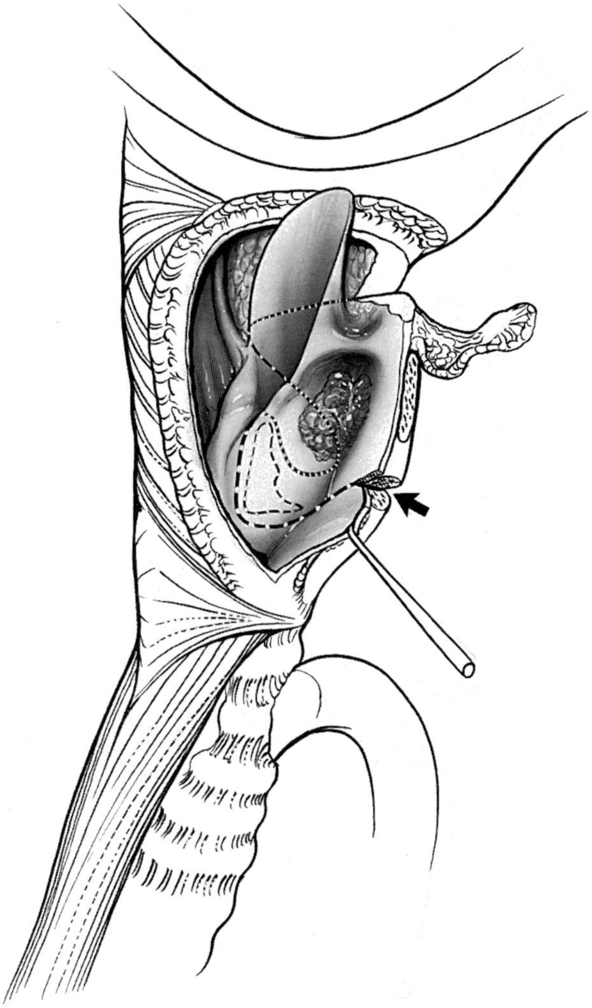

D

Figure 9–3 *Continued* Partial pharyngolaryngectomy for tumor of the pyriform sinus.

Illustration continued on following page

Figure 9–3C. The tumor on the medial wall of the pyriform sinus is exposed through the hypopharyngeal incision.

Figure 9–3D. The pharyngotomy is enlarged superiorly by incision through the valleculae and inferiorly by incision of the lateral pyriform sinus mucosa transversely to correspond with the thyrotomy incision. The incision in the pyriform sinus mucosa will continue around the anterior reflection of the mucosa and then posteriorly on the medial wall of the pyriform sinus, well below the tumor. The incision will curve over the cricoarytenoid joint into the interarytenoid region. This procedure is not indicated for lesions that extend below the cricoarytenoid joint into the apex of the pyriform sinus.

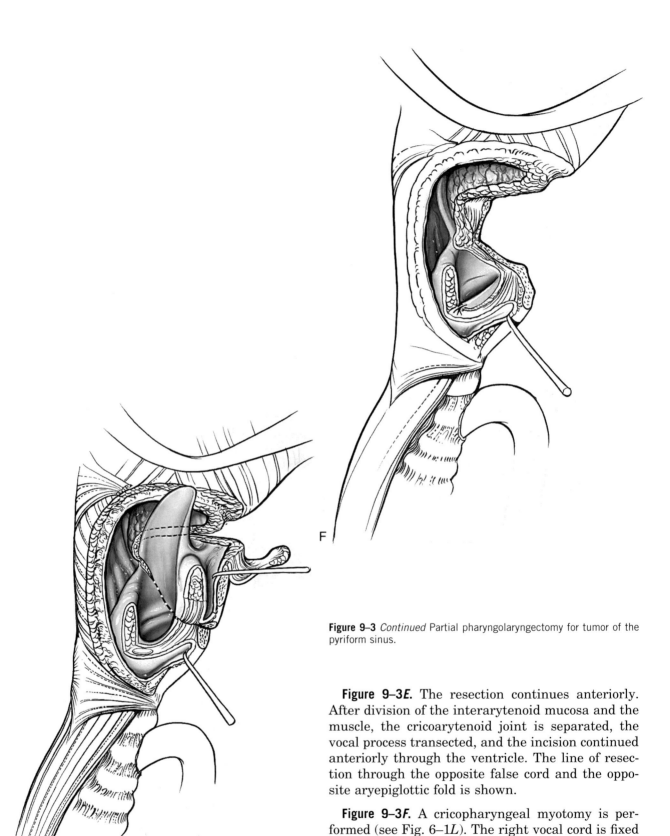

F

E

Figure 9–3 *Continued* Partial pharyngolaryngectomy for tumor of the pyriform sinus.

Figure 9–3E. The resection continues anteriorly. After division of the interarytenoid mucosa and the muscle, the cricoarytenoid joint is separated, the vocal process transected, and the incision continued anteriorly through the ventricle. The line of resection through the opposite false cord and the opposite aryepiglottic fold is shown.

Figure 9–3F. A cricopharyngeal myotomy is performed (see Fig. 6–1*L*). The right vocal cord is fixed to the midline of the cricoid lamina with a suture (see Fig. 6–2*C*).

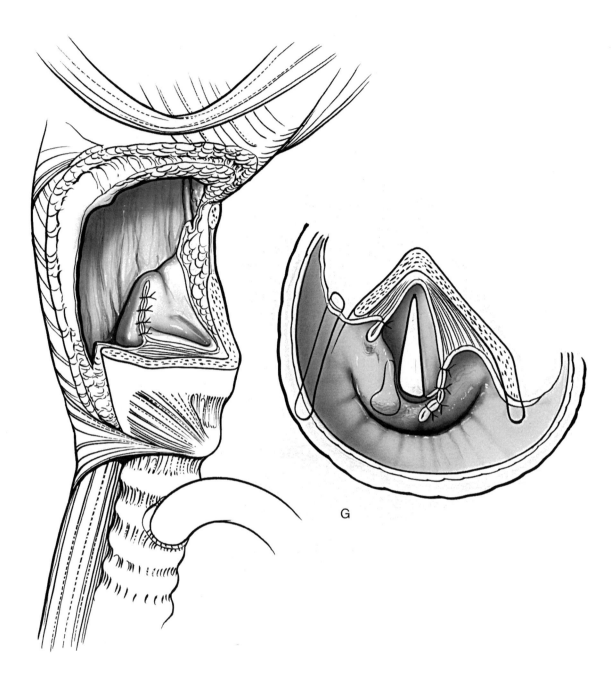

Figure 9–3 *Continued* Partial pharyngolaryngectomy for tumor of the pyriform sinus.

Figure 9–3*G.* The larynx is resurfaced as much as possible by suturing the cut edges of the hypopharyngeal and the pyriform sinus mucosae to the interarytenoid, the false cord, and the ventricular mucosa. The remaining steps in closure are identical to those for SSL (see Figs. 6–1*M* through 6–1*R*).

Partial Pharyngectomy for Posterolateral Hypopharyngeal Wall Tumors

Reference has been made to the series of 13 patients with pyriform sinus tumors treated by Ogura et al.[64] by conservation surgery. Six of these lesions were confined to the lateral or the posterolateral wall and were managed by a different technique than the medial wall lesions. The technique and the results were reported separately.[79] In 1966, we described a similar technique.[72]

The basis for the procedure is the fact that lymphatic drainage from the posterior and the lateral pharynx is lateral to the cervical nodes, rather than toward the larynx. Laryngeal involvement in advanced cases is caused by retrograde lymphatic spread or by local invasion.[79] Thus, in early cases confined to the posterolateral wall, a wide local excision of the tumor without resection of the larynx is feasible without cutting through the potential lymphatic pathway of the lesion.

Preoperative evaluation is most important in the selection of cases for partial pharyngectomy. The procedure is appropriate for tumors on the posterior or the posterolateral wall of the hypopharynx extending from above the cricopharyngeal muscle to the level of the tip of the epiglottis or to a slightly higher position. It is not indicated for lesions involving the oropharynx. Computed tomography (CT) and direct endoscopy are used to determine the superior and inferior extent of the lesion. CT is also helpful in ruling out obvious vertebral invasion. Ogura et al.[79] have emphasized that the tumor must be mobile over the bony posterior wall. This is best determined during the endoscopic examination.

Ogura's group reported good short-term results in five of six cases presented in their original 1960 report. In a later series, reported in 1969 from the same institution,[66] the authors documented only two cases of pharyngeal wall carcinoma treated by partial laryngectomy, with one patient having a 3-year survival. McNeill[37] reported 13 cases of pharyngeal wall carcinoma in 1981, with local control being achieved in only 1 patient. The literature contains other sporadic case reports, mostly to illustrate various methods of reconstruction.

Figure 9–4A. This is a transverse view showing a lesion on the right posterolateral wall of the hypopharynx. The specimen will include the posterior third of the thyroid ala, the lateral wall of the pyriform sinus, and as much of the posterior pharyngeal wall as is required for an adequate resection margin. The greater cornu of the hyoid bone may be included in the surgical specimen or, if more convenient, can be detached and discarded.

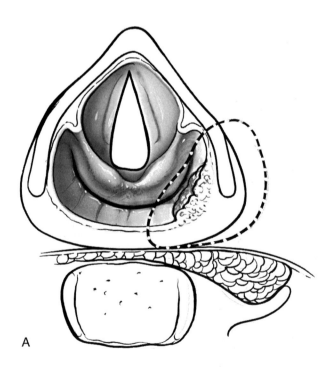

A

Figure 9–4. Partial pharyngolaryngectomy for tumor of the posterolateral hypopharyngeal wall.

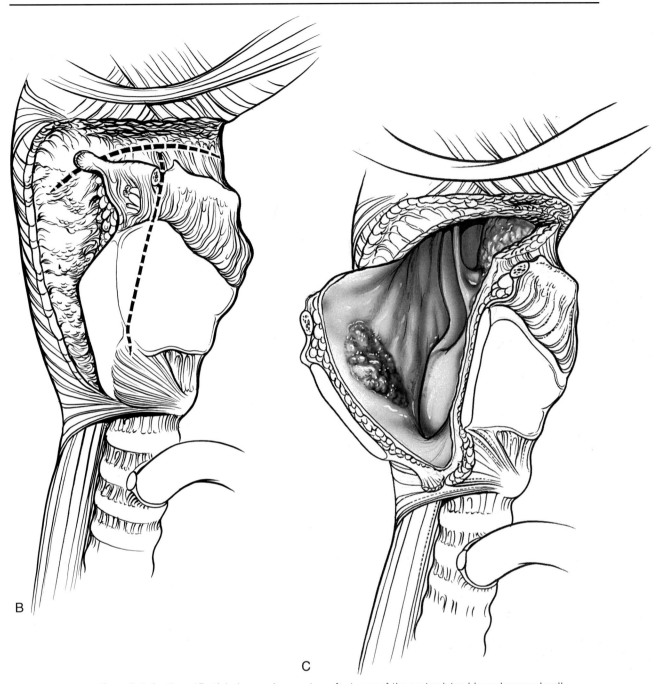

B

C

Figure 9–4 *Continued* Partial pharyngolaryngectomy for tumor of the posterolateral hypopharyngeal wall.

Illustration continued on following page

Figure 9–4B. The bone and cartilage cuts and the line of the mucosal incision are shown. The thyroid ala is incised in a vertical oblique direction, separating the posterior third from the anterior two thirds. The line of incision conforms to the underlying pyriform sinus. The superior cornu of the thyroid ala is discarded for convenience, and the inferior cornu is detached from the cricoid cartilage by avulsing the joint.

Figure 9–4C. The hypopharynx is entered through the valleculae near the anterior midline. This may be facilitated by inserting a finger through the mouth into the valleculae. The incision is extended posteriorly along the bed of the greater cornu, with care taken to maintain an adequate resection margin. The incision is extended inferiorly along the anterior reflection of the pyriform sinus mucosa. The specimen is reflected outward as shown, revealing the tumor.

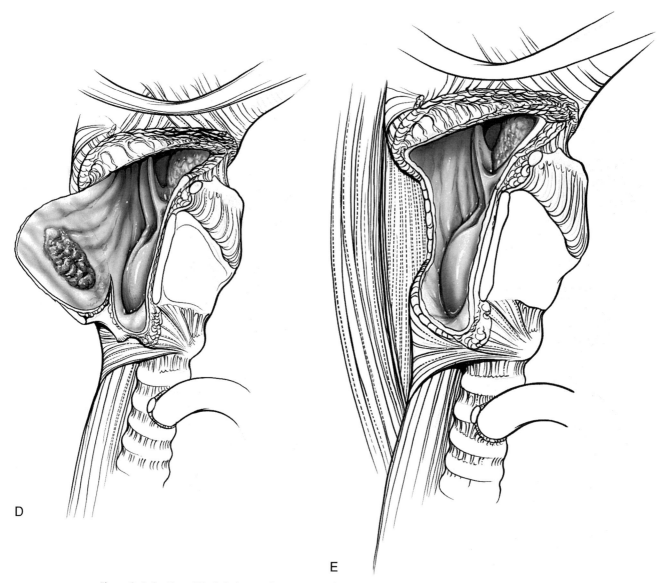

D

E

Figure 9–4 *Continued* Partial pharyngolaryngectomy for tumor of the posterolateral hypopharyngeal wall.

Figure 9–4D. The specimen is further mobilized. The line of resection is indicated by the dotted line. Externally, the pharynx is mobilized by developing the plane between the inferior constrictor muscle and the prevertebral fascia.

Figure 9–4E. The pharyngeal defect after removal of the specimen is shown. If the defect is not too large, primary closure is possible. In the past we have employed stented skin grafts placed over the long muscle of the neck for defects too large for primary closure.[80] These closures would often result in fistulae and could not be used in previously irradiated patients. The major pectoral muscle myocutaneous flap has also been employed for large defects in the posterolateral pharyngeal wall, but in cases in which the larynx has been preserved, the bulky adynamic and insensate flap has precluded swallowing without aspiration.

Use of Vascularized Free Flaps for Reconstruction of Hypopharyngeal Defects

The ability to transfer and revascularize islands of skin or mucosa has provided a more satisfactory means of reconstructing defects in the oral cavity and the pharynx with thin pliant tissue that provides a close match to the resected tissue in shape and thickness. Preservation and restoration of sensory innervation of the flap may help restore normal function. The radial forearm fasciocutaneous free flap is ideal for reconstruction in this region. It is particularly useful in irradiated tissue beds because of its excellent vascularity. Several authors have described the use of the radial forearm flap as a patch graft for hypopharyngeal repair.[81–84] Free segments of jejunum, opened on the antimesenteric border and used as a patch, have also been employed.

The principles of flap revascularization are shown in Figure 9–5. It is our intent not to provide a detailed method for microsurgical free flap transfer, but merely to indicate the sources of blood supply for the reimplanted tissue. All vascular anastomoses are performed under a microscope, and the donor tissue may be harvested from various fasciocutaneous or visceral sites. As will be discussed below, free tissue transfer is of value in complete pharyngoesophageal replacement, as well as in replacement of the large pharyngeal defects that result after total laryngectomy for hypopharyngeal tumors.

Figure 9–5A. The most direct method of graft placement is by anastomosis of the donor artery and the donor vein to adjacent recipient vessels. In this instance, the superior thyroid artery is anastomosed "end-to-end" to the graft artery, while the graft vein is inserted "end-to-side" into the internal jugular vein.

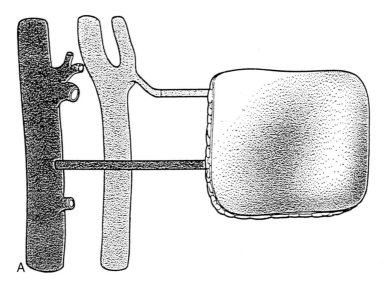

Figure 9–5. Revascularization of free graft. *(A)* "End-to-end."

Illustration continued on following page

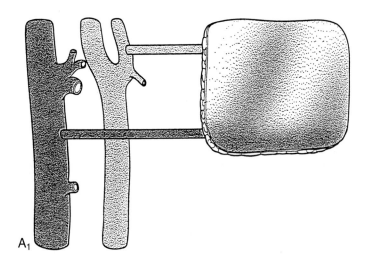

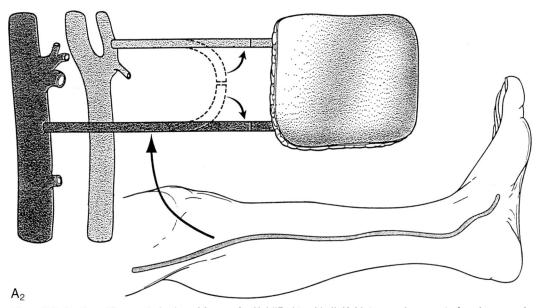

Figure 9–5 *Continued* Revascularization of free graft. *(A₁)* "End-to-side." *(A₂)* Interposed segment of saphenous vein.

Figure 9–5A₁. The graft vessel is anastomosed end-to-side to the external carotid artery, as well as end-to-side to the internal jugular vein. This approach is preferred in many instances where the superior thyroid artery is not accessible or not of adequate length or caliber for satisfactory use.

Figure 9–5A₂. Often the graft needs to be situated too far from the recipient vessels for direct anastomosis. This is less likely with radial forearm flaps, where a generous length of radial artery can be harvested, than with flaps from other donor sites.

Nevertheless, if direct anastomosis of vessels cannot be readily accomplished, pedicle length can be increased by interposing a segment of saphenous vein between the graft and the recipient vessels. The vein segment is harvested from the leg and anastomosed in a loop, end-to-side from the external carotid artery to the internal jugular vein. The venous loop is then occluded at both anastomoses and is divided at an appropriate length. The venous and the arterial ends are anastomosed to the graft vein and the graft artery respectively.

Free Radial Fasciocutaneous Flap for Hypopharyngeal Reconstruction

The procedure shown is a modification of that described by Urken et al.[83] The flap carries with it the medial and the lateral antebrachial cutaneous nerves, which may be anastomosed to branches of the greater auricular nerve to reestablish sensation in the reconstructed defect of the pharyngeal mucosa. A portion of the flap is deepithelialized and connected to a "monitor" segment, which is exteriorized on the skin surface. Testing of the monitor segment establishes the presence of sensation in the flap. At a second stage, the authors resect the exteriorized segment of skin. In a more recent publication,[84] the same group modified the graft so that only a subcutaneous fascial segment intervened between the pharyngeal paddle and the small monitor segment. The subcutaneous fascial segment served to cover the graft and the recipient vessels, producing less bulk than the original deepithelialized portion.

Figures 9–6A and 9–6A₁. The radial flap is harvested from the nondominant forearm because of the availability of a long segment of radial artery; the medial and lateral antebrachial cutaneous nerves are preserved. The donor site is covered with a skin graft.

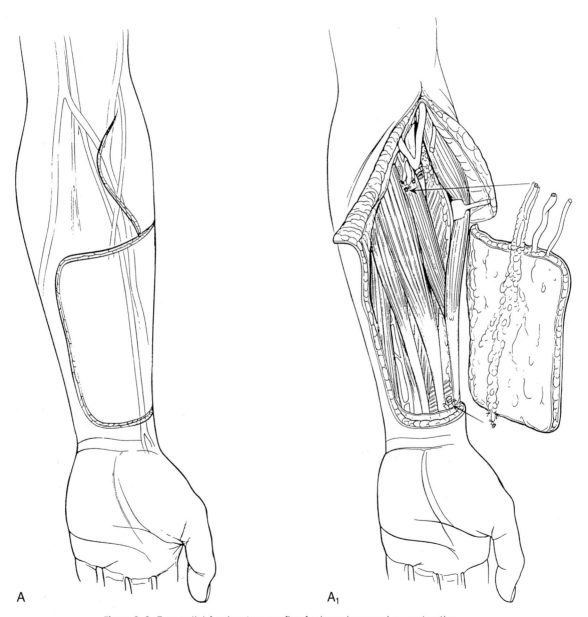

A

A₁

Figure 9–6. Free radial fasciocutaneous flap for hypopharyngeal reconstruction.

Illustration continued on following page

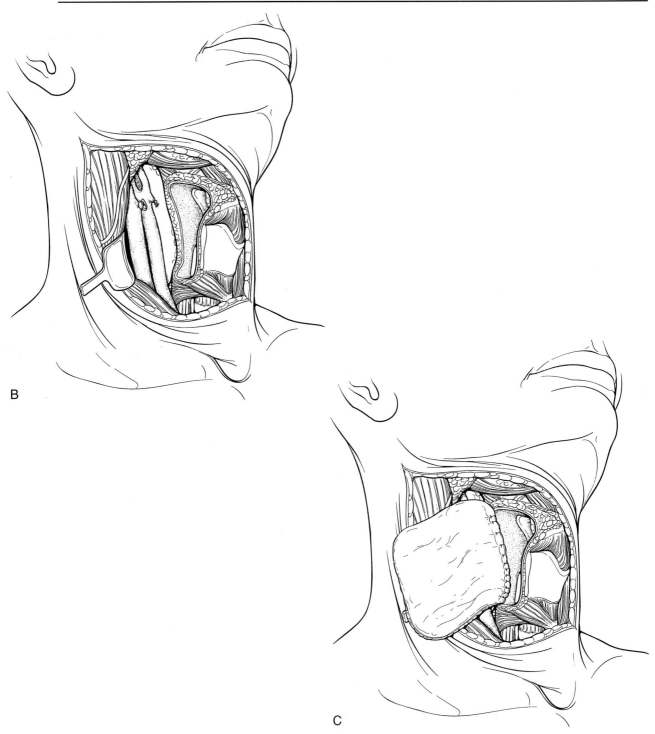

B

C

Figure 9–6 *Continued* Free radial fasciocutaneous flap for hypopharyngeal reconstruction.

Figure 9–6B. The donor site after resection is shown. Note that the superior thyroid artery and the common facial veins have been ligated. The defect is somewhat larger than that shown in Figure 9–4E but represents the same stage of resection.

Figure 9–6C. The skin flap is sutured to the posterolateral wall of the defect.

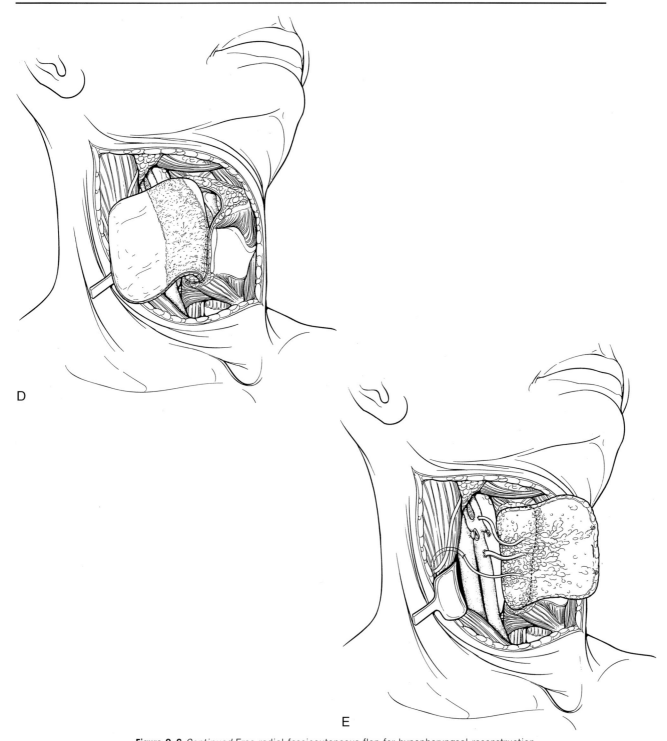

D

E

Figure 9–6 *Continued* Free radial fasciocutaneous flap for hypopharyngeal reconstruction.

Illustration continued on following page

Figure 9–6*D.* The skin lateral to the portion used for pharyngeal closure is deepithelialized. In a more recent modification, this portion of skin is removed completely, creating a bilobed flap with only subcutaneous tissue and fascia between the two skin paddles.

Figure 9–6*E.* The vascular anastomoses are shown: the radial artery anastomosed end-to-side to the external carotid artery, and the antebrachial vein anastomosed end-to-side to the internal jugular vein. The great vessels and the anastomoses will be covered by the deepithelialized or the fascial-subcutaneous portion of the flap.

Figures 9–6*F***, 9–6***G***, and 9–6***H***.** The monitor paddle is trimmed into a small ellipse and is incorporated into the skin wound, where it will reflect the vascular and neurologic status of the buried portion of the flap.

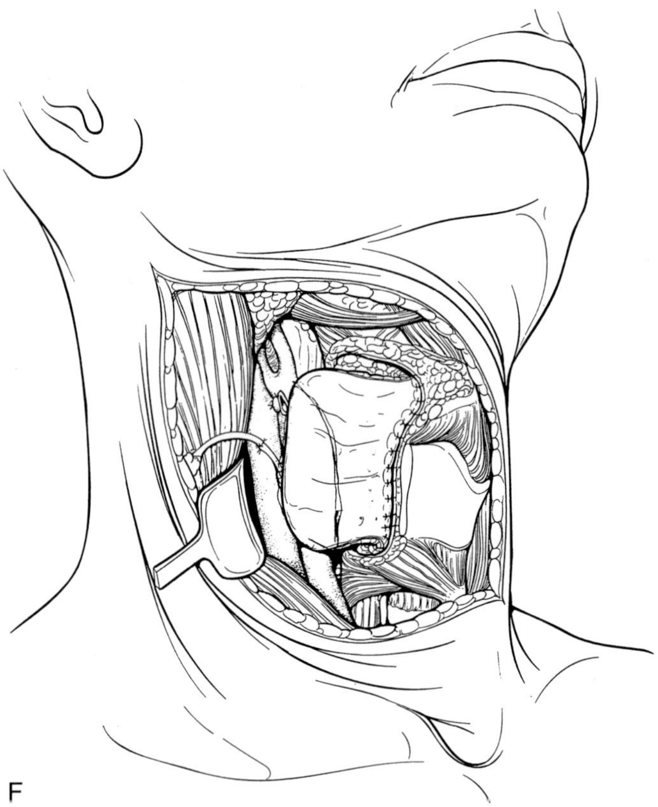

F

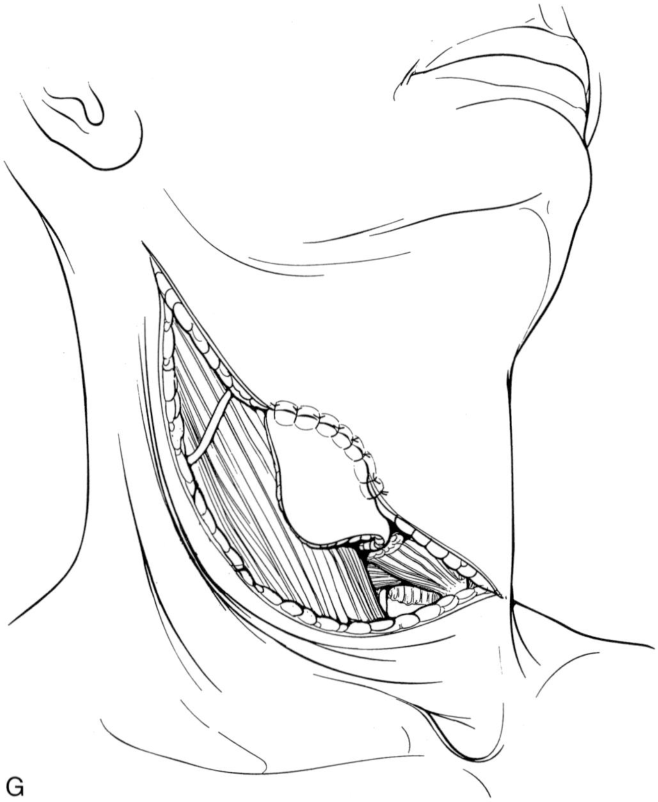

G

Figure 9–6 *Continued* Free radial fasciocutaneous flap for hypopharyngeal reconstruction.

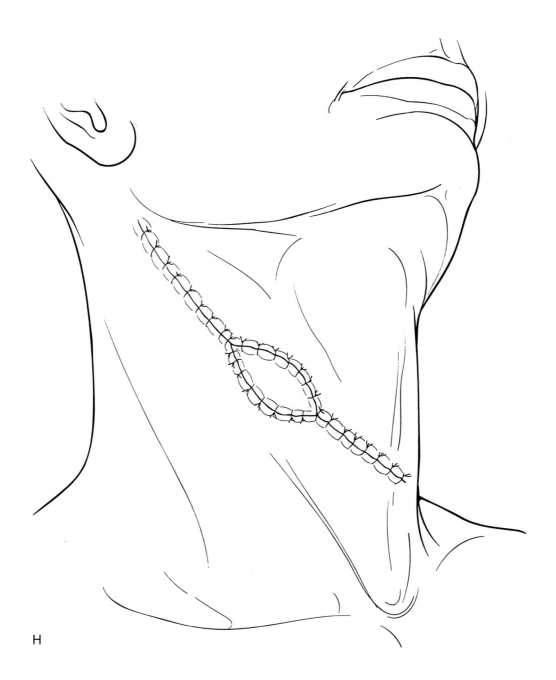

H

Figure 9–6 *Continued* Free radial fasciocutaneous flap for hypopharyngeal reconstruction.

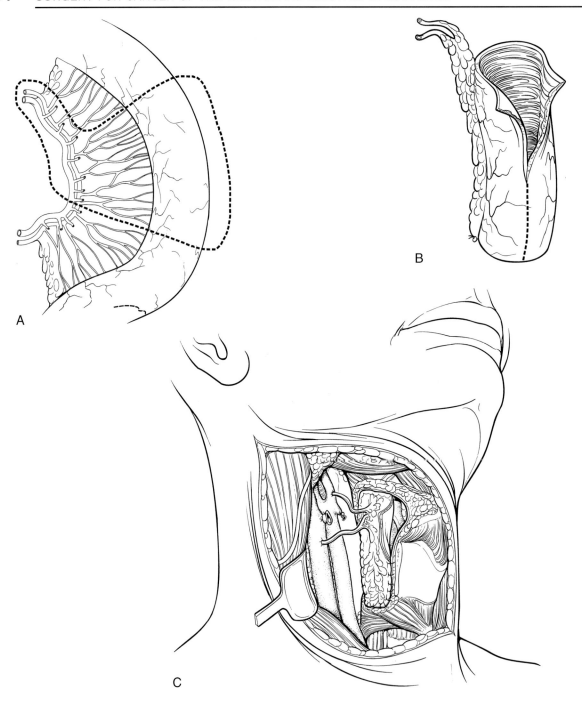

Figure 9–7. Free jejunal patch for hypopharyngeal reconstruction.

Free Jejunal Patch for Closure of Hypopharyngeal Defect

A "patch" of jejunum, pedicled on its mesenteric vessels and opened on the antimesenteric border, may be employed for closure of a defect in the posterolateral pharyngeal wall.

Figure 9–7A. The jejunal segment is harvested with its vascular arcades and mesenteric vessels in a manner similar to that employed for esophageal replacement (see Chapter 10), except that a shorter segment is employed. The defect in the jejunum is closed by end-to-end anastomosis.

Figure 9–7B. The jejunal segment is further trimmed to size and opened along its antimesenteric border.

Figure 9–7C. The pharyngeal defect is closed with the revascularized jejunal patch. Vascular anastomoses are to the external carotid artery and the internal jugular vein.

The Transhyoid Approach: Anterior Transhyoid Pharyngotomy

Perhaps the simplest surgical approach to the hypopharynx is through or adjacent to the body of the hyoid bone. With this approach, the pharynx is entered in the valleculae and, although the exposure provided is limited, access to the epiglottis, the base of the tongue, and the posterior pharyngeal wall is possible. A review of the history of this subject has been presented by Blassingame.[85] According to him, the approach was originally suggested by Vidal de Cassis in 1826. Most of the early experience with anterior pharyngotomy was acquired by the treatment of attempted suicides. Jermitsch, in observations made on these patients, noted minimal bleeding and a favorable tendency for wound healing.[85] By 1906, Spizharny reported good results with the elective use of this procedure for the resection of tumors. He emphasized careful resuturing of the geniohyoid and the mylohyoid median raphe. At the same time, however, the procedure was criticized by Grunwald, an influential writer, who reported a series of six cases.[85] Grunwald did not resuture the pharyngeal mucosa or repair the muscle, and his patients had postoperative deglutitory problems caused by sagging of the larynx. Grunwald's criticism resulted in the abandonment of the procedure for almost 50 years.

In 1949, the approach was revived by Portman[86] for resection of malignant lesions of the valleculae and the base of the tongue. In 1950, Kloop and Delaney[87] noted the technical simplicity of the procedure and the fact that transection of major neurovascular structures was avoided. They used anterior pharyngotomy for resection of a large granuloma of the lateral pharyngeal wall, a carcinoma of the posterior wall, and a small melanoma of the epiglottis. Blassingame,[85] in 1952, refuted the validity of Grunwald's objections to the procedure and demonstrated that satisfactory functional results were obtained with the use of antibiotics and layer suturing of the muscles. He used anterior pharyngotomy for resection of a huge lymphoid tumor of the posterior pharyngeal wall, two carcinomas of the posterior third of the tongue, a lingual thyroid, and a hemangioma of the posterior third of the tongue. The transhyoid approach may also be used for tumors of the base of the skull and the nasopharynx.

Although the exposure obtained by anterior pharyngotomy is more limited than by other approaches, it is possible to resect fairly large benign lesions by proper retraction. For treatment of malignant disease, however, the field of resection afforded by anterior pharyngotomy is rarely adequate. As has been discussed, it is not possible to resect the entire preepiglottic space by this approach, and therefore, it should not be used even for small epiglottic carcinomas.

Figure 9–8A. This is a composite sagittal view showing two lesions suitable for resection by anterior pharyngotomy. These lesions include a small lesion localized to the tip of the epiglottis and a lesion of the posterior pharyngeal wall at the level of the hyoid bone. This approach is applicable for lesions that do not require wide resection margins. It does not usually permit adequate resection of squamous cell carcinoma.

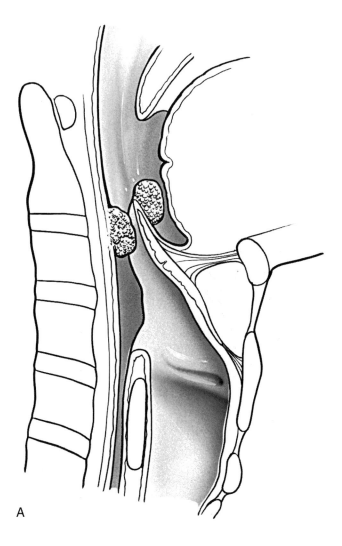

A

Figure 9–8. Anterior transhyoid pharyngotomy.

Illustration continued on following page

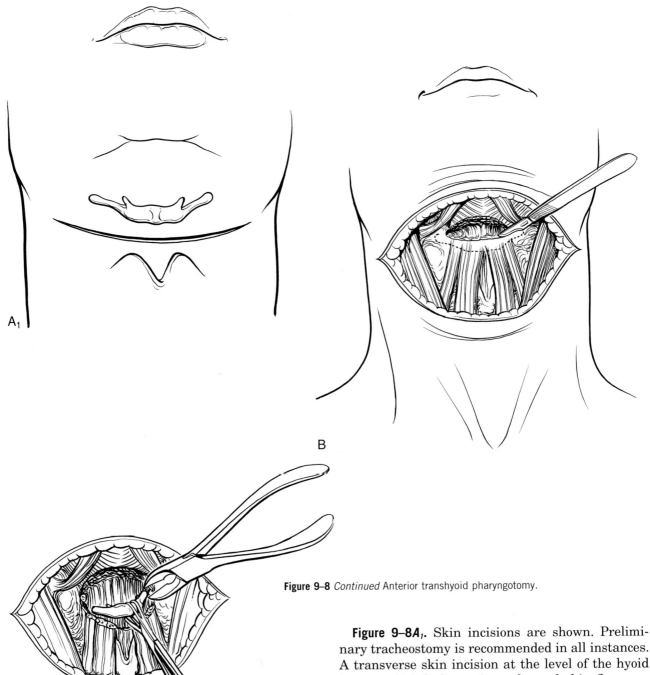

A₁

B

C

Figure 9–8 *Continued* Anterior transhyoid pharyngotomy.

Figure 9–8A₁. Skin incisions are shown. Preliminary tracheostomy is recommended in all instances. A transverse skin incision at the level of the hyoid bone or slightly lower is made, and skin flaps are developed.

Figure 9–8B. A transhyoid or a suprahyoid approach may be chosen. For either approach, the initial step consists of severing the attachments of the suprahyoid muscles from the hyoid bone.

Figure 9–8C. Resection of the body of the hyoid bone (the transhyoid approach) may permit wider retraction of the pharyngotomy opening and easier closure. The infrahyoid muscles are detached from the hyoid bone. Junctions of the body and the greater cornua of the hyoid bone are transected with a bone cutter.

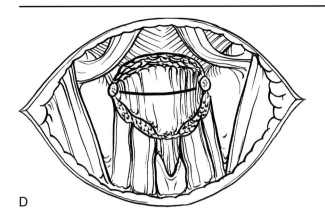

D

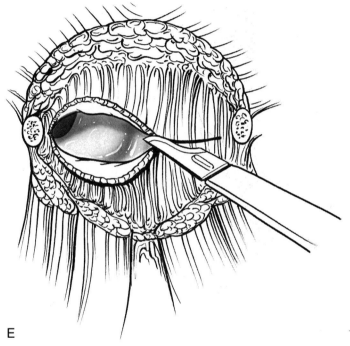

E

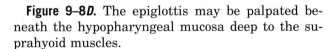
Figure 9–8 *Continued* Anterior transhyoid pharyngotomy.

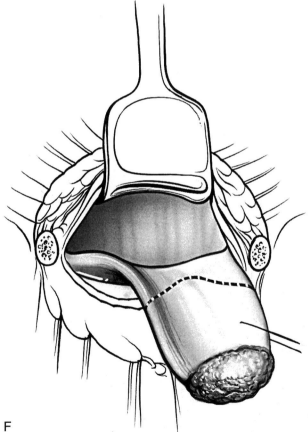

F

Illustration continued on following page

Figure 9–8*D*. The epiglottis may be palpated beneath the hypopharyngeal mucosa deep to the suprahyoid muscles.

Figure 9–8*E*. The hypopharynx is opened into the valleculae, revealing the lingual surface of the epiglottis.

Figure 9–8*F*. The epiglottis is delivered through the mucosal incision. The line of transection is shown.

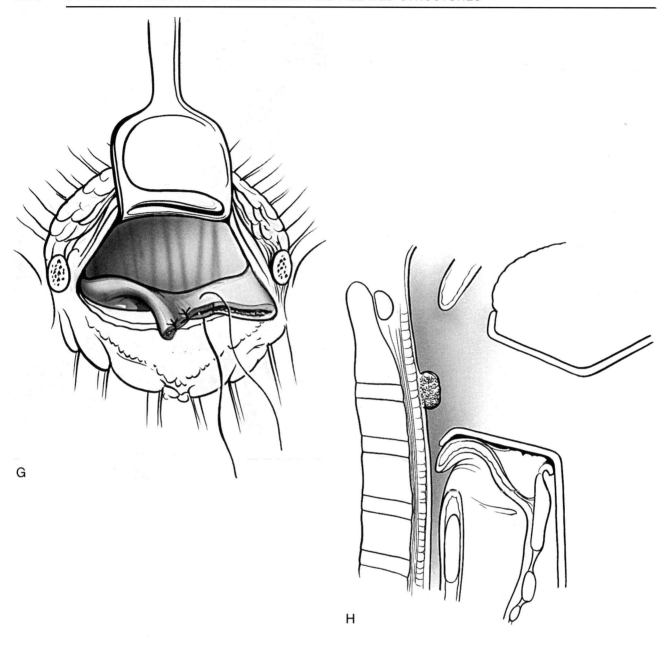

Figure 9–8 *Continued* Anterior transhyoid pharyngotomy.

Figure 9–8G. After resection of the suprahyoid portion of the epiglottis, a few sutures may be placed in the cut surface, approximating the lingual and the laryngeal surface mucosae, if possible.

Figure 9–8H. To approach a lesion of the posterior pharyngeal wall, retractors are placed in the pharyngotomy incision.

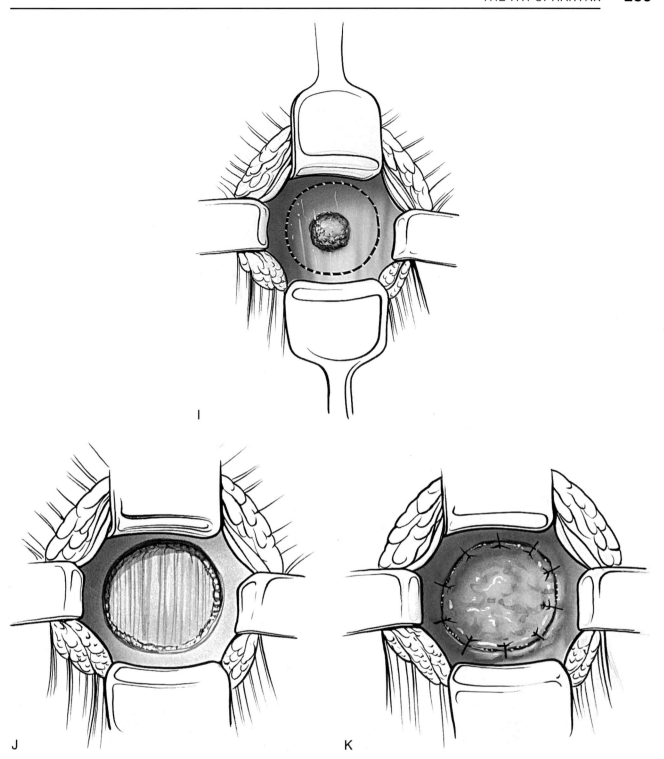

I

J

K

Figure 9–8 *Continued* Anterior transhyoid pharyngotomy.

Illustration continued on following page

Figure 9–8*I***.** The line of circumferential incision in the posterior pharyngeal mucosa is outlined.

Figure 9–8*J***.** The defect in the posterior pharyngeal mucosa after resection is shown. Usually, the resection will have been confined to the mucosal and the submucosal layers. The posterior pharyngeal defect may be left open to granulate.

Figure 9–8*K***.** If preferred, a split-thickness skin graft may be sutured into the defect in the pharyngeal mucosa.

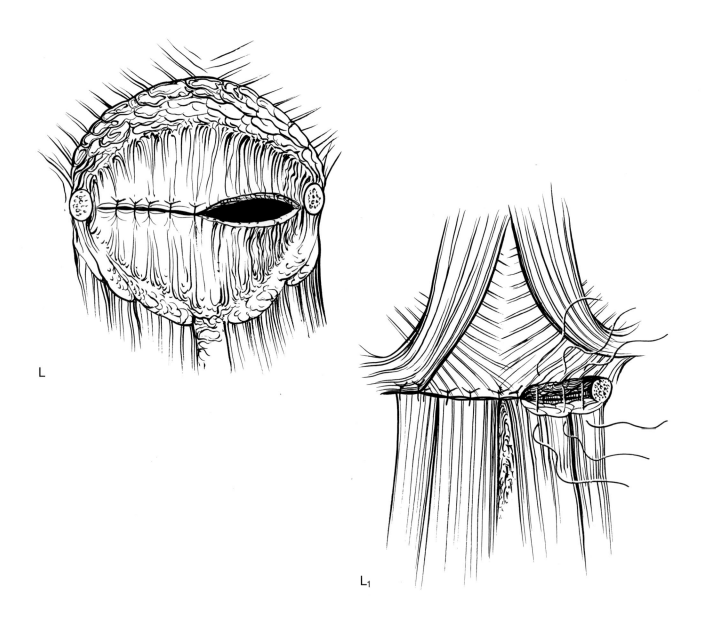

L

L₁

Figure 9–8 *Continued* Anterior transhyoid pharyngotomy.

Figure 9–8*L* and *L₁*. The pharyngotomy is closed in layers. The mucosa is repaired first, after which the infrahyoid muscles are sutured to the suprahyoid muscles.

The Transmandibular Approach

Certain lesions of the posterior pharyngeal wall, the base of the tongue, and the valleculae are best approached by dividing the lower lip and the mandible in the midline. Wilfred Trotter,[88] in 1929, described a median labiomandibular glossotomy that carried the incision through the midline of the tongue, where access was provided to the tongue base, the epiglottis, or the posterior pharyngeal wall. Despite the apparently grotesque nature of this procedure, the cosmetic and functional results were excellent because the midline incision avoided transection of the major neurovascular structures and also avoided entry into the neck on either side. More recently, at Memorial Hospital in New York, Martin et al.[89] and Tollefsen and Spiro[90] employed Trotter's approach for carcinoma of the base of the tongue or carcinoma of the posterior pharyngeal wall. The authors found that the operation was feasible in only 1.5% of the patients with cancer of the base of the tongue (5 out of 330 patients) and 4.3% of the patients with carcinoma of the pharyngeal wall (8 out of 186 patients) treated at that institution during the period under study.

The currently favored "mandibular swing" approach is a variant of the median labiomandibular glossotomy because the soft tissue incision proceeds laterally along the floor of the mouth, rather than through the substance of the tongue. The lingual nerve often must be sacrificed in order to fully mobilize the hemimandible, but there is less tongue edema and morbidity than with the median approach. The midline mandibulotomy is a particularly useful approach for lesions of the tongue base and also provides access to the posterior pharyngeal wall, the nasopharynx, the hypopharynx, and the epiglottis. As with transhyoid pharyngotomy, this approach is not useful for resection of supraglottic laryngeal carcinomas.

Figure 9–9A. Mandibulotomy is useful for the resection of tumors of the base of the tongue and the valleculae. Tumor bulk is not of importance in determining the suitability of this approach, although the amount of tissue resected will determine whether primary closure will be used or whether a flap will be necessary for repair. The lesion shown here is a 4-cm stage T2 tumor of the tongue base, extending posteriorly from the circumvallate papillae on the left side.

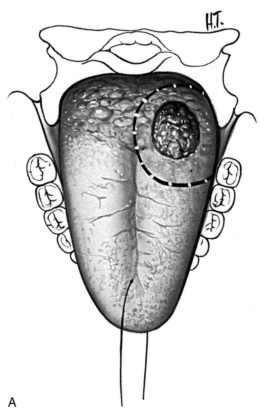

A

Figure 9–9. "Mandibular swing" approach for tumor of the base of the tongue.

Illustration continued on following page

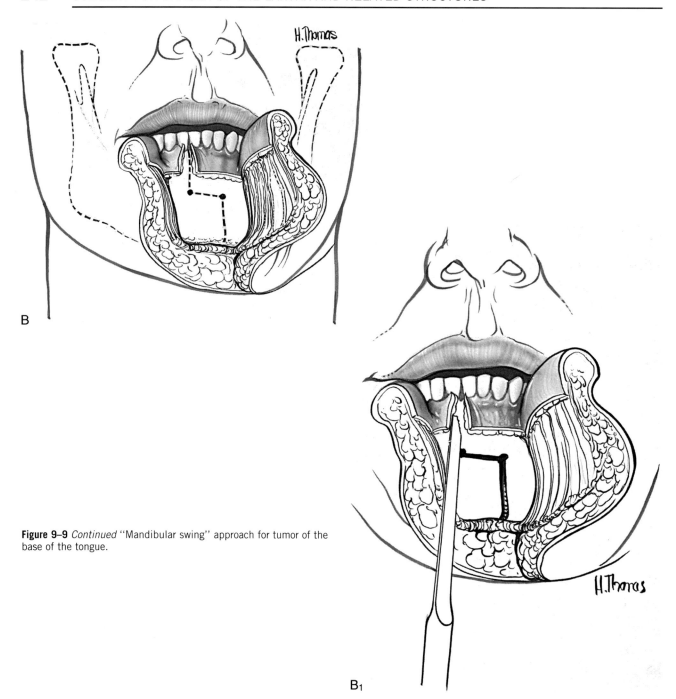

B

B₁

Figure 9–9 *Continued* "Mandibular swing" approach for tumor of the base of the tongue.

Figure 9–9B. The lower lip is bisected in the midline, and the lower cheek flaps are developed in each direction only as far as necessary for mandibulotomy and subsequent application of a reconstruction plate. Preoperative dental films indicate the location of roots of the teeth, and the osteotomy is designed to avoid exposure of either root. If the midline roots are too close together, the osteotomy may be moved laterally between two more favorable teeth, as long as it is medial to the mental nerve.

The incision is made in a steplike manner to provide vertical stability. The reconstruction plate is applied and holes are drilled prior to mandibulotomy, in order to preserve correct occlusion. A "compression" plate would take the teeth out of the occlusion by deviating them medially.

Figure 9–9B₁. A fine osteotome wedged between the roots of the teeth helps complete accurate division of the mandible.

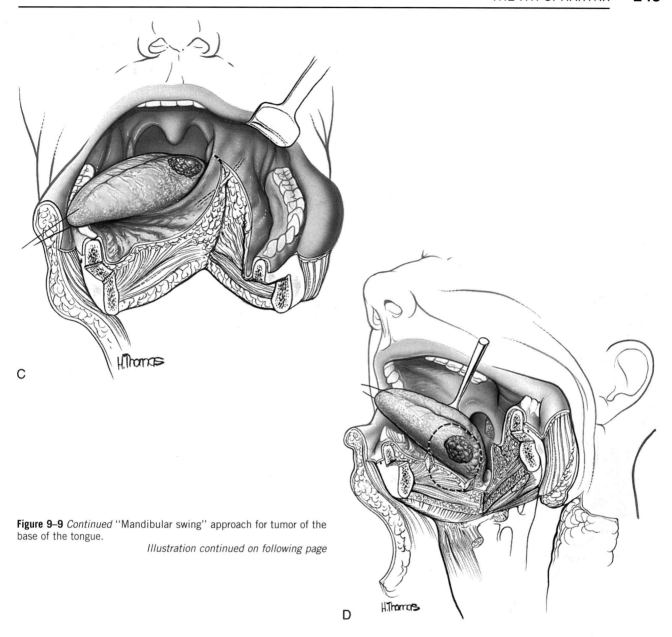

C

H.Thomas

Figure 9–9 *Continued* "Mandibular swing" approach for tumor of the base of the tongue.

Illustration continued on following page

D

H.Thomas

Figure 9–9C. The mucosa and the musculature of the floor of the mouth are incised in the sulcus between the tongue and the mandible. Small gingival flaps may be created to prevent the mucosal suture line from overlapping the osteotomy site. It is not essential to resect the submandibular contents in order to perform this procedure, although in many cases these structures will have been removed during neck dissection. The lingual nerve is shown here crossing from the pterygoid region to the tongue. Although it is possible to preserve this structure by mobilizing and retracting it, this is recommended only for the treatment of benign tumors. For excision of a malignant tumor of the tongue or the hypopharynx, sacrifice of the lingual nerve is essential.

Figure 9–9D. Incision through the tonsillar pillar affords wide exposure of the tongue base with the tumor. The line of resection is outlined. Sizeable tumors are resected in continuity with the hyoglosseal muscle and other deep structures of the submandibular region.

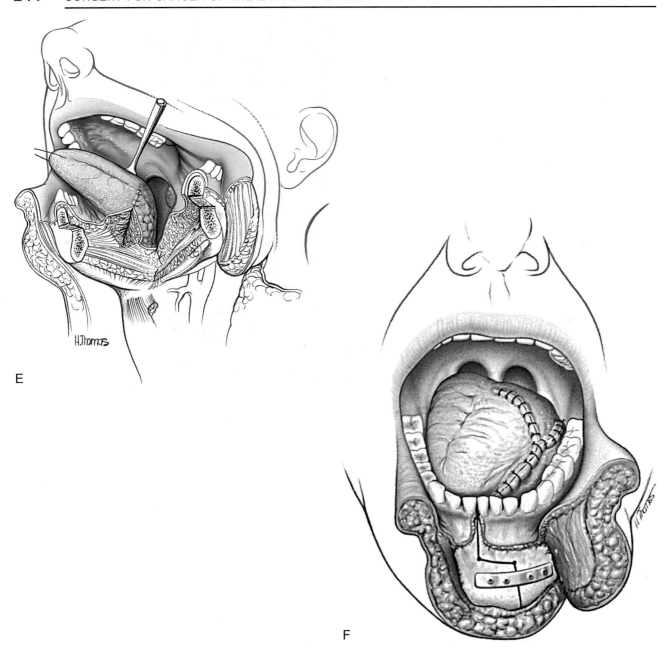

E

F

Figure 9–9 *Continued* "Mandibular swing" approach for tumor of the base of the tongue.

Figure 9–9E. Primary closure of the tongue is demonstrated. The optimal method of closure must be determined for each individual case. A myocutaneous or a revascularized free flap may be used if primary closure cannot be accomplished without excessive tension.

Figure 9–9F. With the mucosal closure completed, the mandible is reapproximated with a reconstruction plate. Inter-maxillary fixation is not necessary.

Procedures Requiring Total Laryngectomy

As previously discussed, the majority of hypopharyngeal tumors (the percentage may vary from institution to institution) are not suitable for conservation surgery and require excision of the entire larynx for adequate removal of the tumor. This surgery entails resection of the larynx in continuity with varying portions of the pharyngeal mucosa. Most hypopharyngeal carcinomas can be resected by total laryngectomy extended to include the involved portion of the hypopharynx with adequate margins of uninvolved mucosa. If more than 3 cm of normal mucosa are preserved, the resultant pharyngeal defect can usually be closed primarily. If less than 3 cm of mucosa remain, a pedicled myocutaneous flap, such as the major pectoral muscle myocutaneous flap, or a microvascular free flap, such as the radial forearm fasciocutaneous flap, is necessary to achieve a tension-free closure and prevent subsequent stenosis. Although the term "pharyngolaryngectomy" is often used to describe this type of procedure, we prefer the term "extended total laryngectomy" in order to distinguish this surgery from the conservation operation (namely, PPL) or from total pharyngolaryngectomy-esophagectomy.

The more advanced hypopharyngeal tumors require excision of the entire hypopharynx, including the cricopharyngeal muscle and the cervical portion of the esophagus. This operation has also been variously termed "total pharyngolaryngectomy," "pharyngolaryngo-esophagectomy," or "laryngoesophagectomy." In previous writings from our service, it has been termed "total pharyngolaryngectomy-esophagectomy" (TPL-E).[91, 92]

Extended Total Laryngectomy

Indications

Extended total laryngectomy is indicated for tumors of the superior hypopharynx, the pyriform sinus, or the pharyngeal wall that are too large to be amenable to conservation surgery but have sufficient uninvolved hypopharyngeal mucosa to be worth preserving. For lesions of the pharyngeal wall and pyriform sinus, at least a third of the circumference of the hypopharynx should remain after excision of the tumor, with adequate margins in order to close primarily. If less than a third of the hypopharynx remains after resection, it is necessary to patch the segment with a pedicled myocutaneous flap or a microvascular free flap or perform a total pharyngolaryngectomy and reconstruct the entire pharyngoesophageal segment. As a general rule, conservation surgery is feasible for tumors 3 cm or smaller. Large tumors not only are more likely to invade the laryngeal framework but will require excision of so much hypopharyngeal mucosa that little function will be possible from the remaining larynx.

Near-total laryngectomy is another option that may be employed for extensive hypopharyngeal carcinoma with involvement limited to only one side of the larynx. Su and Hwang[70] recently reported on 21 patients with advanced hypopharyngeal carcinoma who were treated by near-total laryngopharyngectomy and reconstructed with a major pectoral muscle myocutaneous flap. Patients had successful restoration of phonation and were able to swallow without difficulty.

An older technique has been revived to avoid the need for flap replacement in such tumors, namely, the use of the uninvolved contralateral hemilarynx to supply the mucosa for hypopharyngeal closure. Barzan and Comoretto[93] reported satisfactory results with 34 patients treated in this manner.

Tumors of the superior hypopharynx present a special problem. Smaller lesions are often amenable to conservation surgery. On the other hand, tumors of the base of the tongue that are large enough to require ligation of both lingual arteries present the surgeon with the dilemma of whether to try to preserve the intraoral portion of the tongue. Once an extensive glossolaryngectomy has been performed, the blood supply is often not sufficient to maintain the viability or the function of the anterior two thirds of the tongue. Experience with such tumors has shown that it is better to resect the entire tongue together with the larynx in patients with extensive tumors and to reconstruct the large ventral oral and pharyngeal defect with a microvascular free flap or a pedicled myocutaneous flap. Difficulties will often be encountered, however, with any reconstructive procedure because of the size and location of the defect.

Technique of Extended Total Laryngectomy for Carcinoma of the Pyriform Sinus

Figure 9–10A. This is a transverse view showing a large tumor in the right pyriform sinus. The tumor involves both the medial and the lateral walls of the pyriform sinus and extends to the apex (not shown in this view). The lesion penetrates the mucosa anteriorly, where it extends into the paraglottic space. There is fixation of the right hemilarynx.

Figure 9–10B. Mobilization of the larynx is performed by the technique described in Figures 5–1B to 5–1J. The hypopharynx is entered through the contralateral (left) pyriform sinus. As the mucosal incision is enlarged through the valleculae, the lesion in the right pyriform sinus is visualized. For hypopharyngeal tumors, it is most important to inspect the mucosa prior to incision and to allow as wide a margin of normal mucosa as possible around the tumor. If necessary, the incision should extend well into the base of the tongue to allow an adequate superior margin.

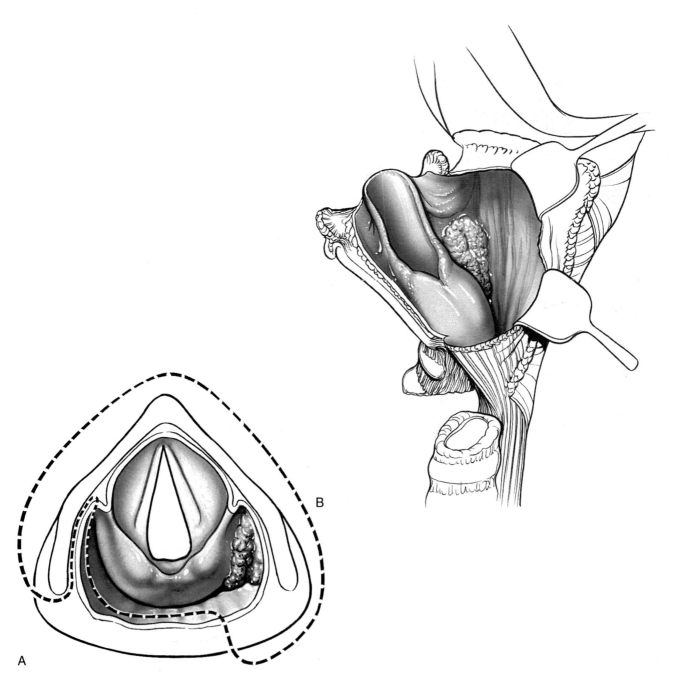

Figure 9–10. Extended total laryngectomy for tumor of the pyriform sinus.

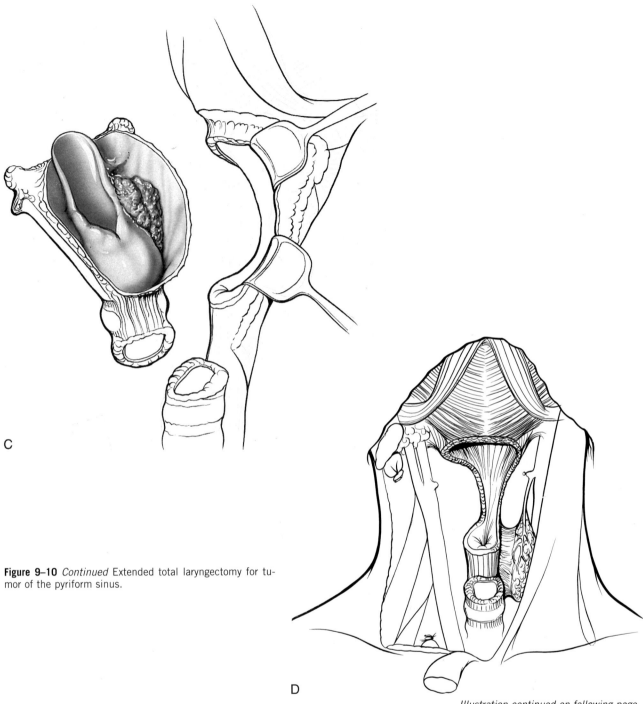

C

D

Figure 9–10 *Continued* Extended total laryngectomy for tumor of the pyriform sinus.

Illustration continued on following page

Figure 9–10C. The resection is completed, taking as much mucosa as necessary to ensure an adequate margin. There should be no concern with the amount of tissue available for closure during the resection phase of the operation.

Figure 9–10D. In general, it will be possible to reconstruct the hypopharynx by primary closure if 50% or more of the circumference of the mucosa remains. The defect will often extend onto the posterior pharyngeal wall. Closure is commenced posteri-

orly, with suturing of the inferior margin to the superior margin of the defect. Interrupted sutures of 2–0 or 3–0 polyglactin are placed, with knots tied inside the lumen. Flexion of the neck will help minimize the defect and reduce tension on the suture line. A nasogastric tube is passed before closure of the mucosa.

A cricopharyngeal myotomy will serve as a relaxing incision in the muscular layer and provide more tissue for closure. It may also prevent certain postoperative swallowing problems.

Figure 9–10E. Closure is continued anteriorly on both sides, toward the midline.

Figures 9–10F and 9–10G. With the large amount of mucosa resected for pyriform sinus carcinoma, a single transverse closure cannot usually be achieved. The hypopharynx is closed as a "T."

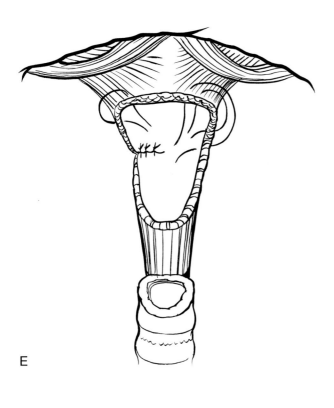

E

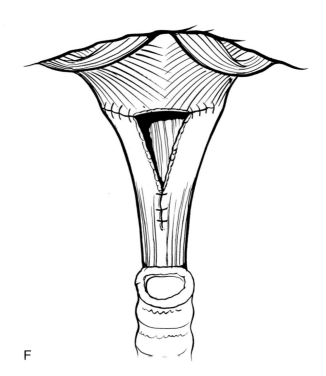

F

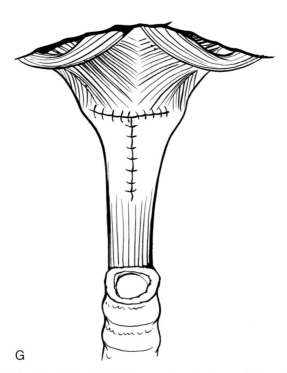

G

Figure 9–10 *Continued* Extended total laryngectomy for tumor of the pyriform sinus.

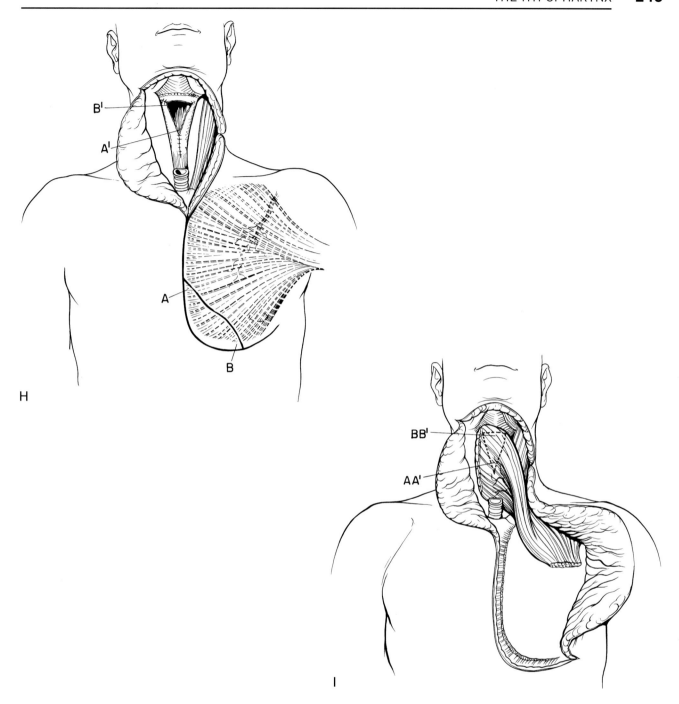

Figure 9–10 *Continued* Extended total laryngectomy for tumor of the pyriform sinus.

Illustration continued on following page

Figure 9–10*H.* If the hypopharyngeal mucosa cannot be completely closed, various alternatives exist for reconstruction. In the past, a temporary pharyngostome was often created, which would be closed during a secondary procedure. With the availability of modern techniques for single-stage reconstruction, this multistage approach is no longer necessary, except in very rare instances.

Use of a major pectoral muscle myocutaneous flap will permit closure in a single stage. The island of skin, sufficient to close the defect, is outlined over the inferior medial portion of the muscle. The cervical skin incision is continued over the chest wall, as shown, to permit exposure of the pectoral muscle.

Figure 9–10*I.* The flap is rotated to cover the defect. Edges of the skin island are sutured to the hypopharyngeal mucosa. The island is inverted when properly rotated so that points A–A′ and B–B′ coincide.

Figure 9–10*J.* Primary closure of the donor site can usually be achieved by advancement of the skin flap. If necessary, a split-thickness skin graft can be applied to the residual defect. Several authors have reported on the effectiveness of the major pectoral muscle myocutaneous flap in patching the hypopharynx.[70, 94–97] Lam et al.[94] reported on 36 pectoral muscle "patch" flaps after resection of hypopharyngeal carcinomas, with only 2 fistulae. Rees et al.[95] reported on 25 patients reconstructed with

a pectoral muscle flap. Six of these patients survived more than 1 year and were evaluated with regard to their functional status. All patients were able to ingest a puréed diet, though none could tolerate a regular diet.

Reconstruction with free tissue transfer (see Figs. 9–5 and 9–6) presents another alternative to the use of myocutaneous flaps for large hypopharyngeal defects after extended total laryngectomy.

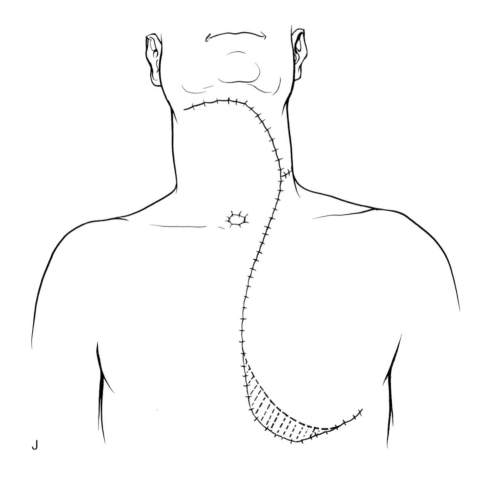

J

Figure 9–10 *Continued* Extended total laryngectomy for tumor of the pyriform sinus.

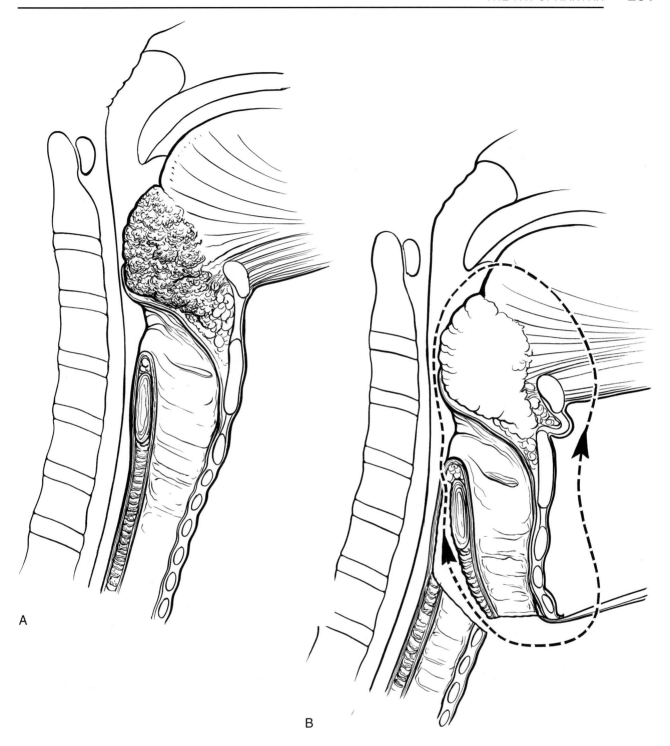

Figure 9–11. Extended total laryngectomy for carcinoma of the superior hypopharynx.

Illustration continued on following page

Technique of Extended Total Laryngectomy
for Carcinoma of the Superior Hypopharynx

Figure 9–11A. This is a longitudinal view showing an extensive tumor involving the valleculae, the lingual surface of the epiglottis, and the base of the tongue.

Figure 9–11B. The resection is outlined. The specimen will include the entire larynx and the contiguous base of the tongue surrounding the tumor. If the lesion is so extensive that both lingual arteries have to be sacrificed, it is preferable to perform a total glossectomy in conjunction with the laryngectomy.

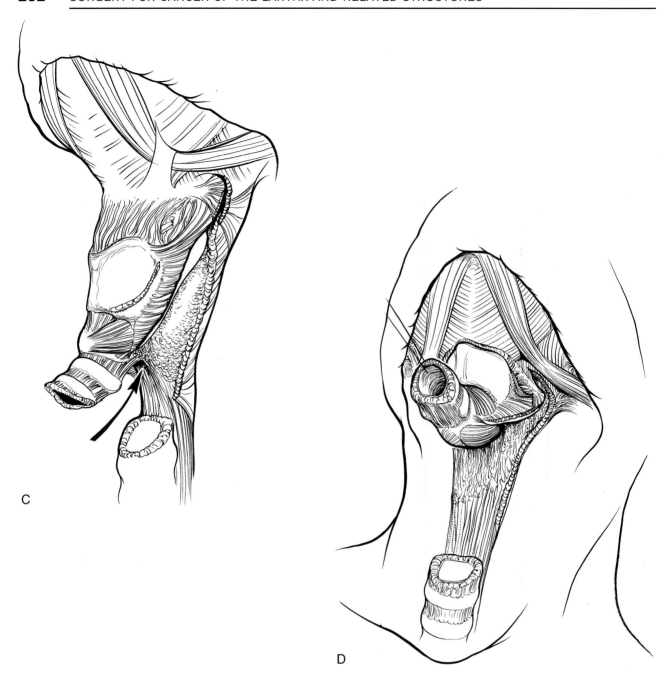

C

D

Figure 9–11 *Continued* Extended total laryngectomy for carcinoma of the superior hypopharynx.

Figure 9–11*C*. The larynx is mobilized according to the previously described technique (see Figs. 5–1*B* to 5–*H*). If there is no involvement of either pyriform sinus, the mucosa may be preserved bilaterally. The hypopharynx will be entered inferiorly through the postcricoid mucosa.

Figure 9–11*D*. Inferior entry of the hypopharynx with maximal preservation of uninvolved mucosa is facilitated by dissecting the hypopharyngeal mucosa from the cricoid lamina and the postarytenoid region while retracting the larynx upward. The mucosa is incised several millimeters inferior to its interarytenoid reflection into the larynx.

Figure 9–11E. The hypopharyngeal incision is enlarged through the pyriform sinuses, eventually exposing the inverted aryepiglottic folds, the epiglottis, the base of the tongue, and the tumor. The mucosa is incised carefully, making certain that an adequate resection margin is maintained.

Figure 9–11F. The base of the tongue is incised last. Exposure is facilitated by traction on the fully mobilized larynx. A margin of 2 cm of uninvolved tongue mucosa and muscle is desirable, although not always possible.

Figure 9–11G. Following resection, there is a large hypopharyngeal defect. It is usually possible to close the defect by direct approximation of tissues as shown in Figures 9–6F and 9–6G. If not, the principles of closure by free tissue transfer or major pectoral muscle myocutaneous flaps are the same as for pyriform sinus or other hypopharyngeal tumors.

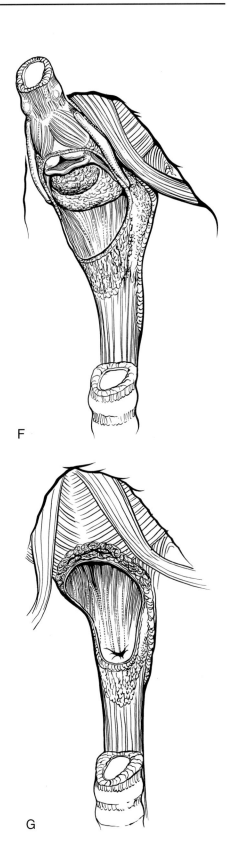

F

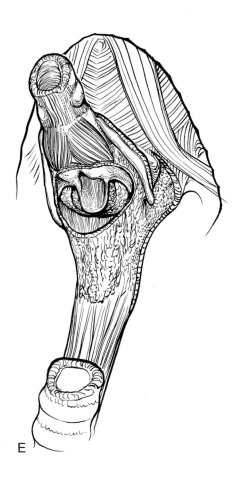

E

G

Figure 9–11 *Continued* Extended total laryngectomy for carcinoma of the superior hypopharynx.

Total Pharyngolaryngectomy-Esophagectomy

Indications

TPL-E is indicated in the following instances: (1) annular postcricoid carcinomas, (2) extensive lesions of the pyriform sinuses with involvement of more than two thirds of the circumference of the hypopharynx, (3) extensive posterior pharyngeal wall lesions with involvement of the larynx, and (4) carcinomas of the cervical esophagus.

Tumors requiring TPL-E are highly symptomatic obstructing lesions. Patients are unable to eat or, eventually, to swallow their own saliva. Little chance for either palliation or cure is offered by radiotherapy.[12, 41, 98, 99] Jacobson[12] collected the results from eight different northern European radiation centers with a total of 1,160 cases, having a mean 5-year cure rate of 7.6%. The highest cure rate reported at any of these centers was 14%. More recently, better results have been reported with radiation therapy, although these are not as good as results obtained with surgery. Stell et al.[100] reported a 38% 5-year survival with radiotherapy for postcricoid carcinoma. The series included three patients who underwent salvage surgery and seven who developed severe esophageal stenosis. Surgical resection of these lesions has consistently produced 3- to 5-year cure rates of approximately 25%[41, 91, 99, 101, 102] and, with effective reconstruction, can produce good palliation.[91, 102, 103] Harrison[104] reported on 68 patients treated by TPL-E in whom the local recurrence rate was only 3%. Thus, surgery must be considered the treatment of choice for patients with these lesions, provided sufficient nutritional and physiologic balance can be restored to permit the procedures to be tolerated. The morbidity and mortality of these procedures must be considered. Harrison et al.[16] determined an 11% perioperative mortality rate in 101 patients treated with TPL-E and pharyngogastric anastomosis.

Reconstruction

After TPL-E, a segmental defect in the alimentary tract remains, which requires total reconstruction of the pharynx and the resected portion of the esophagus. The feasibility and success of the resectional surgery is dependent on the speed and reliability with which alimentary continuity can be restored. Because of the complexity of this problem and the large number of techniques that have been developed to achieve reconstruction, this subject will be discussed separately in detail in the next chapter. The present discussion will focus on the ablative aspects of this surgery.

Preoperative Evaluation

Evaluation of the primary tumor is performed by the usual endoscopic and radiographic techniques. It is important to realize that the hypopharynx is a difficult area to visualize during the barium-swallow examination. Patients who complain of obstruction to swallowing at the cervical level should have an endoscopic as well as a radiographic examination for the initial diagnosis, because a fairly extensive hypopharyngeal tumor may not be recognized by esophagography. In order to evaluate the extent of a lesion, contrast studies, particularly with cineradiography, may be helpful once the diagnosis is known. It may be particularly difficult, however, to determine radiographically the lower extent of an obstructing tumor. This problem may be solved by passing a nasogastric tube distal to the lesion at the time of esophagoscopy so as to permit the lower esophagus to fill with barium. Films taken in the head-down position will then clearly demonstrate the inferior margin of the tumor. Newer imaging techniques, such as CT, are of value in determining the size of the tumor and the extent of laryngeal involvement.

If the anticipated reconstructive procedure will use laparotomy and transfer of an abdominal viscus for esophageal replacement, then contrast studies of the entire upper and lower gastrointestinal tracts should be performed, together with appropriate angiographic studies.

Preparation of the Patient

Patients with an obstructing hypopharyngeal or cervical esophageal neoplasm present numerous and severe management problems. The inability to eat and the aspiration of saliva and food result in starvation and bronchopulmonary infection. Although the preoperative condition of individual patients may vary, attention must be directed to these two factors. If a feeding tube can be inserted through the tumor endoscopically, enteric alimentation with a high-calorie (1.5 calories per milliliter) blenderized or elemental diet is then possible. Intravenous hyperalimentation is most useful if enteric alimentation is not possible or is inadequate. Although gastrostomy or jejunostomy has been used in the past for some patients, intraabdominal procedures for feeding are best avoided if abdominal viscera are to be used for reconstruction. The need for these procedures has been obviated to a large extent by the availability of the intravenous route, which not only avoids the surgical problems attendant on entering the abdomen but usually permits a larger caloric intake than is possible by the enteric route.

Bronchopulmonary sepsis should be controlled by appropriate antibiotics and, if necessary, a tracheostomy. The latter procedure can be performed at the time of initial endoscopic evaluation, if convenient. Definitive surgery should not be performed until the patient has gained some weight and bronchopulmonary sepsis has resolved.

Elective Neck Dissection

The procedure of TPL-E is performed for hypopharyngeal tumors (postcricoid, pyriform sinus, and posterior pharyngeal wall tumors), as well as for tumors of the cervical esophagus.

Tumors of the pyriform sinuses and pharyngeal walls are usually clearly localized to the side of greater involvement. Previous discussion has indicated the high incidence of cervical lymph node metastases associated with these tumors. For these lesions, a neck dissection, at least on the ipsilateral side, should be done in continuity with the pharyngolaryngectomy. Postoperatively, we prefer to administer radiotherapy to both sides of the neck and to the upper mediastinum.

Tumors of the postcricoid region and the cervical esophagus are often annular, and the side of origin or of greater involvement may be difficult to determine. Lymph node metastases in the paratracheal areas and the upper mediastinum are important as a frequent cause of failure after surgical treatment of postcricoid carcinoma. Many authors[5, 41, 105, 106] have advocated manubrial resection and mediastinal node dissection, as well as radical neck dissection for these tumors. Som[106] noted that all six of his patients who survived after laryngotracheal autograft procedures for postcricoid carcinoma had undergone at least one radical neck dissection. Five patients underwent mediastinal node dissections, and positive nodes were found in three. One patient with a positive mediastinal node survived.

More recently, the trend has been to perform bilateral selective neck dissections (in zones II–IV) as well as paratracheal lymph node dissection for these tumors. Weber et al.[35] reported the results of paratracheal dissections on 36 hypopharyngeal carcinomas and 14 cervical esophageal carcinomas. Fewer than 10% of the dissections performed for hypopharyngeal carcinoma revealed positive nodes, but 10 out of 14 of the dissections (71%) for cervical esophageal carcinoma had positive nodes.

Our preference for treatment of annular lesions of the postcricoid and cervical esophageal regions is to employ this combination of procedures in conjunction with postoperative radiation therapy, depending on the exact site of the tumor and the nature of the cervical and the paratracheal nodes

that are found. Manubrial resection and mediastinal dissection are done if the location of the primary tumor and the patient's habitus are such that this will facilitate resection of the gross tumor. Postoperative radiotherapy to both sides of the neck and the mediastinum is used to control subclinical lymph node metastases.

Technique of Total Pharyngolaryngectomy-Esophagectomy

Figure 9–12A. This view is of a postcricoid carcinoma requiring TPL-E.

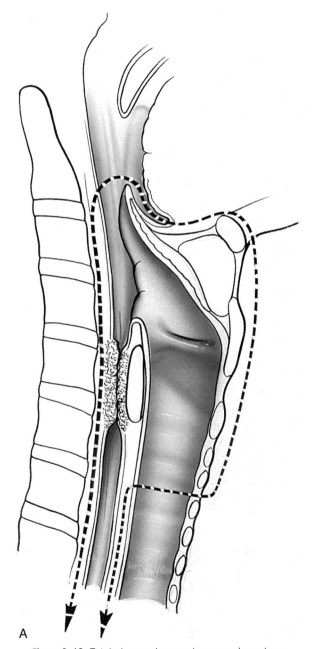

A

Figure 9–12. Total pharyngolaryngectomy-esophagectomy.
Illustration continued on following page

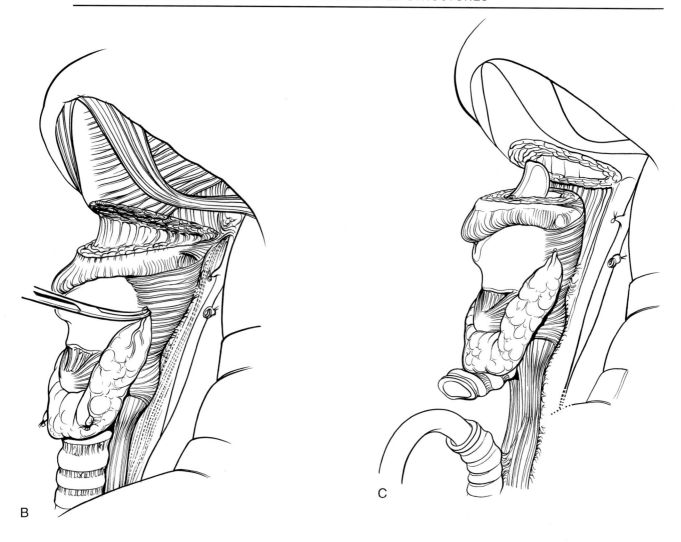

B

C

Figure 9–12 *Continued* Total pharyngolaryngectomy-esophagectomy.

Figure 9–12*B*. The entire pharyngolaryngeal complex is mobilized as a unit. The steps are essentially the same as shown in Figures 5–1*B* to 5–1*F* for total laryngectomy. In some cases, a lobe of the thyroid gland may be preserved on the side of lesser involvement, but most lesions that require TPL-E, particularly postcricoid tumors and cervical esophageal tumors, require total thyroidectomy.

After division of the suprahyoid and the infrahyoid muscles and of the superior and the inferior thyroid vessels, a plane of dissection is begun posteriorly between the inferior constrictor muscles and the prevertebral fascia. The complete development of this plane of dissection and its extension upward and downward as necessary permit complete mobilization of the specimen.

On rare occasions, extension of the tumor posteriorly through the prevertebral fascia may be noted, precluding complete extirpation, although the procedure may be continued for palliation.

Figure 9–12*C*. The trachea is transected at an appropriate level. In many instances, the tumor may extend inferiorly to the level of the tracheal transection. If the tumor does not grossly penetrate the esophageal muscle, it is acceptable to separate the party wall inferiorly so that the point of esophageal transection is well below the point of tracheal resection. A portion of membranous trachea may be left on the esophagus to ensure a thicker margin, if it is felt necessary. The tracheal defect may be sutured directly, producing a somewhat narrower trachea.

If the trachea cannot be transected sufficiently low by a cervical approach, then manubrial resection with a mediastinal tracheostoma may be used.

Following tracheal transection and establishment of airway connections to the anesthesia apparatus, the hypopharynx is entered superiorly through the valleculae, and the entire circumference of the hypopharyngeal wall is transected safely above the tumor.

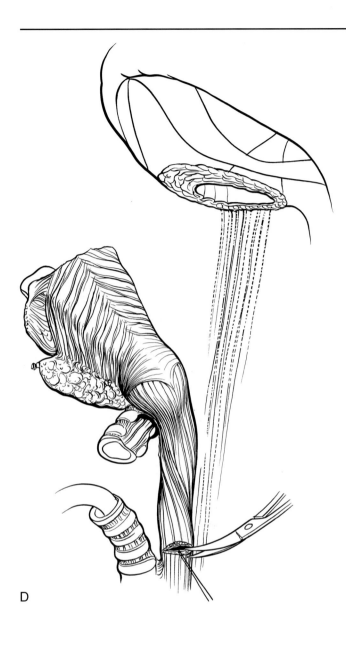

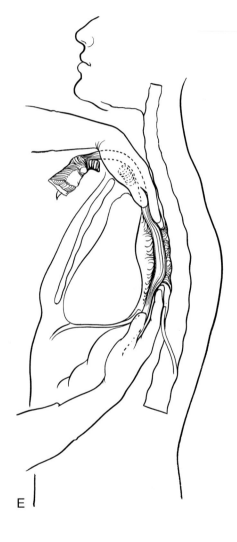

Figure 9–12 *Continued* Total pharyngolaryngectomy-esophagectomy.

Figure 9–12D. The cervical esophagus is transected as far inferior to the tumor as possible. As discussed in the next chapter, the method chosen for reconstruction and the level of inferior transection of the esophagus are interdependent. Procedures requiring a sufficient cuff of distal esophagus to anastomose to a myocutaneous flap or to a transplanted bowel segment are feasible only if an adequate resection margin can be maintained.

Figure 9–12E. If an adequate distal resection margin cannot be achieved with partial esophagectomy, then total blunt extraction of the esophagus through cervical and abdominal incisions is required. This procedure is discussed in detail in the next chapter, as are the numerous procedures used for reconstruction after TPL-E.

REFERENCES

1. Isambert E. Contribution a l'etude du cancer du larynge. *Ann Mal Oreille Larynx* 1876; 2:1–23.
2. Krishaber M. Contribution a l'etude du cancer du larynx. *Gaz Hebd de Med Chirug* 1879; 16:518–535.
3. Sessions DG. Surgical pathology of cancer of the larynx and hypopharynx. *Laryngoscope* 1976; 86:814–839.
4. Carpenter RJ III, DeSanto L, Devine KD, et al. Cancer of the hypopharynx: analysis of treatment and results in 162 patients. *Arch Otolaryngol* 1976; 102:716–721.
5. Harrison DFN. Pathology of hypopharyngeal cancer in relation to surgical management. *J Laryngol Otol* 1970; 84:349–367.
6. Ogura JH, Sessions DG, Ciralsky RH. Supraglottic carcinoma with extension to the arytenoid. *Laryngoscope* 1975; 85:1327–1331.
7. Ogura JH, Sessions DG, Spector GJ. Conservation surgery for epidermoid carcinoma of the supraglottic larynx. *Laryngoscope* 1975; 85:1808–1815.
8. Ogura JH, Spector GJ, Sessions DG. Conservation surgery for epidermoid carcinoma of the marginal area (aryepiglottic fold extension). *Laryngoscope* 1975; 85:1801–1807.
9. Silverberg E, Lubera JA. Cancer statistics. *CA Cancer J Clin* 1989; 39:3–20.
10. Kirchner JA, Owen JR. Five hundred cancers of the larynx and pyriform sinus: results of treatment by radiation and surgery. *Laryngoscope* 1977; 87:1288–1303.
11. Kirchner JA. Pyriform sinus cancer: a clinical and laboratory study. *Ann Otol Rhinol Laryngol* 1975; 84:793–803.
12. Jacobsson F. Carcinoma of the hypopharynx: a clinical study of 322 cases, treated at Radium-Hemmet, from 1939 to 1947. *Acta Radiol* 1951; 35:1–21.
13. Mustard RA, Ibberson O. Carcinoma of the esophagus: a review of 381 cases admitted to the Toronto General Hospital 1937–1953 inclusive. *Ann Surg* 1956; 144:927–940.
14. Carpenter RJ III, DeSanto LW. Cancer of the hypopharynx. *Surg Clin North Amer* 1977; 57:723–735.
15. Ward PH, Hanson DG. Reflux as an etiological factor of carcinoma of the laryngopharynx. *Laryngoscope* 1988; 98:1195–1199.
16. Harrison DFN, Thompson AE. Pharyngolaryngo-esophagectomy with pharyngogastric anastomosis for cancer of the hypopharynx: a review of 101 operations. *Head Neck Surg* 1986; 8:418–428.
17. Olofsson J, van Nostrand AWP. Growth and spread of laryngeal and hypopharyngeal carcinoma with reflections on the effect of preoperative irradiation (139 cases studied by whole organ sectioning). *Acta Otolaryngol Suppl.* (Stockh) 1973; 308:1–84.
18. Wiernik G, Millard PR, Haybittle JL. The predictive value of histological classification into degrees of differentiation of squamous cell carcinoma of the larynx and hypopharynx compared with the survival of patients. *Histopathology* 1991; 19:411–417.
19. Rapoport A, Franco EL. Prognostic factors and relative risk in hypopharyngeal cancer: related parameters concerning stage, therapeutics and evolution. *Revista Paulista de Medicina* 1993; 111:337–343.
20. Beahrs OH, Henson DE, Hutter RVP, et al. *Manual for Staging of Cancer,* 4th ed, pp 34–35. Philadelphia, Lippincott, 1992.
21. Kirchner JA. One hundred laryngeal cancers studied by serial section. *Ann Otol Rhinol Laryngol* 1969; 78:689–709.
22. Laccourreye O, Merite-Drancy A, Brasnu D, et al. Supracricoid hemilaryngopharyngectomy in selected pyriform sinus carcinoma staged as T$_2$. *Laryngoscope* 1993; 103:1373–1379.
23. Florant A, Berreby S, Gilain L, et al. La chirurgie fonctionnelle des cancers de l'hypopharynx: hemi-larygo-pharygectomies postérieures par abord cervical bilatéral. *Ann Otolaryngol Chir Cervicofac* 1986; 103:443–453.
24. Hiroto I. Hypopharyngoesophageal carcinoma, its surgical treatment. *Kurume Med J* 1963; 10:162.

25. Tani M, Amatsu M. Discrepancies between clinical and histopathologic diagnosis in T$_3$ pyriform sinus cancer. *Laryngoscope* 1987; 97:93–96.
26. Tucker GF Jr. The anatomy of laryngeal cancer. *In* Alberti PW, Bryce DP (eds): *Workshops from the Centennial Conference on Laryngeal Cancer,* pp 11–25. New York, Appleton-Century-Crofts, 1976.
27. Willatt DJ, Jackson JR, McCormick MS, et al. Vocal cord paralysis and tumour length in staging postcricoid cancer. *Eur J Surg Oncol* 1987; 13:131–137.
28. Carbone A, Volpe R, Barzan L. Superficial extending carcinoma (SEC) of the larynx and hypopharynx. *Path Res Pract* 1992; 188:729–735.
29. McGavran MH, Bauer WC, Spjut HJ, et al. Carcinoma of the pyriform sinus: the results of radical surgery. *Arch Otolaryngol* 1963; 78:826–830.
30. Wenig BL, Applebaum EL. The submandibular triangle in squamous cell carcinoma of the larynx and hypopharynx. *Laryngoscope* 1991; 101:516–518.
31. Davidson BJ, Kulkarny V, Delacure MD, et al. Posterior triangle metastases of squamous cell carcinoma of the upper aerodigestive tract. *Am J Surg* 1993; 166:395–398.
32. Candela FC, Kothari K, Shah JP. Patterns of cervical node metastases from squamous cell carcinoma of the oropharynx and hypopharynx. *Head Neck Surg* 1990; 12:197–203.
33. Million RR, Cassisi NJ, Wittes RE. Cancer of the head and neck. *In* DeVita VT, Hellman S, Rosenberg SA (eds): *Cancer: Principles and Practice of Oncology,* 2nd ed, Vol 1, pp 407–506. Philadelphia, Lippincott, 1985.
34. Routh A, Hickman BT. Carcinoma of the pyriform sinus. *South Med J* 1987; 80:177–181.
35. Weber RS, Marvel J, Smith P, et al. Paratracheal lymph node dissection for carcinoma of the larynx, hypopharynx, and cervical esophagus. *Otolaryngol Head Neck Surg* 1993; 108:11–17.
36. Farr HW, Arthur K. Epidermoid carcinoma of the mouth and pharynx, 1960–1964. *J Laryngol Otol* 1972; 86:243–253.
37. McNeill R. Surgical management of carcinoma of the posterior pharyngeal wall. *Head Neck Surg* 1981; 3:389–394.
38. Ballantyne AJ. Significance of retropharyngeal nodes in cancer of the head and neck. *Am J Surg* 1964; 108:500–504.
39. Cunningham MP, Catlin D. Cancer of the pharyngeal wall. *Cancer* 1967; 20:1859–1866.
40. Ahlbom HE. Simple achlorhydric anemia. Plummer-Vinson syndrome and carcinoma of the mouth, pharynx and oesophagus in women: observations at Radiumhemmet, Stockholm. *Br Med J* 1936; 2:331–333.
41. Som ML, Nussbaum M. Surgical therapy of carcinoma of the hypopharynx and cervical esophagus. *Otolaryngol Clin North Am* 1969; 2:631–640.
42. Eisbach KJ, Krause CJ. Carcinoma of the pyriform sinus, a comparison of treatment modalities. *Laryngoscope* 1977; 87:1904–1910.
43. Lord IJ, Bright TDR, Rider WD, et al. A comparison of preoperative and primary radiotherapy in the treatment of carcinoma of the hypopharynx. *Br J Radiol* 1973; 46:175–179.
44. Shah JP, Shaha AR, Spiro RH, et al. Carcinoma of the hypopharynx. *Am J Surg* 1976; 132:439–443.
45. Van den Bogaert W, Ostyn F, van der Schueren E. Hypopharyngeal cancer: results of treatment with radiotherapy alone and combinations of surgery and radiotherapy. *Radiotherapy Onc* 1985; 3:311–318.
46. Tandon DA, Bahadur S, Chatterji TK, et al. Carcinoma of the hypopharynx: results of combined therapy. *Ind J Cancer* 1991; 28:131–138.
47. Parsons JT, Mendenhall WM, Stringer SP, et al. Twice-a-day radiotherapy for squamous cell carcinoma of the head and neck: the University of Florida experience. *Head Neck Surg* 1993; 15:87–96.
48. Ahmad K, Fayos JV. High dose radiation therapy in carcinoma of the pyriform sinus. *Cancer* 1984; 53:2091–2094.
49. Alcock CJ, Fowler JF, Haybittle JL, et al. Salvage surgery following irradiation with different fractionation regimes

in the treatment of carcinoma of the laryngopharynx: experience gained from a British Institute of Radiology study. *J Laryngol Otol* 1992; 106:147–153.

50. Vandenbrouck C, Sancho H, LeFur R, et al. Results of a randomized clinical trial of preoperative irradiation versus postoperative in treatment of tumors of the hypopharynx. *Cancer* 1977; 39:1445–1449.

51. Donald PJ, Hayes HR, Dhaliwal R. Combined therapy for pyriform sinus cancer using postoperative irradiation. *Otolaryngol Head Neck Surg* 1980; 88:738–744.

52. El Badawi SA, Goepfert H, Fletcher GH, et al. Squamous cell carcinoma of the pyriform sinus. *Laryngoscope* 1982; 92:357–364.

53. Sasaki TM, Baker HW, Yeager RA, et al. Aggressive surgical management of pyriform sinus carcinoma: a 15-year experience. *Am J Surg* 1986; 151:590–592.

54. Harwick RD. Carcinoma of the pyriform sinus. *Am J Surg* 1975; 130:493–495.

55. Jesse RH, Lindberg RD. The efficacy of combining radiation therapy with a surgical procedure in patients with cervical metastasis from squamous cancer of the oropharynx and hypopharynx. *Cancer* 1975; 35:1163–1166.

56. Persky MS, Daly JF. Combined therapy vs curative radiation in the treatment of pyriform sinus carcinoma. *Otolaryngol Head Neck Surg* 1981; 89:87–91.

57. Yates A, Crumley RL. Surgical treatment of pyriform sinus cancer: a retrospective study. *Laryngoscope* 1984; 94:1586–1590.

58. Driscoll WG, Nagorsky MJ, Cantrell RJ, et al. Carcinoma of the pyriform sinus: analysis of 102 cases. *Laryngoscope* 1983; 93:556–560.

59. Vandenbrouck C, Eschwege F, De La Rochefordiere A, et al. Squamous cell carcinoma of the pyriform sinus: retrospective study of 351 cases treated at the Institut Gustave-Roussy. *Head Neck Surg* 1987; 10:4–13.

60. Ogura JH, Marks JE, Freeman RB. Results of conservation surgery for cancers of the supraglottis and pyriform sinus. *Laryngoscope* 1980; 90:591–600.

61. Ogura JH, Biller HF, Wette R. Elective neck dissection for pharyngeal and laryngeal cancers: an evaluation. *Ann Otol Rhinol Laryngol* 1971; 80:646–650.

62. Stell PM, Dalby JE, Strickland P, et al. Sequential chemotherapy and radiotherapy in advanced head and neck cancer. *Clin Rad* 1983; 34:463–467.

63. Brasnu D, Bassot V, Fabre A, et al. Induction chemotherapy in pyriform sinus carcinoma: analysis of survival. *Proc Am Soc Clin Oncol* 1987; 6:140(abstract 551).

64. Ogura JH, Jurema AA, Watson RK. Partial laryngopharyngectomy and neck dissection for pyriform sinus cancer: conservation surgery with immediate reconstruction. *Laryngoscope* 1960; 70:1399–1417.

65. Ogura JH, Mallen RW. Partial laryngopharyngectomy for supraglottic and pharyngeal carcinoma. *Trans Am Acad Ophthalmol Otolaryngol* 1965; 69:832–845.

66. Ogura JH, Biller H, Calcaterra JC, et al. Surgical treatment of carcinoma of the larynx, pharynx, base of tongue and cervical esophagus. *Int Surg* 1969; 52:29–40.

67. Marks JE, Kurnik B, Powers WE, et al. Carcinoma of the pyriform sinus: an analysis of treatment results and patterns of failure. *Cancer* 1978; 41:1008–1015.

68. Iwai H, Matsuoka I, Nagahara K. Evaluation of total pharyngolaryngectomy for hypopharyngeal cancer. *Arch Otorhinolaryngol* 1975; 209:223–228.

69. Dumich PS, Pearson BW, Weiland LH. Suitability of near-total laryngopharyngectomy in pyriform carcinoma. *Arch Otolaryngol* 1984; 110:664–669.

70. Su CY, Hwang CF. Near-total laryngopharyngectomy with pectoralis major myocutaneous flap in advanced pyriform carcinoma. *J Laryngol Otol* 1993; 107:817–820.

71. Trotter W. A method of lateral pharyngotomy for the exposure of large growths in the epilaryngeal region. *J Laryngol Otol* 1920; 35:289–295.

72. Som ML, Silver CE, Carbajal PG. Surgical approaches to the hypopharynx for benign disease. *Arch Otolaryngol* 1966; 83:222–230.

73. Rubin JS, Silver CE. Surgical approach to submucosal lesions of the supraglottic larynx: the superolateral thyrotomy. *J Laryngol Otol* 1992; 106:416–419.

74. Moisa II, Silver CE. Treatment of neuroendocrine neoplasms of the larynx. *ORL J Otorhinolaryngol Relat Spec* 1991; 53:259–264.

75. Cracovaner AJ, Chodosh PL. The lateral approach to the larynx and hypopharynx. *Arch Otolaryngol* 1960; 71:8–15.

76. Ferguson GB. Experiences in lateral pharyngotomy. *Laryngoscope* 1976; 86:1626–1632.

77. New GB. Congenital cysts of the tongue, the floor of the mouth, the pharynx and larynx. *Arch Otolaryngol* 1947; 45:145–158.

78. New GB. Treatment of cysts of the larynx. *Arch Otolaryngol* 1942; 36:687–690.

79. Ogura JH, Watson RK, Jurema AA. Partial pharyngectomy and neck dissection for posterior hypopharyngeal cancer. Immediate reconstruction with preservation of voice. *Laryngoscope* 1960; 70:1523–1534.

80. Silver CE. *Surgery for Cancer of the Larynx,* pp 177–178. New York, Churchill Livingstone, 1981.

81. Delaere PR, Boeckx WD, Ostyn F, et al. Hypopharyngeal stenosis and fistulas: use of the radial forearm free flap. *Arch Otolaryngol* 1988; 114:1326–1329.

82. Chen HC, Tang YB, Noordhoff MS. Patch esophagoplasty with free forearm flap for focal stricture of the pharyngoesophageal junction and the cervical esophagus. *Plast Reconstr Surg* 1992; 90:45–52.

83. Urken ML, Weinberg H, Vickery C, et al. The neurofasciocutaneous radial forearm flap in head and neck reconstruction: a preliminary report. *Laryngoscope* 1990; 100:161–173.

84. Urken ML, Futran N, Moscoso JF, et al. A modified design of the buried radial forearm free flap for use in oral cavity and pharyngeal reconstruction. *Arch Otolaryngol* 1994; 120:1233–1239.

85. Blassingame CD. Suprahyoid approach to surgical lesions at the base of the tongue. *Ann Otol Rhinol Laryngol* 1952; 61:483–489.

86. Portman G. Surgery at the base of the tongue by transpharyngeal approach. *Arch Otolaryngol* 1949; 50:373–376.

87. Klopp CT, Delaney A. Anterior (median) pharyngotomy. *Arch Surg* 1950; 60:1161–1170.

88. Trotter W. Operations for malignant disease of the pharynx. *Br J Surg* 1929; 16:485–495.

89. Martin H, Tollefsen HR, Gerold F. Median labiomandibular glossotomy: Trotter's median (anterior) translingual pharyngotomy. *Am J Surg* 1961; 102:753–759.

90. Tollefsen HR, Spiro RH. Median labiomandibular glossotomy. *Ann Surg* 1971; 173:415–420.

91. Silver CE. Reconstruction after pharyngolaryngectomy-esophagectomy. *Am J Surg* 1976; 132:428–434.

92. Silver CE. Surgical management of neoplasms of the larynx, hypopharynx and cervical esophagus. *Curr Probl Surg* 1977; 14:2–69.

93. Barzan L, Comoretto R. Hemipharyngectomy and hemilaryngectomy for pyriform sinus cancer: reconstruction with remaining larynx and hypopharynx and with tracheostomy. *Laryngoscope* 1993; 103:82–86.

94. Lam KH, Ho CM, Lau W, et al. Immediate reconstruction of pharyngoesophageal defects: preference or reference. *Arch Otolaryngol* 1989; 115:608–612.

95. Rees RS, Ivey GI III, Shack RB, et al. Pectoralis major musculocutaneous flaps: long-term follow-up of hypopharyngeal reconstruction. *Plast Reconstr Surg* 1986; 77:586–591.

96. Ho CM, Lam KH, Wei WI, et al. Squamous cell carcinoma of the hypopharynx: analysis of treatment results. *Head Neck* 1993; 15:405–412.

97. Fabian R. Pectoralis major myocutaneous flap reconstruction of the laryngopharynx and cervical esophagus. *Sem Thor Cardiovasc Surg* 1992; 4:280–285.

98. Morfit HM, Kloop CT, Neerken AJ. Bridging of laryngopharyngeal and upper cervical esophageal defects. *Arch Surg* 1957; 74:667–674.

99. Mustard RA. The use of the Wookey operation for carcinoma of the hypopharynx and cervical esophagus. *Surg Gynecol Obstet* 1960; 111:577–592.

100. Stell PM, Carden EA, Hibbert J, et al. Postcricoid carcinoma. *Clin Oncol* 1978; 4:215–226.

101. Grimes OF, Stephens HB. The treatment of carcinoma of the hypopharynx and cervical esophagus. *Arch Surg* 1956; 72:742–755.

102. Harrison DF. Rehabilitation problems after pharyngogastric anastomosis. *Arch Otolaryngol* 1978; 104:244–246.

103. Akiyama H, Hiyama M, Miyazono H. Total esophageal reconstruction after extraction of the esophagus. *Ann Surg* 1975; 182:547–552.

104. Harrison DFN. Surgical repair in hypopharyngeal and cervical esophageal cancer: analysis of 162 patients. *Ann Otolaryngol* 1981; 90:372–375.

105. Som ML. Surgical treatment of carcinoma of postcricoid region. *NY State J Med* 1961; 61:2567–2576.

106. Som ML. Laryngotracheal autograft for postcricoid carcinoma: a reevaluation. *Ann Otol Rhinol Laryngol* 1974; 83:481–486.

Chapter 10

Reconstruction of the Cervical Esophagus

Carl E. Silver and Roger J. Levin

Chapter 9 discussed the technique and indications for ablation of the entire larynx, the hypopharynx, and the cervical esophagus (total pharyngolaryngectomy-esophagectomy). This massive surgical resection will produce cure rates of approximately 25% for appropriate lesions. Although this figure is low, it is considerably higher than that obtained with radiotherapy. In addition, radiotherapy rarely gives relief from hypopharyngeal or upper esophageal obstruction, whereas surgery, if successful, will restore the patient's ability to swallow. This palliative aspect of treatment is extremely important because extensive symptoms are produced by these obstructive lesions. Patients not only are unable to eat, but eventually cannot even swallow their saliva.

Effective palliation, however, is possible only if reconstruction of the pharyngoesophageal segment is accomplished rapidly and consistently. Unfortunately, this is not an easy task. A recapitulation of the experience of the past 40 years with pharyngoesophageal reconstruction demonstrates numerous instances of prolonged hospitalization, multiple operations, and persistent salivary fistulae. All too often the tumor recurred before reconstruction of the esophagus was completed.

With pharyngoesophageal reconstruction, as with all difficult surgical problems when no single approach has offered an ideal solution, a large number of different techniques have been used. Over time, older techniques, with their inherent difficulties, have been supplanted by new procedures that have produced more consistently successful results with greater rapidity and with less morbidity than was previously feasible. The advent of free tissue transfer procedures and one-stage procedures involving transfer of abdominal viscera has revolutionized the reconstruction of the hypopharynx and the cervical esophagus. Several feasible options are now available for reconstruction of these massive defects, all of which have good success when performed properly.

The methods that have been used for pharyngoesophageal reconstruction include the following: use of local tissues, grafts, and prostheses; use of regional skin flaps or pedicled myocutaneous flaps; free transplantation of abdominal viscera or fasciocutaneous flaps; and transposition of abdominal viscera carrying their own blood supply. A classification of some of the more popular procedures that have been used is given in Table 10–1. It would be unlikely, as well as unnecessary, for a single surgeon to have acquired experience in the use of all of the reconstructive procedures that have been re-

ported. In this chapter we will attempt to present the procedures that have been found useful in current surgical practice.

Table 10–1. METHODS OF PHARYNGOESOPHAGEAL RECONSTRUCTION
Skin grafts and local tissues
Skin graft
Rob and Bateman[1]
Edgerton[2]
Negus[3]
Laryngotracheal autograft
Som[8, 18]
Barzan and Comoretto[20]
Cook et al.[19]
Regional skin flaps
Cervical skin
Wookey[24]
Deltopectoral flap
Bakamjiam[27]
Fredrickson et al.[37]
Pedicled myocutaneous flaps
Lateral trapezius
Guillamondegui and Larson[41]
Demergasso and Piazza[42]
Greater pectoral
Cusumano et al.[43]
Rees et al.[47]
Theogaraj et al.[48]
Lee et al.[49]
Lam et al.[52, 54]
Transposed abdominal viscera
Reversed gastric tube
Gavrilu and Georgescu[60]
Heimlich[62, 63]
Colon
Carlson et al.[36]
Goligher and Robin[76]
Mannings et al.[78]
Entire stomach
Ong and Lee[88]
Le Quesne and Ranger[89]
Stell[90]
Silver[92]
Microvascular tissue transfer
Gastric antrum
Heibert and Cummings[117]
Panje et al.[141]
Sigmoid colon
Nakayama et al.[121]
Jejunum
Seidenberg et al.[109]
Som and Silver[110]
Coleman et al.[124]
Biel and Maisel[125]
Surkin et al.[126]
Petruzzelli et al.[127]
Radial forearm
Harii et al.[135]
Takato et al.[136]
Chen et al.[138]
Lateral cutaneous thigh
Hayden[139]
Hayden and Fredrickson[140]

HISTORICAL CONSIDERATIONS

Skin Grafts and Prostheses

Free grafts of fascia lata wrapped around a cylinder of tantalum mesh were used by Rob and Bateman[1] for immediate reconstruction of both the trachea and the esophagus in 1949. Edgerton,[2] in 1952, and Negus[3] and Conley,[4] in 1953, used split-thickness skin grafts wrapped over cone-shaped stents of tantalum mesh or plastic for one-stage reconstruction of the cervical esophagus. Full-thickness tubular grafts of penile skin have been successfully used by some authors.[5-7] These types of reconstruction are prone to contracture and incomplete healing, resulting in a high incidence of stricture and fistula formation at both the proximal and the distal anastomoses.[8,9] Attempts have been made to restore pharyngoesophageal continuity by implantation of plastic prostheses, but the results have not been encouraging.[10-13] The results of laboratory evaluations of the use of homografts, such as aorta, pericardium, and lyophilized dura, for reconstruction were similarly far from ideal.[14,15]

Laryngotracheal Autograft

Certain small postcricoid carcinomas may be adequately excised without resecting the entire larynx. The unresected portion of the larynx can be used for restoration of pharyngoesophageal continuity. Asherson,[16] in 1954, first used this type of procedure for an early carcinoma of the posterior wall of the hypopharynx. After separation of the larynx from the pharynx by peeling the anterior esophageal mucosa from the cricoid cartilage, the pharynx was resected, and the entire preserved larynx was sutured into the defect. A similar operation was described in 1955 by Wilkins,[17] differing from Asherson's procedure only in that most of the cartilaginous framework of the larynx was removed.

In 1956 Som[8] described a "laryngotracheal autograft" procedure that included resection of the posterior half of the larynx and the first few tracheal rings in continuity with the pharyngoesophagus. Only the anterior half of the laryngotracheal segment was used to reconstruct the anterior and lateral walls of the pharyngoesophageal defect. The posterior wall was replaced by a stented split-thickness skin graft. Because the graft lay on the anterior surface of the spine, the tendency for graft contracture and stricture formation was minimized. The procedure was performed in one stage.

In 1974 Som[18] reported the results of 23 operations. Six of the 23 patients survived 5 years or more, with only 1 instance of stricture formation.

Som emphasized that laryngotracheal autograft reconstruction was feasible in only 27% of the patients in his series of postcricoid cancers and other related lesions, most lesions being too extensive for the limited resection. The procedure was most suitable for small postcricoid cancers in women with Plummer-Vinson syndrome. More recently, Cook et al.[19] reported on 4 patients in whom they used this procedure, arguing that the method was simple and saved the patients from a more extensive procedure. Barzan and Comoretto[20] reported on 34 patients in whom the remaining hemilarynx and hemipharynx were used to reconstruct defects from pyriform sinus carcinoma resections, obviously necessitating permanent tracheostomies. No cases of hypopharyngeal stenosis were observed.

Cervical Skin

The use of cervical skin for reconstruction after resection of carcinoma of the cervical esophagus was first suggested by Mikulicz[21] in 1886. Bircher,[22] in 1907, described a procedure for esophageal reconstruction with cervical skin, and in 1908 Von Hacker[23] successfully used a long cervical skin flap for reconstruction of a pharyngoesophageal defect. Wookey developed this concept into the relatively reliable method of reconstruction that bears his name, and in 1942 he published details of the technique and the results of treatment in four patients.[24] In 1960 his colleague, Mustard,[25] summarized their combined experience with 44 patients. He reported a 24% 5-year survival and satisfactory reconstructive results. Wookey's procedure consisted of the development of a laterally based rectangular skin flap that was interposed between the stumps of transected oropharynx and cervical esophagus. At a second stage, this skin-lined tube was closed longitudinally, thus creating a new esophageal segment. In 1967 Silver and Som[26] described various modifications of the original Wookey procedure and reported satisfactory results in a series of patients.

Despite these improvements, the inherent shortcomings of this procedure remained. The laterally based cervical skin flap, which crossed the midline, tended to have marginal circulation at its tip, and partial flap loss occurred frequently. The fact that many patients had undergone previous radiotherapy enhanced the possibility of this complication. Once necrosis occurred, many weeks of hospitalization and, often, further surgery were required before the patient was ready for the second stage. During this frequently prolonged period, patients would suffer from the constant aspiration of saliva, which would drip into the dependent tracheostoma from the large, superiorly placed oropharyngostoma. Another disadvantage of the Wookey operation, which remained despite the slightly increased length of the flap provided by the Silver-Som modification, was the limitation of the length of esophagus that could be resected.

Deltopectoral Flap

One of the outstanding contributions to progress in the field of oncologic surgery of the head and neck was the description, in 1965, by Bakamjian[27-29] of a medially based flap of skin from the upper chest. This versatile flap, which receives its blood supply from the perforating branches of the internal mammary artery, has proved useful for a variety of reconstructive problems, including simple resurfacing of the neck, reconstruction of oral and oropharyngeal defects, and pharyngoesophageal reconstruction. Bakamjian noted that the flap was strikingly resistant to necrosis and could often be used without preliminary delay. He attributed the success of this procedure both to the abundant arterial supply and to the good venous drainage afforded by the dependent final position of the pedicle of the flap. Although the deltopectoral flap is not an "arterialized" flap throughout its length, it is rarely necessary to exceed a 2:1 ratio (length/width) by more than a small factor when using this flap for pharyngoesophageal reconstruction. In his original report, Bakamjian[27] described the successful use of the deltopectoral flap for a two-staged pharyngoesophageal reconstruction. Subsequently, numerous authors have confirmed the reliability of the flap for this purpose,[30-33] and until the advent of myocutaneous flaps and free tissue transfer, the deltopectoral flap has proved to be the most reliable method of pharyngoesophageal reconstruction with skin.

Despite the improvements afforded by the deltopectoral flap, the procedure had its limitations. The chief disadvantage was the limitation posed by the length of esophagus that could be resected distally. Because it was necessary to anastomose the end of the esophageal stump to the side of the skin tube, a length of at least 2 to 3 cm of distal cervical esophagus was necessary to employ the procedure. Thus the procedure was useful only for lesions that could be adequately resected within that margin. In addition, strictures and fistulae, although correctable, would occur with some frequency.

Although the use of the deltopectoral flap for head and neck reconstruction has been largely abandoned in favor of newer techniques, some authors continue to find it valuable for hypopharyngeal and esophageal reconstruction. In 1988, Chaffoo and Goode[34] reported on 65 cases of head and neck re-

construction that were accumulated over a 20-year period. Despite the modifications in flap design that they presented, complete reconstruction usually required three stages. Guillamondegui and colleagues[35] described 41 patients who underwent deltopectoral flap reconstructions out of a total of 78 patients with defects of the hypopharynx and cervical esophagus. On average, four procedures were needed to close the fistula and restore the normal continuity of the digestive tract. In 15 out of the 41 patients, the fistula was never closed. Overall, the patients required 62 days of hospitalization, and an average of 91 days elapsed between resection and the restoration of feedings. An update of this series in 1992 included 4 more cases, with similar results.[36] Fredrickson et al.[37] compared the results of deltopectoral flap reconstruction to gastric transposition after total laryngopharyngectomy. The average number of days until resumption of swallowing was 90 for patients receiving the deltopectoral flaps, and 12 for patients undergoing gastric transposition. Patients with deltopectoral flaps averaged 7 admissions each for the duration of their follow-up. The authors concluded that for patients who might die within a year of their surgery, deltopectoral flap reconstruction was clearly inferior to gastric transposition.

MYOCUTANEOUS FLAPS

One of the great advances in head and neck reconstruction has been the development and application of myocutaneous flaps for replacement of substantial tissue defects. McCraw et al.[38, 39] showed that various large muscles provided the blood supply to well-defined areas of the overlying skin, known as vascular territories. Elevation of a compound flap consisting of the muscle with its intact blood supply, together with an overlying "paddle" of skin within the vascular territory of the muscle, can provide well-vascularized skin for reconstruction. Myocutaneous flaps can usually be transferred without preliminary delay and can be used for one-stage reconstruction because the paddle of skin is transferred as an "island." Myocutaneous flaps based on the trapezius muscle, the sternocleidomastoid muscle, the latissimus dorsi muscle, the platysma muscle, and the greater pectoral muscle have been used successfully in head and neck surgery.

Myocutaneous flaps have been used for reconstruction of the pharyngoesophageal segment after total pharyngolaryngectomy. Ariyan[40] used both sternocleidomastoid muscle and trapezius muscle myocutaneous flaps to close a large esophageal defect in a heavily irradiated patient. Guillamondegui and Larson[41] reported on 11 trapezius muscle flaps, 5 of which were tubed for reconstruction after laryngopharyngectomy. Demergasso and Piazza[42] presented 85 trapezius muscle myocutaneous and osteomyocutaneous flap reconstructions in the head and neck, including 5 complete reconstructions of the hypopharynx. In 1992, Carlson and colleagues[36] reported on 13 of 148 reconstructions of the hypopharynx using a lateral trapezius muscle flap. They included 21 pectoral muscle flaps in their cohort when evaluating the effectiveness of myocutaneous flaps for replacement of the hypopharynx and cervical esophagus. Though more reconstructions were performed with pectoral muscle flaps, the authors felt that the thinness of the trapezius muscle flap made it more suitable than the pectoral muscle flap for forming a tube.

Greater Pectoral Muscle Myocutaneous Flap

Although we have used various other myocutaneous flaps in our patients, we have found the greater pectoral muscle flap to be the most reliable and consistently useful.[43] This flap has great length and can provide generous amounts of well-vascularized skin for reconstruction. Most reconstructions can be accomplished in a single stage and the donor site can usually be closed primarily without a skin graft. The greater pectoral muscle, when transposed to the neck, provides cosmetically useful bulk and also covers the carotid artery.

The use of the greater pectoral muscle myocutaneous flap in head and neck reconstruction was described by Ariyan.[44] Withers et al.[45] reported one case of reconstruction with a greater pectoral muscle myocutaneous flap after a near-total pharyngolaryngectomy. Baek et al.[46] have used this flap successfully for a variety of purposes, including hypopharyngeal reconstruction.

Advocates of reconstruction using the pectoral muscle flap claim several advantages when compared with either older techniques, such as use of the deltopectoral flap, or newer techniques, such as visceral transposition or free flap reconstruction. The flaps are easy to raise, do not require two surgical teams, and are very hardy. More importantly, major body cavities are not entered, thereby limiting the morbidity. Reported disadvantages of this

method include a high rate of fistula formation, stricture formation at the distal anastomosis site, and dysphagia attributed to the bulkiness of the flap.[42, 43, 47–55]

Rees et al.[47] reported on 25 patients who underwent pectoral muscle flap reconstruction of the hypopharynx, although they did not specify what percentage had complete tubing of the flap. Gullane et al.[50] presented their results with hypopharyngeal and esophageal replacement, including 3 tubed pectoral muscle flaps. The majority of their reconstructions, however, were done with a free jejunal flap or by gastric transposition. In 1981 Baek et al.[53] used the tubed pectoral muscle flap exclusively in 14 patients with pharyngoesophageal defects and, at that time, stated that it was their reconstruction of choice. Lam et al.[54] opted for the tubed pectoral muscle flap in 18 out of 97 hypopharyngeal-esophageal reconstructions and a "patch-on" pectoral muscle flap in 36 more patients.

Several authors have modified the reconstructive method to decrease stricture formation and enhance swallowing. Lee and Lore[49] reported on using a dermal graft to form the posterior pharyngeal wall and then partially tubing a pectoral muscle flap to complete the neopharynx-esophagus. Excellent swallowing ability was achieved in three of four patients. Lam et al.[52] suggested making three longitudinal 2-cm slits in the proximal esophagus, as well as in the adjacent distal end of the tubed pectoral muscle flap, to allow interdigitation. This lessened the tendency for cicatricial scarring and stenosis. Su and Hwang[51] applied the concept of the near-total laryngectomy to their hypopharyngeal reconstructions, utilizing the uninvolved laryngeal remnant to create an innervated vocal shunt and partially tubing a pectoral muscle flap. Their 4 patients obtained intelligible shunt speech along with satisfactory deglutition.

In 1988 we reported our experience with 10 cases of pharyngoesophageal replacement with the tubed pectoral muscle myocutaneous flap.[43] We have accumulated several more cases since that time. The interval to swallowing was 10–21 days in non-radiated patients and 3–13 weeks in radiated patients. Eight patients achieved satisfactory and lasting deglutatory function. Although four patients developed fistulae, two closed with conservative management. We do not feel that the flap is too bulky to tube, especially given the tendency of these patients with an obstructing malignancy to be cachectic.

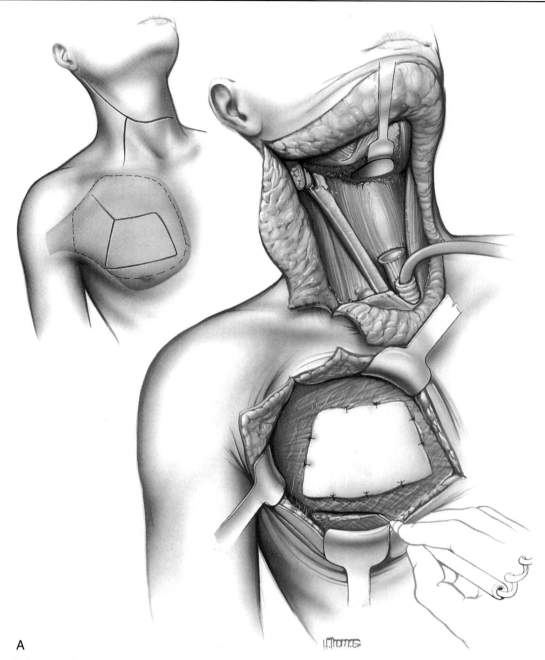

A

Figure 10–1. Major pectoral muscle myocutaneous esophagoplasty. (From Cusumano R, Silver C, Brauer R, et al. Pectoralis myocutaneous flap for replacement of cervical esophagus. *Head Neck* 1989; 11:450–456. Copyright ©1989. Reprinted by permission of John Wiley & Sons, Inc.)

Illustration continued on following page

Technique of Greater Pectoral Muscle Myocutaneous Esophagoplasty

Figure 10–1A. A greater pectoral muscle myocutaneous flap of adequate size is designed. The flap is placed directly over the greater pectoral muscle and is trapezoidal to conform to the diameters of the proximal pharyngeal and the distal esophageal anastomoses. Anastomotic tension and narrow cir-

cumference of anastomosis are important causes of postoperative stenosis. These factors are eliminated by creating a flap of adequate length and width. Absence of a "random" portion of skin improves the blood supply to the flap.

The major pectoral muscle is mobilized by dividing the costal and humeral attachments. The defect in the cervical pharyngoesophagus is shown.

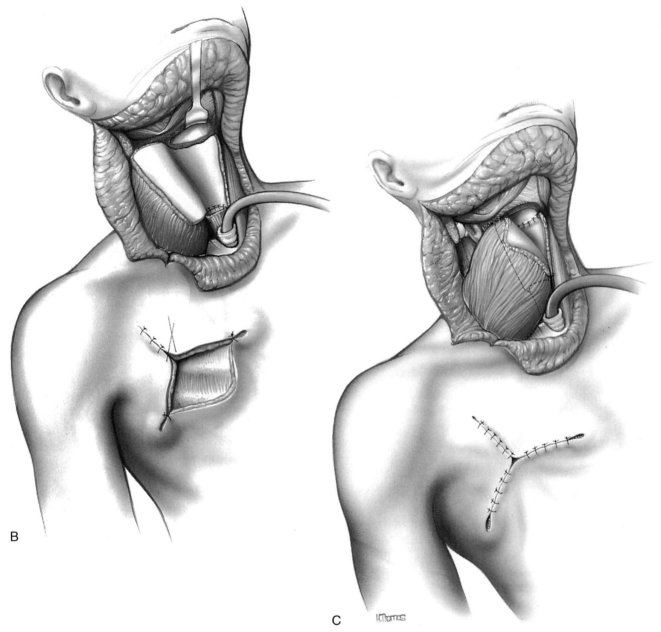

B

C   H.Thomas

Figure 10–1 *Continued* Major pectoral muscle myocutaneous esophagoplasty. (From Cusumano R, Silver C, Brauer R, et al. Pectoralis myocutaneous flap for replacement of cervical esophagus. *Head Neck* 1989; 11:450–456. Copyright © 1989. Reprinted by permission of John Wiley & Sons, Inc.)

Figure 10–1B. The flap is rotated into its cervical position. Sutures are placed for proximal and distal anastomoses. The longitudinal suture line will assume a lateral or anterolateral or anterolateral position on the contralateral side of the neck.

Figure 10–1C. The superior (pharyngeal) anastomosis and longitudinal suture line are completed. We have found no advantage to exteriorizing any portion of the reconstructed pharyngoesophagus and employ a single-stage closure. Despite its large size and awkward shape, the donor site on the chest wall can usually be closed primarily, even in male patients.

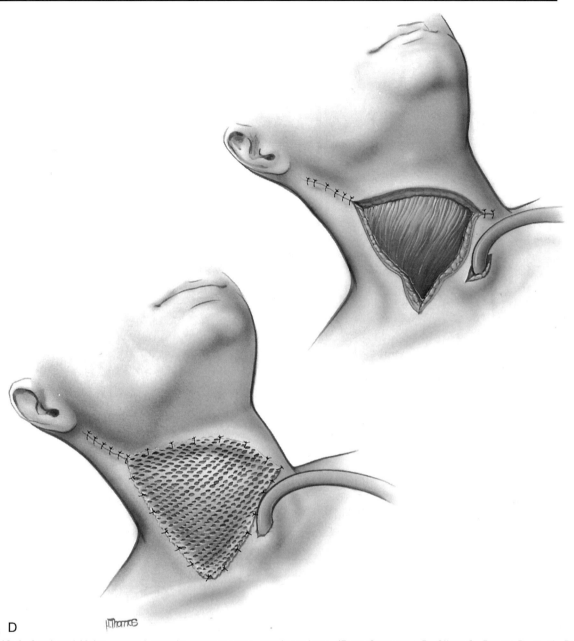

D

Figure 10–1 *Continued* Major pectoral muscle myocutaneous esophagoplasty. (From Cusumano R, Silver C, Brauer R, et al. Pectoralis myocutaneous flap for replacement of cervical esophagus. *Head Neck* 1989; 11:450–456. Copyright © 1989. Reprinted by permission of John Wiley & Sons, Inc.)

Figures 10–1*D.* It may often prove difficult to close the cervical skin over the pectoral muscle without constricting the flap pedicle or subjecting the closure to excessive tension. A meshed split-thickness skin graft applied over the muscle will eliminate these problems and provide excellent resurfacing of the neck.

TRANSPOSED AND PEDICLED ABDOMINAL VISCERA

Reversed Gastric Tube Esophagoplasty

The concept of using a tubed pedicle of stomach for esophageal bypass was suggested by Jianu[56] in 1912. In 1920 Kirschner[57] described a method of esophageal bypass using the stomach, which was advanced by the Roux-en-Y technique to the neck, with reimplantation of the distal esophagus near the pyloric region. Kirschner's procedure was revived by Ong[58] in 1973, who found it useful for palliative bypass of unresectable intrathoracic lesions. In 1948 Mes[59] modified Kirschner's procedure to produce a longer substitute esophagus. An isoperistaltic gastric tube was created and pedicled at the pyloric end, receiving its blood supply from the right gastroepiploic vessels. The fundic end was anastomosed to the cervical esophagus. Gavrilu and Georgescu,[60] in Bucharest, developed an antiperistaltic tube, pedicled at the fundic end of the stomach and vascularized by the left gastroepiploic vessels. This conduit was a convenient esophageal substitute that could readily be developed to sufficient length and was used with success clinically. Their procedure remained essentially unknown in the United States until it was popularized and modified by Heimlich.[61] A splenectomy permitted access to the fundic region of the stomach, allowing the pedicle to be placed as high as possible. This enabled creation of a tube of almost any length desired. Working in conjunction with our service, Heimlich[62, 63] reported successful use of the reversed gastric tube for replacement of the cervical esophagus after total pharyngolaryngectomy-esophagectomy (TPL-E). Although the gastric tube could be passed by either the substernal or the subcutaneous route to the neck, we preferred the subcutaneous route for cervical esophageal replacement, because the consequences of complications such as anastomotic leakage would thus be minimized, and an opportunity would be afforded to use skin if further reconstruction were required. For secondary reconstruction, the subcutaneous route is mandatory because the substernal route is no longer easily available.

Some authors[64, 65] have recently reported the use of isoperistaltic gastric tubes based on the right gastroepiploic vessels, similar in principle to the procedure described by Mes. Nevertheless, the antiperistaltic or reversed gastric tube has been more widely used in both one- and two-stage operations for esophageal reconstruction.

Indications

Reversed gastric tube esophagoplasty has recently been used more frequently and is considered by many authors to be the procedure of choice for esophageal replacement in infants and children.[66-68] It is an excellent procedure for bypass of benign esophageal strictures.[69] Although the procedure has been employed for thoracic esophageal carcinomas with some frequency, it has not been widely used for cervical esophageal replacement after pharyngolaryngectomy-esophagectomy. Our interest in the procedure for this purpose was stimulated by our association with Heimlich, and we have reported the successful use of the operation for both primary and secondary reconstruction of the cervical esophagus.[70]

We feel that a greater length of new esophagus can be developed from the stomach than from the colon. This permits easier transfer by the safer subcutaneous route to the level of the oropharynx. The gastric tube operation is also simpler, requiring only a single anastomosis in the neck. Longitudinal closure of the tube is usually done with a stapling device.[71] Esophagocoloplasty requires three major anastomoses, consequently with a longer operating time and a greater opportunity for complications.

In the past we have used reversed gastric tube esophagoplasty for cases that were not suitable for immediate reconstruction but that required the resection of a length of esophagus too great for skin flap reconstruction. The tubed pectoral muscle myocutaneous flap or transposition of the entire stomach is our procedure of choice if immediate reconstruction is desired. For the two-staged procedure, the tumor is resected, and the trachea and oropharynx are exteriorized at the first operation. The distal esophagus is transected and closed as low in the mediastinum as possible. After the initial resection, the patient is nourished by intravenous hyperalimentation or by a gastrostomy placed high on the lesser curvature of the stomach. When the patient has gained sufficient weight and when pulmonary sepsis has been resolved completely, a reversed gastric tube is transferred subcutaneously and anastomosed to the oropharyngeal stump.

Technique of Reversed Gastric Tube Esophagoplasty

Figure 10–2A. This procedure may be performed in a single stage with a two-team approach. We prefer to use the gastric tube for secondary reconstruction. Exposure of the stomach is obtained through a large

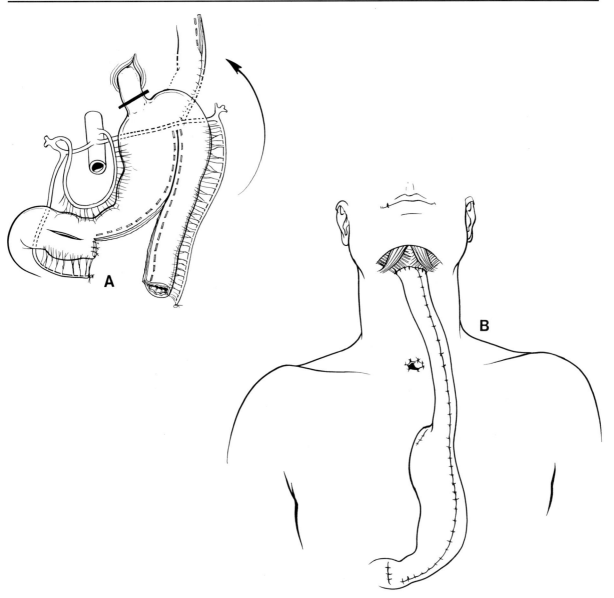

Figure 10–2. Reversed gastric tube esophagoplasty.

upper midline abdominal incision. The greater curvature of the stomach is mobilized by dividing the gastrocolic and gastrosplenic ligaments. The vessels in these ligaments are clamped and transected as far from the greater curvature of the stomach as possible, to avoid encroachment on the gastroepiploic vessels. A splenectomy is done to enhance exposure of greater curvature superiorly.

The reversed gastric tube is created along the greater curvature of the stomach. A small incision is made in the greater curvature about 3 to 4 cm from the pylorus, and a 28 Fr rectal tube is inserted and held against the curvature. The rectal tube serves as a template for the neoesophagus. A stapling instrument is pressed against the rectal tube,

and a double row of staples is inserted through the gastric wall. The gastric tube is created by incision between the staples. A pyloroplasty is performed to facilitate gastric emptying.

Figure 10–2B. The long line of staples in the greater curvature and the gastric tube is buried with a continuous seromuscular suture of nonabsorbable material. If used for secondary reconstruction, the subcutaneous route is the only available route for transfer of the tube to the pharynx. Mobilization of the tail of the pancreas enhances the available length of the tube and facilitates approximation to the pharynx.

Complications

Anastomotic fistulae are the most frequent complications of reversed gastric tube esophagoplasty.[64, 67] Most fistulae will close spontaneously in response to conservative treatment. Anastomotic strictures requiring dilatations occurred in 43% of cases reported by Ein et al.[67] Necrosis of a significant portion of the tube and disruption of the longitudinal suture line rarely occur, although we have noted these complications in some of our patients. Gozner et al.[72] reported two cases of peptic ulcer occurring in presternal reversed gastric tubes.

Esophagocoloplasty

Segments of colon have been used for esophageal replacement since the work of Kelling[73] and Vulliet[74] in 1911. The principle of this operation is based on the function of the marginal artery, which, if intact, can transport blood along a length of bowel after transection of one or more main mesenteric arterial branches. Thus, the bowel can be pedicled on a single arterial branch and transposed, either substernally or subcutaneously, to the neck. In 1944 Yudin[75] reported 80 cases of esophagocoloplasty for bypass or replacement of the thoracic esophagus. The use of colon for reconstruction after pharyngolaryngectomy and cervical esophagectomy was first reported in the English language literature by Goligher and Robin[76] in 1954. By the 1960s, both the right and the left colon were used for this purpose with increasing frequency.[77] Mannings et al.[78] reported the results of treatment of a series of patients at the Mayo Clinic with some good results but a high overall morbidity rate. In 1992 Carlson and colleagues[36] at the M.D. Anderson Cancer Center reported on 19 cases of esophagocoloplasty, 3 cases using the right colon and 16 cases using the left colon. Though only 1 flap was lost, 42% of the patients had functional failure. Interestingly, only 3 cases of esophagocoloplasty were performed after 1983, coinciding with the introduction of gastric transposition.

Both the right and the left colon have been used for esophagocoloplasty. The right colon possesses the theoretical advantage of assuming an isoperistaltic orientation when interposed into the esophageal defect. However, this apparent advantage is negated by the greater length of the left colon that can be mobilized and pedicled on the middle colic vessels. In addition, angiographic evidence has indicated that the marginal artery is more consistently present on the left side than on the right side of the colon.[79]

The antiperistaltic orientation of the left colon is not functionally significant. Although manometric and radiographic studies have demonstrated conflicting results concerning the presence or absence of actual peristalsis within interposed colonic segments, there is little question that antiperistaltic left colon segments function well, despite some delay in passage of ingested material from the mouth to the stomach.[80, 81]

Indications

At the present time, esophagocoloplasty is employed mainly when alternatives such as gastric transposition or microvascular reimplantation cannot be employed. Usually this will occur when a single-stage reconstruction cannot be accomplished, or when previous surgery has rendered the stomach unuseable. The choice between esophagocoloplasty and reversed gastric tube esophagoplasty often depends on the personal experience and comfort with each procedure of the individual surgeon.

The recent popularity of the technique of blunt pull-through esophagectomy without thoracotomy has led to the clinical observation that the posterior mediastinum is the shortest of all routes for esophageal substitution. Some authors[82–84] have used this route for colon interposition, as well as for gastric transposition after esophagectomy. This type of procedure will be discussed in more detail in relation to gastric transposition. Although we have feared risking necrosis of the colon within the mediastinum, the oncologic advantage of total esophagectomy, combined with the shortness of the route, would appear to make this procedure worthwhile in cases in which one-stage resection and reconstruction are desired and gastric transposition is not feasible.

Technique of Esophagocoloplasty (Using the Left Colon)

Figure 10–3A. This semischematic drawing shows the blood supply of the colon and the points of vascular transection for esophagocoloplasty with the left colon. The superior left colic artery and the anastomotic connections between the middle colic and the right colic arteries and between the superior and the inferior branches of the left colic artery are divided, creating an isolated loop of bowel supplied by the middle colic artery.

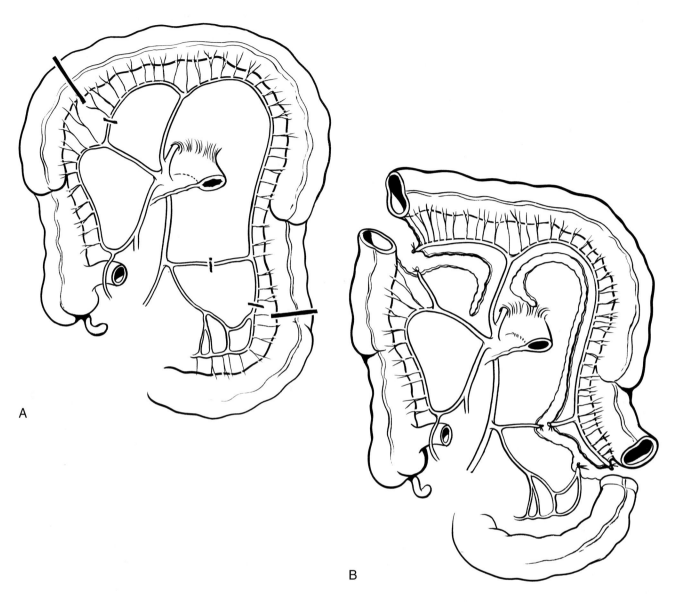

A

B

Figure 10–3. Esophagocoloplasty.

Illustration continued on following page

Figure 10–3B. Actual mobilization of the bowel is performed by dissecting the greater omentum from the colon and dividing the gastrocolic and the phrenocolic ligaments, as well as the lateral peritoneal reflections of the colon. When liberated, the vascular anatomy is examined by transillumination and palpation of arterial pulsations. The mesentery and the arteries are divided at a distance from the bowel sufficient to prevent interruption of the marginal arterial circulation.

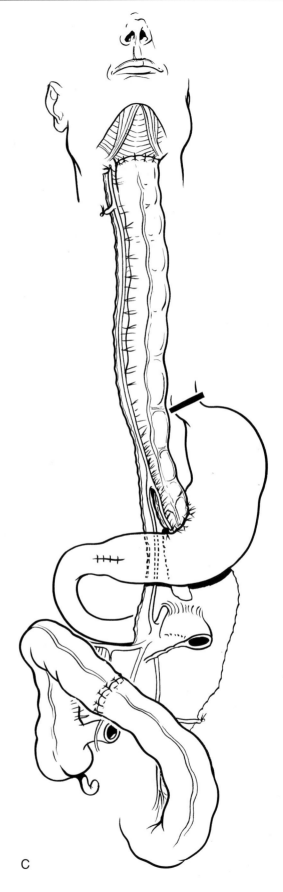

Figure 10–3C. The bowel is transposed to the neck with an antiperistaltic orientation by one of the routes described in Figure 10–3D. It is important to pass the mobilized loop and its vascular pedicle posterior to the stomach; otherwise the pedicle will form an obstructing band across the pyloric region. The distal (right) end of the colon is anastomosed to the aspect of the stomach with smaller curvature, on either the anterior or the posterior wall, depending on where it can be placed most conveniently without torsion or kinking. The gastrolic anastomosis should be placed as close to the fundic end of the stomach as possible.

A pyloroplasty is mandatory if vagectomy has been performed with the esophagectomy. Many surgeons, including ourselves, perform pyloroplasty in all cases to enhance gastric emptying.

Alimentary continuity is restored by colocolostomy.

C

Figure 10–3 *Continued* Esophagocoloplasty.

Figure 10–3D. Three alternative routes for transfer of the left colon to the neck are shown. These alternatives are also applicable to reversed gastric tube esophagoplasty.

The subcutaneous route is the safest because the consequences of necrosis of the transposed segment are relatively minimal in comparison to the other routes. The subcutaneous route, however, is the longest route to the neck, and it may be difficult to mobilize a segment of colon that is sufficiently long for this approach.

We often use a substernal tunnel for transfer of the left colon to the neck. The tunnel is created by blunt dissection, working from both the abdominal and the cervical incisions. Passage of a strong tape beneath the sternum and upward traction on the tape facilitate enlargement of the tunnel and transfer of the bowel. The substernal route cannot be used for secondary reconstruction of the esophagus if pharyngolaryngectomy has been performed previously.

In cases in which total esophagectomy has been performed, the colon may be transferred through the posterior mediastinum in the bed of the resected esophagus. This is the shortest of all the routes to the neck. This route is used for gastric transposition combined with blunt extrathoracic esophagectomy, but it may be used for the left colon or the gastric tube in cases in which gastric transposition is not feasible. The posterior mediastinal route cannot be used for secondary reconstruction.

Complications

The complications of esophagocoloplasty are the same as those of other visceral transpositions, differing only in degree, as reported by various authors. Necrosis of the colon and leakage or dehiscence at the cervical anastomosis are the major problems.

Gastric Transposition

Replacement of the esophagus by transposition of the entire stomach through the posterior mediastinum into the neck with direct pharyngogastric anastomosis has proved to be a satisfactory procedure in selected cases. Resection of the pharynx and the larynx is combined with closed resection of the thoracic esophagus. The stomach is transposed through the posterior mediastinum, in the bed of the previously resected esophagus. The operation is performed in one stage, and only one anastomosis is required. The blood supply of the transposed stomach is superior to that of other organs used as esophageal substitutes, and the pharyngogastric

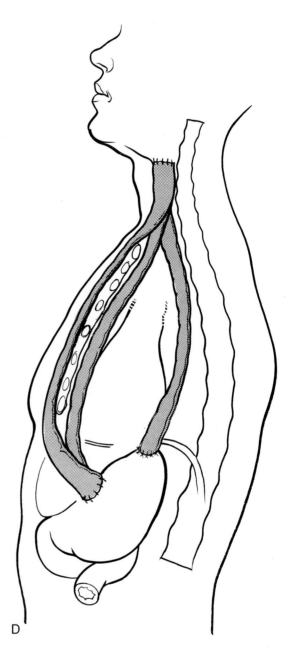

D

Figure 10–3 *Continued* Esophagocoloplasty.

anastomosis is particularly resistant to stricture formation or leakage.

The idea of performing blunt total esophagectomy through cervical and abdominal incisions was suggested by Denk[85] who in 1913 performed the procedure in cadavers and experimental animals. Turner,[86, 87] in 1936, was the first to use this approach successfully for resection of intrathoracic esophageal carcinoma. Limitations in exposure and control of bleeding, however, rendered the technique unsuitable for that purpose. In 1960 Ong and Lee[88] reported three cases of tranposition of the stomach through the posterior mediastinum for esophageal replacement after pharyngolaryngectomy. LeQuesne and Ranger,[89] in 1966, reported their experience with 14 cases of gastric transposition for esophageal replacement. The first three patients had undergone a three-incision procedure with laparotomy and thoracotomy, as well as cervical dissection. Because of poor results obtained with these patients, the authors began to use the technique of closed chest blunt dissection of the normal thoracic esophagus. Elimination of the thoracotomy lessened the morbidity and mortality of the procedure and produced a great improvement in the results. Further modifications and improvements in the procedure were subsequently reported by Stell,[90] Leonard and Maran,[91] Silver,[92] and Akiyama et al.[82]

More recently, interest has been revived in Turner's original concept of closed chest blunt esophagectomy for resection of intrathoracic esophageal carcinoma. Several authors[83, 84, 93] have successfully used this procedure for resection of tumors at all levels of the thoracic esophagus. Advocates of this approach feel that the incidence of complications and mortality is significantly lower than for conventional thoracotomy, particularly when surgery is primarily intended for palliation. This application of the procedure, however, has been controversial. When dealing with postcricoid lesions or tumors of the cervicothoracic segment of the esophagus, the portion of esophagus that has to be dissected blindly is normal and, therefore, less problematic.

Indications

Gastric transposition combined with blunt closed chest total esophagectomy is most suitable for postcricoid and cervical esophageal carcinomas, particularly when these lesions extend inferiorly below the thoracic outlet. Removal of the entire esophagus helps to ensure adequate margins for these tumors, as well as to open the posterior mediastinal route for esophageal replacement. For the reasons already stated, transposed stomach is a better esophageal substitute than are other viscera and should be used if technically feasible.

Gastric transposition is less suitable for hypopharyngeal tumors that extend upward rather than inferiorly. This is most often encountered with posterior pharyngeal wall lesions that rarely extend below the cricopharyngeal muscle but may extend upward into the nasopharynx. Although transposed stomach reaches easily to the level of the base of the tongue, posterior pharyngeal wall anastomosis farther superiorly would be difficult. Additional mobilization and traction on the stomach or creation of a flap of gastric fundus might permit an anastomosis, but such a procedure would be technically complex and prone to postoperative morbidity. In the past, we preferred the deltopectoral flap or the tubed pectoral muscle myocutaneous flap as an esophageal substitute for this type of lesion.[70] More recently, we have employed microvascular free flaps.

Although various authors[82, 94] have indicated their preference for gastric transposition for all pharyngoesophageal replacements, their papers are unclear as to what limitations are placed on the use of this technique for lesions with upward extension. Our approach has been to individualize cases on the basis of general health, habitus, prior radiotherapy, and other factors. Gastric transposition is quite successful in heavily irradiated patients[70, 94] and is preferred in these instances. Patients who are not in sufficiently good condition to withstand the rather extensive operation required for one-stage gastric transposition should undergo reconstruction with a tubed pectoral muscle myocutaneous flap or another flap not requiring invasion of a body cavity.

Occasionally, gastric transposition is technically impossible. A gastroduodenal ulcer or a tumor or scarring and tissue loss from previous gastric surgery may preclude the use of the stomach for esophageal replacement. The right gastric and gastroepiploic vessels must be intact, and there should be no interruption of the vascular arcades along the greater or lesser curvatures in order to ensure an adequate blood supply of the transposed stomach. Previous thoracic, mediastinal, or upper abdominal surgery may make blunt esophagectomy without thoracotomy impossible.

Technique of Total Esophagectomy with Gastric Transposition (Gastric "Pull-Up")

Figure 10–4A. A carcinoma of the cervical esophagus situated entirely below the cricopharyngeal muscle and extending inferiorly into the mediasti-

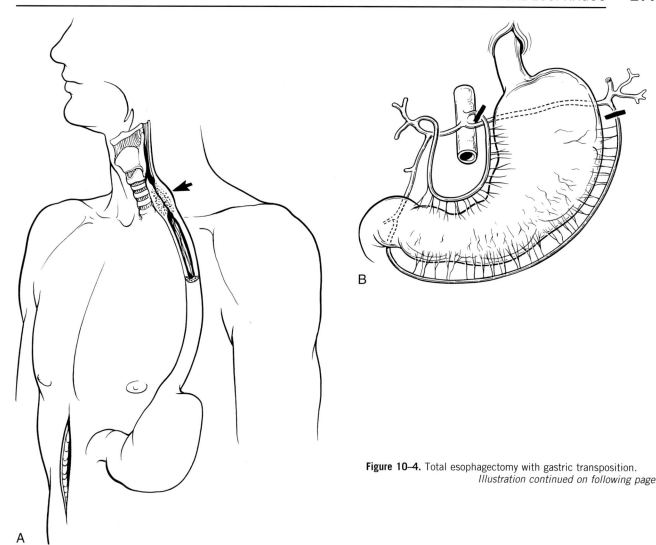

A

B

Figure 10–4. Total esophagectomy with gastric transposition.
Illustration continued on following page

num is shown. This lesion will require considerable resection of the distal esophagus and is best managed by total esophagectomy.

Figure 10–4B. A two-team approach is used for this operation. While the cervical team performs the pharyngolaryngectomy as shown in Figure 9–12, the abdominal team will mobilize the stomach. It is wise to give the cervical team a sufficient "head start" to establish the resectability of the tumor before opening the abdomen.

A generous upper midline laparotomy incision is made. The transposed stomach will receive its blood supply from the right gastric and the right gastroepiploic vessels. The left gastric, the short gastric, and the left gastroepiploic vessels are divided.

The stomach is mobilized by dividing the gastrosplenic ligaments at a sufficient distance from the stomach to avoid compromising the arcade of gastroepiploic vessels on the greater curvature. The greater curvature vessels should be suture ligated. Preservation of venous drainage is as critical as is

ensuring adequate arterial flow. Thus, it is important not to injure or divide the right gastroepiploic vein near its origin.

The gastroesophageal junction is mobilized by dividing the left triangular ligaments of the liver and dissecting the peritoneal and ligamentous attachments around the esophageal hiatus. A tape is passed around the distal esophagus, and both vagus nerves are divided between clips. The esophageal hiatus is enlarged by dilatation and transection of the muscle until the surgeon's hand can be easily passed into the posterior mediastinum.

In order to permit transposition of the entire stomach into the posterior mediastinum, it is necessary to free most of the duodenum from its posterior attachments. This is done by the Kocher technique, which consists of incising the posterolateral peritoneal attachments and sweeping the entire duodeno-pancreatic-biliary complex anteromedially.

A gastric drainage procedure is mandatory. We prefer a small Heineke-Mikulicz pyloroplasty for this purpose.

Figure 10–4C. After completion of the pharyngolaryngectomy and the mobilization of the stomach and the duodenum, dissection of the intrathoracic esophagus is commenced. Both the cervical and the abdominal surgeons work by blunt digital dissection. About two thirds of the esophagus will be mobilized from below and about one third from the cervical incision. The posterior plane is established first, after which the lateral and then the anterior attachments are separated. The lateral attachments of the esophagus may be visualized and clipped before transection for a certain distance in both directions, but at the midthoracic level avulsion of these attachments is necessary. Although some bleeding will occur from this dissection, it is generally only a diffuse ooze and will be controlled by tamponade when the bulky stomach fills the posterior mediastinum.

Various maneuvers facilitate manual esophageal dissection. We have found that in the final stages of the mobilization it is most convenient to have a single surgeon, working with one hand inserted through the abdominal incision and the other through the cervical, to divide the remaining attachments of the esophagus to complete its liberation. Insertion of a No. 28 rubber rectal tube into the esophagus may facilitate dissection and will be helpful in the delivery of the stomach through the mediastinum.

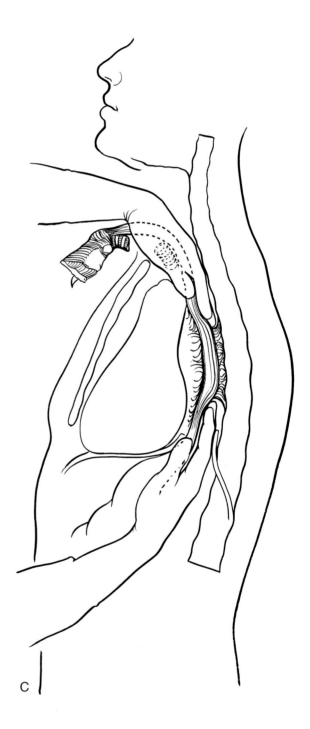

C

Figure 10–4 *Continued* Total esophagectomy with gastric transposition.

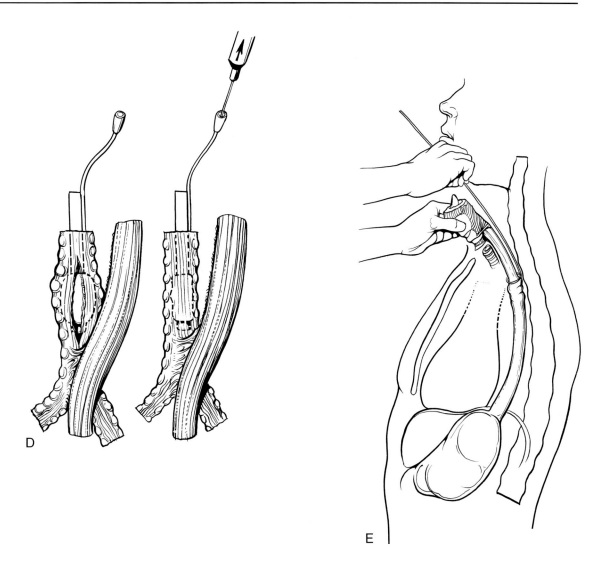

Figure 10–4 *Continued* Total esophagectomy with gastric transposition.

Illustration continued on following page

Figure 10–4D. The most difficult aspect of the esophageal mobilization involves the management of the posterior tracheal wall. As the esophagus is being separated from the trachea, the delicate membranous posterior wall may tear easily. The expansile force exerted by the pneumatic cuff of the endotracheal tube contributes to the tendency of the tracheal wall to split. The endotracheal cuff should be decompressed before separating the esophagus and the trachea.

A tear in the posterior tracheal wall tends to extend rapidly, even below the carina, and severe ventilatory difficulties, resulting from the uncontrolled leakage of air, may be encountered. The laceration should be repaired by continuous suture as quickly as possible. On one occasion we found it necessary to remove a wedge of manubrium rapidly in order to gain adequate exposure of the posterior tracheal wall. If, after suture, a relatively small air leak persists, it will be tamponaded when the stomach is transposed. Immediate thoracotomy has been successfully used for repair of an otherwise unmanageable air leak.[84]

Figure 10–4E. Alternative methods for esophageal extraction have been reported by Akiyama et al.[82] The method depicted here uses a ring dissector and may be useful when employed in combination with the digital technique.

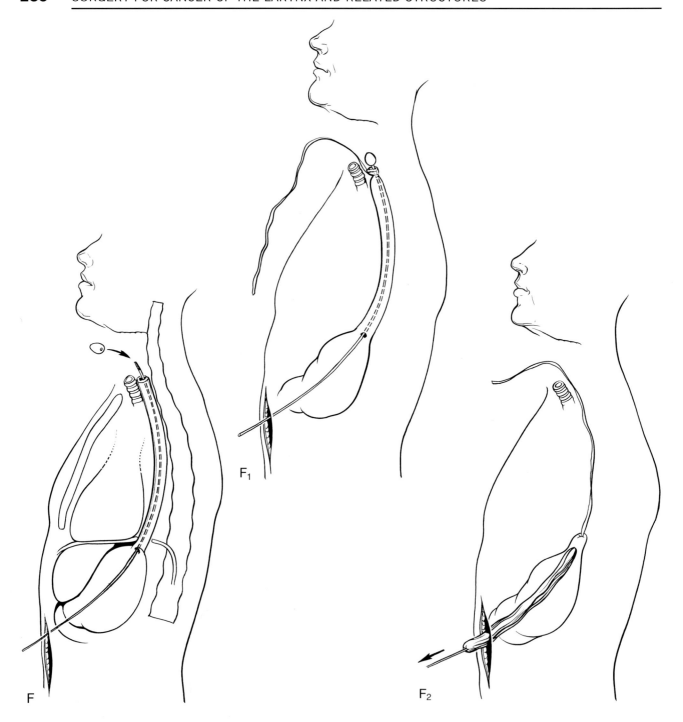

Figure 10–4 *Continued* Total esophagectomy with gastric transposition.

Figure 10–4F. A second alternative method uses an internal vein stripper that may be employed when the esophagus can be transected below the tumor at a relatively high level. The stripper is inserted through a small incision in the lower esophagus and is passed upward.

Figure 10–4F₁. The head of the stripper is placed on the threaded end and secured with a ligature around the esophagus. Before stripping the esophagus, a length of tape is tied to the stripper to serve as a guide for the stomach.

Figure 10–4F₂. The stripper is withdrawn through the abdominal incision, thus extracting and inverting the esophagus. The guide tape is secured to the esophageal stump after the lower end of the esophagus is transected.

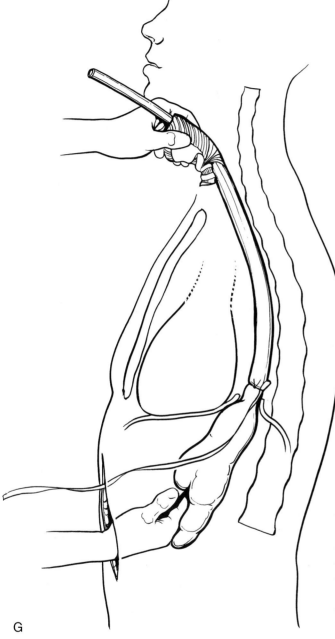

G

Figure 10–4 *Continued* Total esophagectomy with gastric transposition.

Illustration continued on following page

Figure 10–4G. The stomach is now transposed through the posterior mediastinum into the neck. Before commencing this step, it is wise to create as much of the tracheostoma as possible by suturing the trachea to the cervical skin. Otherwise, once the stomach is transposed, it tends to envelop and obscure the tracheal stump, making the stump difficult to control and suture.

The abdominal surgeon feeds the stomach into the mediastinum inferiorly, while the neck surgeon gently pulls on the esophagus. An intraesophageal No. 28 rubber rectal tube secured to the distal esophagus may permit greater traction without tearing the esophagus. A 1-inch Penrose drain is temporarily fixed to the lower esophagus before transposition, so that it will be positioned through the mediastinum. The lower end of the drain will be brought out through an abdominal stab wound before closure.

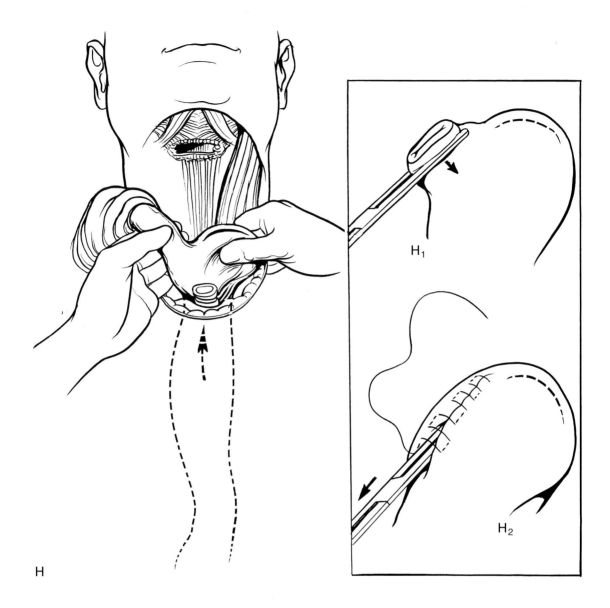

Figure 10–4 *Continued* Total esophagectomy with gastric transposition.

Figures 10–4H, 10–4H₁, and 10–4H₂. The cardio-esophageal junction will eventually reach the lower cervical region. The gastric fundus tends to be tucked posteriorly against the spine because it trails the cardioesophageal junction when the stomach is pulled up. Gentle traction on the prolapsed fundus will deliver a generous portion of the stomach into the cervical wound, sufficient to reach the oropharynx.

The cardioesophageal junction is transected (Fig. 10–4H₁) and the defect closed by the Parker-Kerr technique (Fig. 10–4H₂). A stapling instrument may also be used for this purpose.

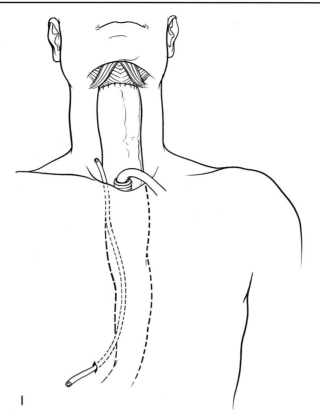

Figure 10–4 *Continued* Total esophagectomy with gastric transposition.

Figure 10–4*I*. The pharyngogastric anastomosis is created using a two-layer technique. The pharynx is anastomosed to an incision placed in the dome of the fundus. A nasogastric tube is placed through the anastomosis.

While the closure of the cardioesophageal junction and the pharyngogastric anastomosis proceeds, the abdomen is closed. Before abdominal closure, the pyloroplasty should be inspected to be certain it remains intact, and the duodenum and bile ducts should be inspected for torsion, leaks, or obstruction. A jejunostomy tube is often inserted as a precaution.

Complications and Sequelae

Gastric transposition is an extensive procedure. Although some authors[82, 84, 94] have noted the relative paucity of complications with this procedure compared to other reconstructive methods, significant morbidity and mortality can and do occur.

Perioperative Mortality and Length of Hopitalization

In 1989 our group reported on 15 cases of gastric transposition for replacement of esophageal and pharyngoesophageal defects.[95] Satisfactory and last-ing deglutition was achieved in 12 of the 15 patients. Oral feeding was begun, on average, 2 weeks after surgery. In all cases, surgical margins were free of tumor. Three patients (20%) died of surgical complications. Perrachia et al.[96] reported an operative mortality of 12.9% in a series of 85 gastric transpositions. Lau and colleagues[55] reported perioperative mortality of 6% in 48 patients with hypopharyngeal carcinoma who had reconstruction by gastric pull-up. Mehta et al.[97] described 75 patients who underwent gastric transposition for replacement of the pharyngoesophagus. The peri-operative mortality rate was below 10%. Fifty-three patients were able to resume a soft diet within 21 days. The average hospital stay for uncomplicated cases was 18 days, and, for complicated cases, 40 days.

In 1981, Harrison[98] reported 62 cases of TPL-E with gastric pull-up as part of a larger series of 162 patients with hypopharyngeal and esophageal carcinoma. Though he initially noted a mortality rate of 12%, this was reduced to 8.7% with the later cases. In 1986, he updated this series to 101 cases.[99] The hospital mortality rate was 11%. Minor postoperative complications, such as pleural effusion and bile regurgitation, were seen in all patients. Successful swallowing occurred in all patients before they left the hospital, usually within 2 weeks.

Respiratory and Intrathoracic Problems

We have encountered several instances of tears in the posterior tracheal wall that have been successfully repaired intraoperatively and then effectively tamponaded when the stomach was transposed. An uncontrolled air leak from the membranous trachea may require immediate repair through a right thoracotomy approach, as reported by Szentpetery et al.[84] Pneumothorax may occur from entry into the pleural cavity during the dissection, particularly around the esophageal hiatus. Orringer and Sloan[83] reported the development of pneumothorax, either unilateral or bilateral, in 8 out of 26 patients after blunt esophagectomy without thoracotomy.

Lau and colleagues[55] reported a 23% incidence of intrathoracic infection in a series of 48 cases that resulted in death in 2 patients. The authors reported transient bradycardia, arrhythmia, and hypotension in all patients during the mediastinal dissection, without any permanent sequelae.

An immediate postoperative radiograph of the chest should always be taken and an intercostal tube placed if necessary.

Hemorrhage

The most likely source of severe immediate postoperative bleeding is the gastric vasculature.[84, 90] Stell[90] has suggested suture transfixion of the greater curvature vessels in order to prevent dislodgment of ligatures when the stomach is pulled through the mediastinum.

Although it is not possible to directly control many of the bleeding points in the mediastinum along the bed of the resected esophagus, the transposed stomach will adequately tamponade vessels and raw surfaces within the posterior mediastinum. Bleeding from these sites does not pose a clinical problem.

Delayed rupture of major vessels, particularly the innominate artery, is an occasional postoperative catastrophe. Two of our 15 patients died from innominate artery hemorrhage.[95] Both patients had developed necrosis and infection of the adjacent tracheal wall. We have also encountered one instance of severe hemorrhage from a lingual artery at the site of an anastomotic fistula in an irradiated patient, which was controlled by ligation. Orringer and Sloan[83] reported 2 fatalities from innominate artery rupture in their series of 28 cases, both in patients who had required anterior mediastinal tracheotomies.

Anastomotic Disruption and Fistula

Because of the limited extent of entry into the gastrointestinal tract, anastomotic disruption oc-curs less frequently after gastric transposition than after other methods of esophageal replacement. One patient from our series of 15 patients reported in 1989[95] experienced transient drainage of bilious fluid from the mediastinum in the immediate postoperative period, which cleared without sequelae. Another patient developed mediastinitis secondary to disruption of the pyloroplasty. This disruption had occurred as a result of traction on the stomach during the transposition. We have subsequently learned to inspect the pyloroplasty closure carefully after transposing the stomach.

Our 1989 report included three pharyngogastrostomy fistulae in 15 cases. Two fistulae healed with conservative management. The third fistula occurred in a patient who had required fundoplasty because the transposed stomach was not sufficiently long to reach the superior resection margin. Additional reconstructive surgery was required to correct that situation. Orringer and Sloan[83] reported four instances of anastomotic leakage in their series of 26 patients. Carlson et al.[36] reported on data from 23 patients accumulated over a 9-year period. No cases of gastric necrosis occurred, and only 2 patients died in the postoperative period. Gastrointestinal complications, such as prolonged ileus or bowel obstruction occurred in 5 patients. Six mucocutaneous fistulae developed, 3 of which were closed. Gullane and colleagues[50] evaluated 17 gastric transpositions, 2 with feeding gastrostomies in place. There was 1 instance of subtotal gastric necrosis, treated with débridement and controlled pharyngostomy.

Gastric Function

Because gastric transposition entails a complete vagotomy, a gastric drainage procedure is necessary. Although digital dilatation of the pylorus and pyloromyotomy have been used with apparent success by other authors, we prefer to perform a small Heineke-Mikulicz pyloroplasty because of dissatisfaction with the simpler procedures.

Several authors have noted that good gastric function and no swallowing problems result after this operation,[82, 84, 94] and this has been confirmed by our own experience. Harrison[94] reported that good reservoir function is retained and that acid regurgitation is not a problem because of the vagotomy. There were occasional complaints of discomfort after bulky meals. Lam et al.[100] found atrophic gastritis in 13 out of 19 patients with an intrathoracic stomach for esophageal replacement. Although the mechanical response to distension by food was retained, basal and maximal acid output were markedly reduced. Serum gastrin levels were elevated. Wei et al.[101] noted regurgitation in 23% of the patients. The majority were able to take solid food without difficulty.

Digestive problems after gastric transposition are minimized by encouraging the patients to eat small amounts, to eat slowly, and to remain seated quietly, in an erect position, for a short period after eating.

Endocrine Deficiencies

A significant incidence of hypocalcemia has been reported after resection of the hypopharynx and cervical esophagus.[94, 102–105] At least 50% of our patients have had either hypothyroidism or hypoparathyroidism after total pharyngolarygectomy-esophagectomy. In many cases, adequate oncologic surgery requires the resection of the entire thyroid-parathyroid complex en bloc with the pharygolaryngectomy specimen. Even when efforts are made to preserve a certain amount of thyroid and parathyroid tissue, functional loss may occur because of devascularization. Wei and colleagues[101] discussed the late complications resulting from TPL-E and pharyngogastric anastomosis in a review of 136 patients. They noted that the incidence of hypothyroidism and hypoparathyroidism reflected whether a thyroidectomy was performed. Two thirds of the patients who had a total thyroidectomy as part of the extirpative procedure required both thyroxine replacement and calcium or vitamin D replacement. A majority of their cohort also underwent external beam radiation therapy, which probably contributed to a significant degree of hypothyroidism, even in patients with both lobes of the thyroid preserved.

Thyroid and parathyroid function should be monitored postoperatively in these patients. Clinical manisfestations of endocrine deficiencies may be subtle and may go undetected by physicians preoccupied with other problems. Hypocalcemia may cause such unusual manifestations as mental depression, headache, and abdominal pain, as well as the more common digital and circumoral paresthesias. Unrecognized chronic hypocalcemia may produce cataracts, convulsive disorders, and psychosis.[105]

Communication

Wei et al[101] found that only 11% of the patients developed an alaryngeal mode of oral communication, with 6.6% developing "gastroesophageal" speech, and 4.4% speaking with an electrolarynx. Harrison[94] observed that well-motivated patients were able to develop good "esophageal" speech. Our experience has been similar and we believe that the patients who would develop good speech after ordinary total laryngectomy would also be the ones to be able to speak after gastric transposition.

The matter of alaryngeal speech in 5 patients with TPL-E was addressed by Maniglia et al.,[106] who performed delayed tracheogastric punctures. Although there were no complications related to the procedure, voice quality was characterized by a lower pitch, a reduced intensity, a slower rate, and a "wet" quality. Nonetheless, speech intelligibility and fluency were adequate for conversational speech.

Comparison with Other Reconstructive Methods

Several studies have compared other methods of reconstruction of the pharyngoesophagus to gastric transposition and pharyngogastric anastomosis. In 1980, Frederickson et al.[37] examined reconstructions using the older staged deltopectoral flap in contrast to gastric pull-up. It is not surprising that the latter operation resulted in more effective reconstructions, with an average operation-to-swallow time of 12 days for the gastric pull-up group versus 90 days for the deltopectoral flap group. Lam et al.[54] compared the tubed greater pectoral muscle myocutaneous flap to gastric pull-up. Although they favored the latter procedure, they also cautioned that the procedure traversed three anatomic regions of the body and had a higher perioperative mortality. However, they felt that as cancer of the hypopharynx and cervical esophagus carries a poor prognosis, successful palliation necessitates immediate, functional reconstruction, best provided by gastric pull-up. By contrast, de Vries et al.[107] felt that a free jejunal interposition graft was better than TPL-E with gastric pull-up. They cited a shorter hospital stay, quicker time to swallowing, and fewer problems with regurgitation and the dumping syndrome in the jejunal interposition group. Nevertheless, the choice of a free jejunal graft is contingent on the level of the inferior extent of the resection. The distal esophageal stump must be accessible for safe anastomosis.

Results

The results of several reported series of gastric transposition are summarized in Table 10–2. The number of cases tabulated is 479. Approximately 8% of the patients died in the early postoperative period. Results were considered "satisfactory" in 63% of the patients. This is, of course, a vague criterion, because of the differing interpretations of the requirements for success. As with most complicated procedures, results have tended to improve as surgical teams have developed more experience in technique and in selection of patients.

Table 10–2. RESULTS OF GASTRIC TRANSPOSITION			
Author	Number of Patients	Early Postoperative Death	Results
Silver et al.,[95] 1989	15	3	Satisfactory palliation in 80% of patients; 6 patients disease free 3 or more years
Stell,[90] 1979	19	5	11 patients alive 6–18 months after surgery
Akiyama et al.,[82] 1978	24	0	Good palliation in all patients; longest survival, 3 years 7 months
Fredrickson,[37] 1981	9	0	2 patients alive at 4 and 10 years
Harrison,[99] 1986	101	1	58% 5-year survival
Wei et al.,[101] 1984	136	—	Longest follow-up—13 years 3 months; median follow-up—18 months
Lau et al.,[55] 1987	48	3	12 patients free of disease
Schusterman et al.,[131] 1988	15	1	Longest follow-up—64 months
Mehta et al.,[97] 1990	75	7	70.6% success rate; long-term follow-up not reported
Carlson et al.,[36] 1992	23	2	44% 2-year survival; 6% 4-year survival
Total	465	22	295 patients (62.5%) with good to satisfactory results

Cure rates are generally considered better for hypopharyngeal than for esophageal cancers. For example, in a series of 103 TPL-Es studied by Perrachia et al.,[96] a 5-year survival of 43% was achieved in patients with primary carcinoma of the hypopharynx, as compared with 17% survival for patients with carcinoma of the cervical esophagus.

By contrast, in our series reported in 1989,[95] 10 patients had carcinoma involving the cervical esophagus that required pharyngolaryngectomy as well as esophagectomy. Only 3 patients (30%) remained disease free for 3 years or longer. Three out of 5 patients (60%) remained disease free after resections of the cervicothoracic esophagus that did not require a laryngectomy.

An interesting objection to the gastric transposition operation was raised by Stell,[33] who noted a high incidence of early tumor recurrence in patients who had undergone successful gastric transposition operations. Patients reconstructed with deltopectoral flaps had better survival statistics. Stell opined that the extensive dissection and opening of tissue planes required for gastric transposition might facilitate the spread of the tumor. This experience, however, is not substantiated by the experience of others. The crude 3-year survival rate of 29% recently reported by Harrison[103] is at least as high as that reported with any other method of

reconstruction. Shepperd,[108] in his series of 23 cases, found that recurrent tumor almost always occurred within the lymph nodes. Recurrence at the primary site occurred in only one case, and in no instance was there evidence of extensive implantation of the tumor as a result of the dissection. We feel that the effect of a surgical procedure on the cure rate is influenced chiefly by the adequacy of the resection and not by the method used for reconstruction.

FREE TRANSPLANTATION OF VISCERA

The advent of microvascular surgery has revived interest in the replacement of the esophagus by freely transplanted revascularized segments of the intestinal tract. A technique for transplantation of jejunum in dogs and human beings was developed at our institution and reported in 1959 by Seidenberg et al.[109] Our interest in this technique continued through the next 10 years, but although early results appeared promising,[110] subsequent experience was disappointing.[70] Similar results at other institutions resulted in loss of enthusiasm for this approach.

Sporadic success was nevertheless achieved by various surgeons who used jejunum and ileum,[111–116] gastric antrum,[117] sigmoid colon,[118–121] and ileocolic sements.[122] During this era, vascular anastomosis was most often performed with a stapling device. The most successful work was that of Nakayama et al.[121] who, in 1964, reported a series of 20 sigmoid colon and iliac transplants. There were only 5 failures in the series, mostly in the early cases. Nakamura et al.[115] reported successful esophageal replacement with revascularized segments of jejunum in 11 out of 13 cases using a vascular stapler. Excellent palliation was obtained in all their cases, but 8 patients died from recurrent cervical tumor that, the authors felt, resulted from inadequate lymph node dissection. The procedure was felt to be most suitable for tumors that measured less than 5 cm longitudinally and that were confined to the cervical region. Grange and Quick[122] employed ileocolic segments successfully in 2 cases. These authors noted that the ileocolic artery was sufficiently large for anastamosis to the external carotid without the aid of a stapling device or a microscope.

Nevertheless, with the evolution of the operating microscope and of microsurgical technique, reliable transfer of revascularized segments of tissue by this technique became feasible. The microscope was used with success by Baudet et al[118, 123] and by McKee and Peter[114] and is almost universally employed at the present time, as this seems to be the most dependable way of ensuring vascular anastomotic patency.

In addition to the technical difficulty and length of the operations, an important limitation of the visceral transplant method is in the amount of esophagus that can be resected distally. An adequate cuff of distal esophagus must be available in order to perform an anastomosis. A greater length of esophagus, up to the point of a total esophagectomy, can be resected if transposed, rather than transplanted, stomach or bowel is used for replacement. The presence of a vascular anastomosis in the neck, particularly to a major vessel, also constitutes a risk, although hemorrhage from disrupted anastomoses is rare.

Free Jejunal Transplantation

Of all the free visceral transplants that have been employed, the greatest experience has been gained with the jejunal autograft. It can be used to reconstruct defects up to 20 cm in length. In 1992, Carlson et al.[36] reported on 26 flaps in 25 patients. There were only 3 abdominal complications, including prolonged ileus, gastrointestinal bleeding, and jejunostomy leak. There was a 20% fistulization rate, but the majority closed with conservative management. Perracchia and colleagues[96] reviewed 152 resections for cervical esophageal or hypopharyngeal carcinoma performed between 1975 and 1988. Thirty patients underwent free intestinal loop interposition with an operative mortality of 6.1%. Coleman et al.[124] reported on 96 microvascular jejunal transfers in 88 patients, with initial success in 78 patients. Five of the 10 initial failures were then successfully repaired with a second free jejunal flap, for a final reconstruction rate of 94.3%. Fifty-five patients underwent primary reconstruction and 24, secondary reconstruction.

Numerous series have now been compiled, all of which demonstrate a high success rate accompanied by low morbidity and mortality.[36, 50, 94, 124–131] Biel and Maisel[125] presented 17 patients with free jejunal interposition and analyzed the literature on this method of reconstruction from Seidenberg's first account of this procedure to 1987. They compiled 347 cases. The authors calculated rates of 3.5% for mortality, 11.5% for graft loss, 10.6% for fistula formation, and 5.5% for stricture formation among these cases.

Monitoring of free flaps is mandatory in order to detect early signs of ischemia. Indirect methods include implantable Doppler and surface temperature probes. Direct methods of observation, however, are prefered. If the flap extends into the oropharynx, it can be inspected transorally. If not, repeated endoscopies may be necessary using either a laryngoscope or a fiberoptic nasopharyngoscope. All these methods are inherently limited because of postoperative edema, which makes evaluation cumbersome and difficult to interpret.

The most direct method of inspection relies on exteriorization of a portion of the free jejunal graft. In 1980, Hester et al.[132] described a technique in which a small window covered by a sheet of Silastic was left open in the skin closure, allowing repeated visual inspection. Katsaros et al.[133] were the first to exteriorize a segment of jejunum for postoperative monitoring. They isolated the distal 2 cm of the graft as a small island flap based on the terminal branches of the vascular arcade. This smaller segment was brought out through the incision and sutured to the skin. After 5 days, the exteriorized segment was excised under local anesthesia. Urken et al.[134] modified this by stapling both ends of the exteriorized segment, opening the antimesenteric border to expose the mucosal surface, and suturing the serosal surface to the skin to decrease the risk of neck infection. The exteriorized segment was removed and its mesentery ligated on the fifth postoperative day.

Technique of Free Jejunal Transplantation

Figure 10–5A. Two surgical teams perform the procedure. The abdominal team makes a small midline laparotomy incision through which a segment of jejunum is isolated. A loop is chosen that has well-developed mesenteric vessels and will conform to the cervical defect and available vessels when oriented in an isoperistaltic direction.

Various methods of hypothermia have been used to minimize damage to the graft during the period of ischemia. We have flushed the graft with cold heparinized saline through the artery and then placed the loop in a basin of the same solution.

The jejunal graft is handed to the cervical team while the abdominal surgeons restore continuity of the jejunum by anastomosis. A temporary tube gastrostomy is often performed, if not previously done, and the abdomen is closed.

Figure 10–5B. Several alternatives exist regarding which vessels to use for revascularization at the recipient site. In the instance shown, the mesenteric vessel is anastomosed end-to-end to a branch of the external carotid. End-to-side anastomosis may be done as an alternative.

The illustration shows a branch of the common facial vein anastomosed to the mesenteric vein. The external jugular vein may be used, if more suitable.

In our experience, the condition of the cervical vessels rather than of the mesenteric vessels is the limiting factor. The mesenteric vessels are usually thin-walled, soft, and pliant, whereas the cervical vessels may be quite sclerotic, brittle, and thick-walled, particularly in irradiated patients.

The procedure is first to secure the graft into the defect by placing a few seromuscular sutures in the proximal and distal anastomoses. This will prevent excessive motion of the graft during vascular anastomosis or traction on the vascular anastomoses while the bowel anastomoses are completed. The vein is then anastomosed, after which the arterial anastomosis is performed. The bowel anastomoses are then completed.

Figure 10–5C. An alternative method of vascularization is to the inferior thyroid artery and external jugular vein. Other cervical vessels may be used, if suitable.

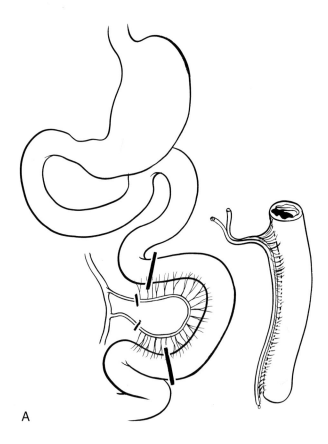

A

Figure 10–5. Free jejunal transplantation.

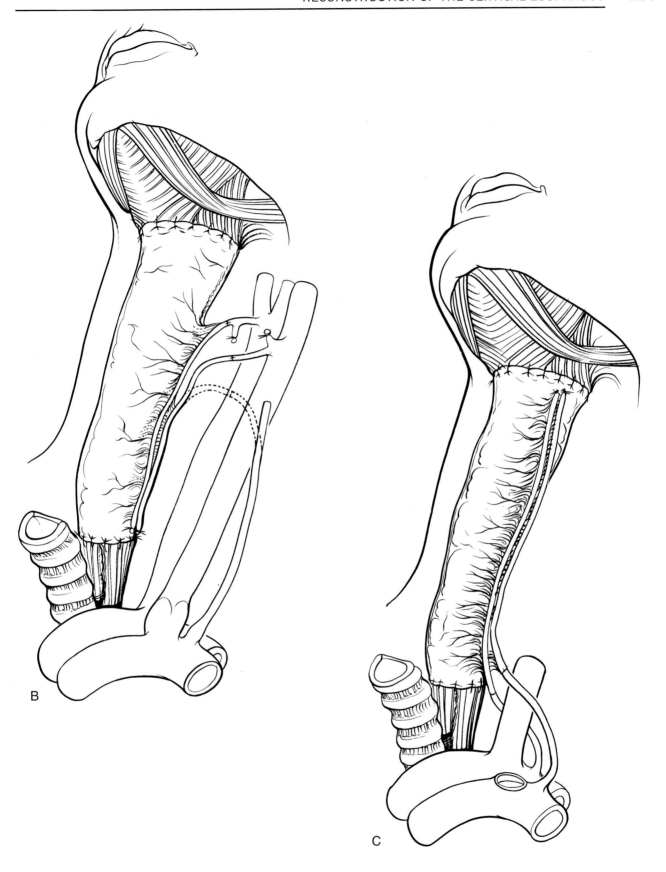

Figure 10–5 *Continued* Free jejunal transplantation.

Free Fasciocutaneous Flaps

Because the free jejunal transplants and the gastric pull-up procedure necessitate an abdominal procedure and are also associated with morbidity and because of the functional limitations of the various myocutaneous flaps, several authors now advocate the use of free fasciocutaneous flaps for reconstruction of the hypopharynx and cervical esophagus. The three flaps described for reconstruction of the pharyngoesophagus are the scapular-parascapular flap, the radial forearm flap, and the lateral cutaneous thigh flap. Experience has been gained principally with the latter two procedures because the scapular-parascapular system of flaps requires either an awkward positioning of the patient during the primary resection or complete repositioning of the patient once the tumor has been removed.

Free Radial Forearm Flap

In 1985, Harii and colleagues[135] reported the use of 12 free radial forearm flaps for reconstruction of the pharyngoesophagus. Nine of these were circumferential defects. All the patients were able to swallow postoperatively, although three could tolerate only liquids. The longest defect repaired with this flap was 15 cm in diameter. The donor graft was harvested under tourniquet control without heparinization, and the operation was performed within 3½ hours. The authors felt the procedure was ideal for elderly patients. The limited functional deficit incurred at the donor site enabled early ambulation and reduced morbidity for these patients.

Takato et al.[136] employed 33 radial forearm free flaps to reconstruct the hypopharynx and esophagus, without major complications. They relied on a Z-plasty at the posterior skin-mucosal junction between the flap and the esophagus to prevent stricture formation. This free flap can also be used for patch repair of esophageal-hypopharyngeal strictures.[137, 138]

The free radial forearm flap is based on the radial artery and the cephalic vein. Patency of both the radial and the ulnar arteries must be ensured by preoperative testing. An Allen test (manual occlusion and sequential release of the radial and the ulnar vessels at the wrist) is a good clinical indicator of normal arterial supply to the hand, although many surgeons prefer to confirm this with angiography.

Technique of Free Radial Forearm Flap

Figures 10–6A and 10–6A₁. Harvesting of the flap is conducted with the same principles as shown in Figure 9–6 for the patch grafting of pharyngeal defects, except that a larger area of skin may be required for complete pharyngoesophageal replacement, and it is not necessary to include cutaneous nerves in the graft. The radial flap is harvested from the nondominant forearm, based on a long segment of radial artery, under tourniquet control. The donor site is covered with a skin graft.

Figures 10–6B, 10–6B₁, and 10–6B₂. The skin flap is now tubed and sutured into the segmental defect in the pharyngoesophagus. The same principles apply to this procedure as to free jejunal transplantation with regard to selection of donor vessels. A saphenous vein graft (see Fig. 9–5A₂) may be employed to enhance the length of available vessels.

Lateral Cutaneous Thigh Flap

The lateral cutaneous thigh flap has many characteristics that make it suitable for reconstruction of the pharyngoesophagus: (1) it can be harvested comfortably by a second team relatively far-removed from the ablative team; (2) it provides a large amount of thin skin with uniform subcutaneous tissue; and (3) it has minimal donor site morbidity. The pedicle vessels are of a large caliber, ranging from 2 to 5 mm. This flap is easily tubed for circumferential defects and can replace a segment of up to 25 cm in length without flap necrosis. It is based on the third perforating branch of the deep femoral artery and its accompanying veins. Hayden and Fredrickson[139, 140] have used this flap in 14 cases of pharyngoesophageal reconstruction with excellent results and without major morbidity.

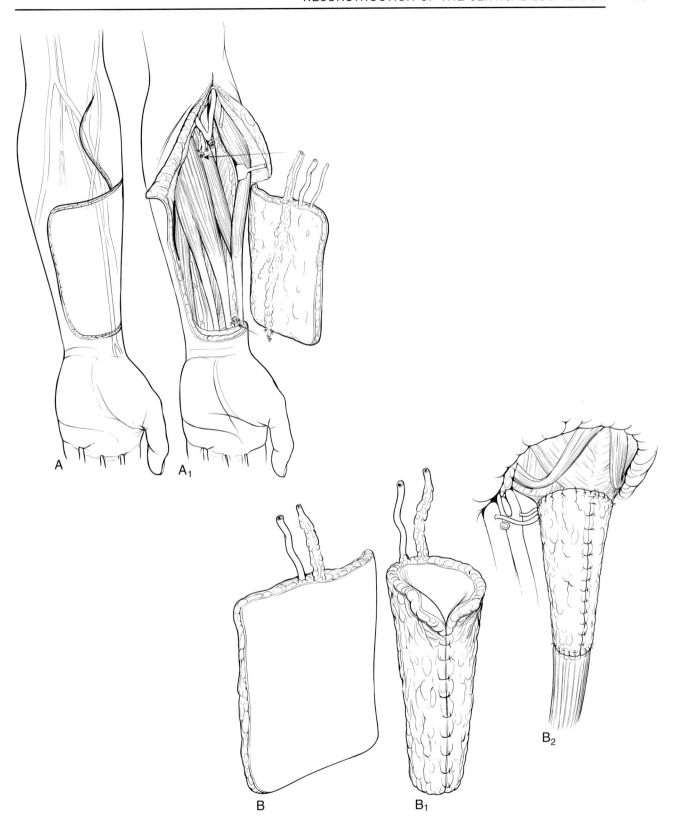

Figure 10–6. Free radial forearm flap.

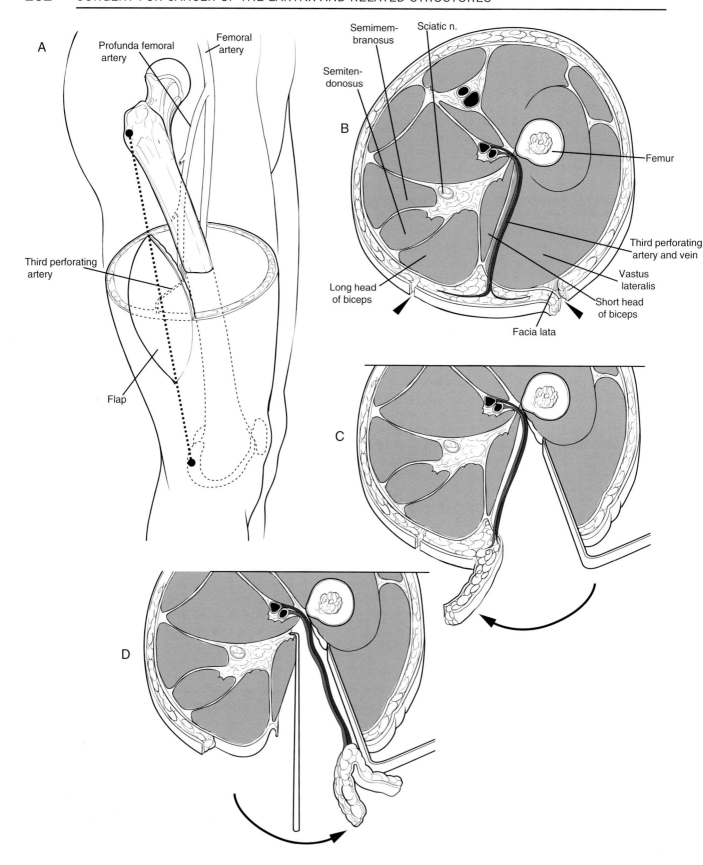

Figure 10–7. Lateral cutaneous thigh flap.

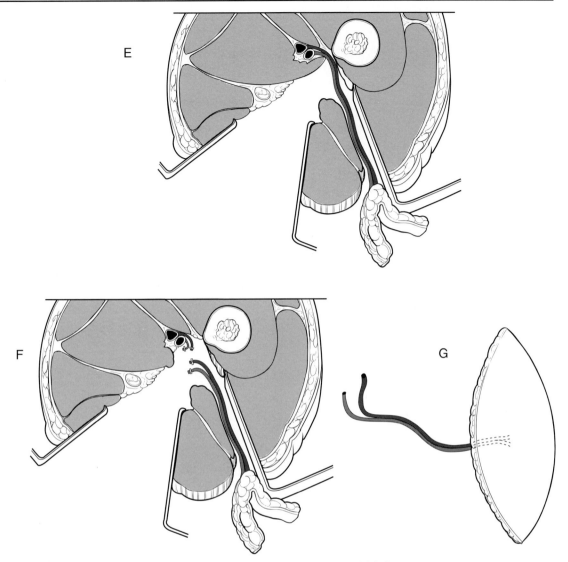

Figure 10–7 *Continued* Lateral cutaneous thigh flap.

Technique of Lateral Cutaneous Thigh Flap

Figure 10–7*A*. The vascular territory of the third perforating branch of the deep femoral artery is the skin on the lateral midportion of the thigh. An elliptical flap is designed in this region to conform to the esophageal defect to be replaced.

Figure 10–7*B*. The third perforating branch of the deep femoral artery travels between the great adductor muscle and the short head of the biceps muscle of the thigh. The anterior border of the incision is made through the skin and the fascia lata over the great adductor muscle. The posterior incision is over the long head of the biceps muscle of the thigh.

Figure 10–7*C*. The fasciocutaneous flap is reflected posteriorly from the surface of the great adductor muscle until the vascular pedicle can be traced medially between the muscle bellies.

Figure 10–7*D*. Posteriorly, the flap is reflected anteriorly from the surface of the long head of the biceps muscle.

Figure 10–7*E*. In order to obtain a greater length and diameter of the vessel, the perforating branch can be traced to its origin from the deep femoral artery. The long head of the biceps muscle is reflected medially, and the vascular pedicle is identified perforating through the tendon of the great adductor muscle.

Figure 10–7*F*. The site of perforation is enlarged by incising the tendonous tissue, creating a window through which the vessels can be transected as far proximally as possible.

Figure 10–7*G*. The skin flap is now freed and can be shaped to conform to the esophageal defect. The donor site is closed primarily.

CHOICE OF PROCEDURE

It is not possible to choose an ideal method of pharyngoesophageal reconstruction applicable in all situations. Nevertheless, we can define optimal procedures for various indications.

It seems evident that gastric transposition is the most satisfactory method for reconstruction in one stage after resection of postcricoid and cervical esophageal carcinomas that extend below the thoracic inlet. For this approach to be successful, however, the patient must be sufficiently healthy to withstand the fairly extensive operation. If, at exploration, the stomach is found to be unsuitable for use, the posterior mediastinal route can be used for left colon interposition.

After hypopharyngeal resections that extend above the level of the hyoid bone, reconstruction with myocutaneous flaps or free microvascular grafts is preferable to attempted transposition of abdominal viscera. Revascularized jejunum is an excellent substitute for cervical esophagus, but it requires laparotomy, with its associated morbidity. For elderly and debilitated patients, free fasciocutaneous or pedicled myocutaneous flaps are preferable, when feasible.

Esophagocoloplasty and reversed gastric tube esophagoplasty are more suitable for secondary than for primary reconstruction, either as planned staged procedures or after the failure of other methods. The choice between using the colon or the gastric tube is determined more by the individual preference of the surgeon than by any intrinsic advantage of one procedure over the other. The subcutaneous route is safer and, for secondary reconstruction, is much simpler than the substernal route but is the longest route from the abdomen to the neck.

REFERENCES

1. Rob CG, Bateman GH. Reconstruction of the trachea and cervical esophagus: preliminary report. *Br J Surg* 1949; 37:202–205.
2. Edgerton MT. One-stage reconstruction of the cervical esophagus or trachea. *Surgery* 1952; 31:239–250.
3. Negus VE. Reconstruction of pharynx after pharyngoesophagolaryngectomy. *Br J Plast Surg* 1953; 6:99–101.
4. Conley JJ. One-stage radical resection of cervical esophagus, larynx, pharynx and lateral neck with immediate reconstruction. *Arch Otolaryngol* 1953; 58:645–654.
5. Kaplan I, Markowicz H. One-stage primary reconstruction of the cervical esophagus by means of a free tubular graft of penile skin. *Br J Plast Surg* 1964; 17:314–319.
6. Lim RY, Ponce F. Reconstruction of cervical esophagus with penile skin. *W Va Med J* 1975; 71:34–36.
7. Shanon E, Plaschkes J. Reconstruction of the pharynx using a penile skin graft. *Arch Otolaryngol* 1967; 86:453–455.
8. Som ML. Laryngoesophagectomy. *Arch Otolaryngol* 1956; 63:474–480.
9. Som ML, Nussbaum M. Surgical therapy of carcinoma of the hypopharynx and cervical esophagus. *Otolaryngol Clin North Am* 1969; 2:631–640.
10. Morfit HM, Klopp CT, Neerken AJ. Bridging of laryngopharyngeal and upper cervical defects. *Arch Surg* 1957; 74:667–674.
11. Chu W, Ries G, Jaurigu VG, et al. Restoration of pharyngeal continuity with a replaceable prosthetic conduit: a new method. *Am J Surg* 1978; 135:269–271.
12. Montgomery WW. Salivary bypass tube. *Ann Otol Rhinol Laryngol* 1978; 87:159–162.
13. Javor PA. A new suction obturator to control saliva after laryngopharyngectomy. *Plast Reconstr Surg* 1976; 57:106–109.
14. Mattes P, Meister H. Esophageal replacement with lyophilized dura. *Langenbecks Arch Chir* 1977; 343:93–105.
15. Salomon J, Nudelman I, Kissin L, et al. Experimental segmental replacement of esophagus by biological tissues. *Isr J Med Sci* 1977; 13:272–277.
16. Asherson N. Pharyngectomy for postcricoid carcinoma: one stage operation with reconstruction of the pharynx using the larynx as an autograft. *J Laryngol Otol* 1954; 68:550–559.
17. Wilkins SA. Immediate reconstruction of the cervical esophagus: a new method. *Cancer* 1955; 8:1189–1197.
18. Som ML. Laryngotracheal autograft for postcricoid carcinoma: a reevaluation. *Ann Otol Rhinol Laryngol* 1974; 83:481–486.
19. Cook DW, Canepa C, Winek T, et al. Laryngeal flap for hypopharynx reconstruction. *Head Neck* 1991; 13:318–320.
20. Barzan L, Comoretto R. Hemipharyngectomy and hemilaryngectomy for pyriform sinus cancer: reconstruction with remaining larynx and hypopharynx and with tracheostomy. *Laryngoscope* 1993; 103:82–86.
21. Mikulicz J. Ein Fall von Resektion des Carcinomatosen Oesophagus mit Plastichem Ersatz des Excidirten Stuckes. *Prager Med Wochenschr* 1886; 11:93.
22. Bircher E. Ein Beitrag zur Plastischen Bildung eines neuen Oesophagus. *Zentralbl Chir* 1907; 34:1479–1482.
23. Von Hacker V. Uber Resection und Plastik am Halsabschnitt der Speiseröhre insbesondere beim Carcinom. *Arch Klin Chir* 1908; 82:257–323.
24. Wookey H. The surgical treatment of carcinoma of the pharynx and upper esophagus. *Surg Gynecol Obstet* 1942; 75:499–506.
25. Mustard RA. The use of the Wookey operation for carcinoma of the hypopharynx and cervical esophagus. *Surg Gynecol Obstet* 1960; 111:577–592.
26. Silver CE, Som ML. Reconstruction of the cervical esophagus after total pharyngolaryngectomy: a modified Wookey operation. *Ann Surg* 1967; 165:239–243.
27. Bakamjian VY. A two-stage method for pharyngoesophageal reconstruction with a primary pectoral skin flap. *Plast Reconstr Surg* 1965; 36:173–184.
28. Bakamjian VY. Total reconstruction of pharynx with medially based deltopectoral skin flap. *NY State J Med* 1968; 68:2771–2778.
29. Bakamjian VY. Experience with the medially based deltopectoral flap in reconstructive surgery of the head and neck. *Br J Plast Surg* 1971; 24:174–183.
30. Lodish EM. The use of the deltopectoral flap in reconstruction for pharyngoesophageal carcinoma. *J Am Osteopath Assoc* 1977; 76:89–96.
31. Petty CT, Theogaraj SD, Cohen IK. Secondary reconstruction of the cervical esophagus. *Plast Reconstr Surg* 1975; 56(1):70–76.
32. Ramadan MF, Stell PM. Reconstruction after pharyngolaryngoesophagectomy using delto-pectoral flaps. *Clin Otolaryngol* 1979; 4:5–11.
33. Stell PM. Pharyngeal reconstruction using the deltopectoral flap. *ORL J Otorhinolaryngol Relat Spec* 1973; 35:317–323.
34. Chaffoo R, Goode R. Modification of the deltopectoral flap

for pharyngoesophageal reconstruction. *Laryngoscope* 1988; 98:460–462.

35. Guillamondegui O, Geoffray B, McKenna R. Total reconstruction of the hypopharynx and cervical esophagus. *Am J Surg* 1985; 150:422–426.
36. Carlson G, Schusterman M, Guillamondegui O. Total reconstruction of the hypopharynx and cervical esophagus: a 20-year experience. *Ann Plast Surg* 1992; 29:408–412.
37. Fredrickson J, Wagenfeld J, Pearson G. Gastric pull-up vs deltopectoral flap for reconstruction of the cervical esophagus. *Arch Otolaryngol* 1981; 107:613–616.
38. McCraw JB, Dibbell DG. Experimental definition of independent myocutaneous vascular territories. *Plast Reconstr Surg* 1977; 60:212–220.
39. McCraw JB, Dibbell DG, Carraway JH. Clinical definition of independent myocutaneous vascular territories. *Plast Reconstr Surg* 1977; 60:341–352.
40. Ariyan S. One-stage repair of a cervical esophagostome with two myocutaneous flaps from the neck and shoulder. *Plast Reconstr Surg* 1979; 63:426–429.
41. Guillamondegui O, Larson D. The lateral trapezius musculocutaneous flap: its use in head and neck reconstruction. *Plast Reconstr Surg* 1981; 67:143–150.
42. Demergasso F, Piazza M. Trapezius myocutaneous flap in reconstructive surgery for head and neck cancer: an original technique. *Am J Surg* 1979; 138:533–536.
43. Cusumano R, Silver C, Brauer R, Strauch B. Pectoralis myocutaneous flap for replacement of cervical esophagus. *Head Neck* 1989; 11:450–456.
44. Ariyan S. The pectoralis major myocutaneous flap: a versatile flap for reconstruction in the head and neck. *Plast Reconstr Surg* 1979; 63:73–81.
45. Withers EH, Franklin JD, Madden JJ, et al. Pectoralis major musculocutaneous flap: a new flap in head and neck reconstruction. *Am J Surg* 1979; 138:537–543.
46. Baek SM, Biller HF, Krespi YP, et al. The pectoralis major myocutaneous island flap for reconstruction of the head and neck. *Head Neck Surg* 1979; 1:293–300.
47. Rees R, Ivey G, Shack RB, et al. Pectoralis major musculocutaneous flaps: long-term follow-up of hypopharyngeal reconstruction. *Plast Reconstr Surg* 1986; 77:586–590.
48. Theogaraj SD, Merritt W, Acharya G, et al. The pectoralis major musculocutaneous island flap in single-stage reconstruction of the pharyngoesophageal region. *Plast Reconstr Surg* 1980; 45:267–276.
49. Lee K, Lore J. Two modifications of pectoralis major myocutaneous flap. *Laryngoscope* 1986; 96:363–367.
50. Gullane P, Patterson A, Boyd B. Pharyngeal reconstruction: current controversies. *J Otolaryngol* 1987; 16:169–173.
51. Su C, Hwang C. Near-total laryngopharyngectomy with pectoralis major myocutaneous flap in advanced pyriform carcinoma. *J Laryngol Otol* 1993; 107:817–820.
52. Lam K, Wei W, Lau W. Avoiding stenosis in the tubed greater pectoral flap in pharyngeal repair. *Arch Otolaryngol Head Neck Surg* 1987; 113:428–431.
53. Baek S, Lawson W, Biller H. Reconstruction of hypopharynx and cervical esophagus with pectoralis major island myocutaneous flap. *Ann Plast Surg* 1981; 7:18–24.
54. Lam K, Ho C, Lau W, et al. Immediate reconstruction of pharyngoesophageal defects. *Arch Otolaryngol Head Neck Surg* 1989; 115:608–612.
55. Lau W, Lam K, Wei W. Reconstruction of hypopharyngeal defects in cancer surgery: do we have a choice? *Am J Surg* 1987; 154:374–380.
56. Jianu A. Gastrotomie u Oesophagoplastik. *Dtsch Ztschr* 1912; 118:383–390.
57. Kirschner MB. Ein neues Verfahren der Oesophagoplastik. *Langenbecks Arch Klin Chir* 1920; 114:606–663.
58. Ong GB. The Kirschner operation: a forgotten procedure. *Br J Surg* 1973; 60:221–227.
59. Mes GM. New method of esophagoplasty. *J Int Coll Surg* 1948; 11:270–277.
60. Gavrilu D, Georgescu L. Esophagoplastic direction a material gastric. *Rev Stiintelor Med* (Bucur) 1955; 3:33.

61. Heimlich HJ. Reconstruction of the entire esophagus and restoration of swallowing with reversed gastric tube. *NY State J Med* 1961; 61:2478–2482.
62. Heimlich HJ. Carcinoma of the cervical esophagus. *J Thorac Cardiovasc Surg* 1970; 59:309–318.
63. Heimlich HJ. Reversed gastric tube esophagoplasty for failure of colon jejunum and prosthetic interpositions. *Ann Surg* 1975; 182:154–160.
64. Postlethwait RW. Technique for isoperistaltic gastric tube for esophageal bypass. *Ann Surg* 1976; 186:673–676.
65. Yamato T, Hamanaka Y, Hirata S, et al. Esophagoplasty with an autogenous tubed gastric flap. *Am J Surg* 1979; 137:597–602.
66. Anderson KD, Randolph JG. Gastric tube interposition: a satisfactory alternative to the colon for esophageal replacement in children. *Ann Thorac Surg* 1978; 25:521–525.
67. Ein SH, Shandling B, Simpson JS, et al. Fourteen years of gastric tubes. *J Pediatr Surg* 1978; 13:638–642.
68. Ionescu GO, Tuleasca I, Viasu V, et al. Reversed gastric tube oesophagoplasty in children. *Chir Pediatr* 1979; 20:47–51.
69. Yannopoulos P, Marselos A. Total bypass of the oesophagus for benign strictures using a reversed gastric tube. *Thorax* 1977; 32:729–733.
70. Silver CE. Reconstruction after pharyngolaryngectomy-esophagectomy. *Am J Surg* 1976; 132:428–434.
71. Steichen FM. The creation of autologous substitute organs with stapling instruments. *Am J Surg* 1977; 134:659–673.
72. Gozner A, Stanciu D, Kirilla A, et al. Ulcer on the presternal tube after esophagoplasty of the greater curvature of the stomach. *Rev Chir* 1978; 27:213–217.
73. Kelling G. Oesophagoplastik mit Hilfe des Querkolon. *Zentralbl Chir* 1911; 38:1209–1212.
74. Vulliet H. De l'oesophagoplastie et des diverses modifications. *Sem Med* 1911; 31:529.
75. Yudin S. Surgical construction of 80 cases of artificial esophagus. *Surg Gynecol Obstet* 1944; 78(6):561–583.
76. Goligher JC, Robin IG. Use of left colon for reconstruction of the pharynx and esophagus after pharyngectomy. *Br J Surg* 1954; 42:283–290.
77. Scanlon EF, Staley CJ. Reconstruction of cervical esophagus by use of colon transplants. *Surg Clin North Am* 1963; 43:3–10.
78. Mannings PC Jr, Beahrs OH, Devine KD. Pharyngoesophagoplasty: interposition of right colon. *Arch Surg* 1964; 88:939–946.
79. Ventemiglia R, Khalil KG, Frazier OH, et al. The role of preoperative mesenteric arteriography in colon interposition. *J Thorac Caraciovasc Surg* 1977; 74:98–104.
80. Corazziari E, Mineo TC, Anzini F, et al. Functional evaluation of colon transplants used in esophageal reconstruction. *Am J Dig Dis* 1977; 22:7–12.
81. Rodgers BM, Talbert JL, Moazam F, et al. Functional and metabolic evaluation of colon replacement of the esophagus in children. *J Pediatr Surg* 1978; 13:35–39.
82. Akiyama H, Hiyama M, Miyazono H. Total esophageal reconstruction after extraction of the esophagus. *Ann Surg* 1975; 182:547–552.
83. Orringer MB, Sloan H. Esophagectomy without thoracotomy. *J Thorac Cardiovasc Surg* 1978; 76:643–654.
84. Szentpetery S, Wolfgang T, Lower RR. Pull-through esophagectomy without thoracotomy for esophageal carcinoma. *Ann Thorac Surg* 1979; 27:399–403.
85. Denk W. Zur Radikaloperation des Oesophaguskarzinoms. *Zentralbl Chir* 1913; 40:1065–1068.
86. Turner GG. Carcinoma of the oesophagus: the question of its treatment by surgery. *Lancet* 1936; 1:67–74.
87. Turner GG. Carcinoma of the oesophagus: the question of its treatment by surgery. *Lancet* 1936; 1:130–134.
88. Ong GB, Lee TC. Pharyngogastric anastomosis after oesophagopharyngectomy for carcinoma of the hypopharynx and cervical oesophagus. *Br J Surg* 1960; 48:193–200.
89. Le Quesne LP, Ranger D. Pharyngolaryngectomy with immediate pharyngogastric anastomosis. *Br J Surg* 1966; 53:105–109.

90. Stell PM. Esophageal replacement by transposed stomach. *Arch Otolaryngol* 1970; 91:166–170.

91. Leonard JR, Maran AG. Reconstruction of the cervical esophagus via gastric anastomosis. *Laryngoscope* 1970; 80:849–862.

92. Silver CE. Gastric pull-up operation for replacement of the cervical portion of the esophagus. *Surg Gynecol Obstet* 1976; 142:243–245.

93. Hattori T, Hamai Y, Ishii T. A new procedure for transabdominal resection of esophagocardial cancer and cervical anastomosis obviating thoracotomy. *Jap J Surg* 1975; 5:211–221.

94. Harrison DFN. Rehabilitation problems after pharyngogastric anastomosis. *Arch Otolaryngol* 1978; 104:244–246.

95. Silver CE, Cusumano RJ, Fell SC, et al. Replacement of upper esophagus: results with myocutaneous flap and with gastric transposition. *Laryngoscope* 1989; 99:819–821.

96. Peracchia A, Bardini R, Ruol A, et al. Surgical management of carcinoma of the hypopharynx and cervical esophagus. *Hepatogastroenterology* 1990; 37(4):371–375.

97. Mehta S, Sarkar S, Mehta A, et al. Mortality and morbidity of primary pharyngogastric anastomosis following circumferential excision for hypopharyngeal malignancies. *J Surg Oncol* 1990; 43:24–27.

98. Harrison DFN. Surgical repair in hypopharyngeal and cervical esophageal cancer. *Ann Otol* 1981; 90:372–375.

99. Harrison DFN, Thompson AE. Pharyngolaryngoesophagectomy with pharyngogastric anastomosis for cancer of the hypopharynx: review of 101 operations. *Head Neck Surg* 1986; 8:418–428.

100. Lam KH, Lim ST, Wong J, et al. Gastric histology and function in patients with intrathoracic stomach replacement after esophagectomy. *Surgery* 1979; 85:283–290.

101. Wei W, Lam KH, Choi S, et al. Late problems after pharyngolaryngoesophagectomy and pharyngogastric anastomosis for cancer of the larynx and hypopharynx. *Am J Surg* 1984; 148:509–513.

102. Buchanan G, West TE, Woodhead JS, et al. Hypoparathyroidism following pharyngolaryngo-oesophagectomy. *Clin Oncol* 1975; 1:89–96.

103. Harrison DFN. Surgical management of hypopharyngeal cancer. Particular reference to the gastric "pull-up" operation. *Arch Otolaryngol* 1979; 105:149–152.

104. Isaacson SR, Lowy LD, Snow JB. Hypoparathyroidism secondary to surgery for carcinoma of the pharynx and larynx. *Trans Am Acad Ophthalmol Otolaryngol* 1977; 84:584–591.

105. Isaacson SR, Snow JB. Etiologic factors in hypocalcemia secondary to operations for carcinoma of the pharynx and larynx. *Laryngoscope* 1978; 88:1290–1297.

106. Maniglia A, Leder S, Goodwin WJ, et al. Tracheogastric puncture for vocal rehabilitation following total pharyngolaryngoesophagectomy. *Head Neck* 1989; 11:524–527.

107. de Vries E, Stein D, Johnson J, et al. Hypopharyngeal reconstruction: a comparison of two alternatives. *Laryngoscope* 1989; 99:614–617.

108. Shepperd HW. Surgery for the postcricoid carcinoma. Report on 23 cases in which replacement by stomach was attempted. *J Otolaryngol* 1977; 6:271–276.

109. Seidenberg B, Rosenack SS, Hurwitt ES, et al. Immediate reconstruction of the cervical esophagus by a revascularized isolated jejunal segment. *Ann Surg* 1959; 149:162–171.

110. Som ML, Silver CE. Vascular surgical techniques in head and neck surgery and transplantation of the canine larynx. *Bull NY Acad Med* 1968; 44:523–531.

111. Harrison DFN. The use of colonic transplants and revascularized jejunal autografts for primary repair after pharyngolaryngo-oesophagectomy. *Proc R Soc Med* 1964; 57:1104–1109.

112. Jurkiewicz MJ. Vascularized intestinal graft for reconstruction of the cervical esophagus and pharynx. *Plast Reconstr Surg* 1965; 36:509–517.

113. Keminger K, Roka R. Complications after oesophageal replacement. *Zentralbl Chir* 1977; 102:1136–1147.

114. McKee DM, Peters CR. Reconstruction of the hypopharynx and cervical esophagus with microvascular jejunal transplant. *Clin Plast Surg* 1978; 5:305–312.

115. Nakamura T, Inokuchi K, Sugimachi K. Use of revascularized jejunum as a free graft for cervical esophagus. *Jap J Surg* 1975; 5:92–102.

116. Peters CR, McKee DM, Berry BE. Pharyngoesophageal reconstruction with revascularized jejunal transplants. *Am J Surg* 1971; 121:675–678.

117. Hiebert CA, Cummings GO. Successful replacement of the cervical esophagus by transplantation and revascularization of a free graft of gastric antrum. *Ann Surg* 1961; 154:103–106.

118. Baudet J, Traissac L, Laisne D, et al. Reconstruction of the cervical esophagus after circular pharyngolaryngectomy, using a transplanted sigmoid loop with vascular microsuture. *Rev Laryngol Otol Rhinol* (Bord) 1977; 98:481–485.

119. Chrysospathis P. The contribution of vascular surgery to oesophageal replacement. *Br J Surg* 1966; 53:122–126.

120. Maillet P, Gaillard J, Sisteron A, et al. Cancer de l'oesophage cervical. Pharyngolaryngectomie totale. Retabissement du transit par transplant sigmoidien revascularise. *Lyon Chir* 1965; 61:420–433.

121. Nakayama K, Yamamoto K, Tamiya T, et al. Experience with free autografts of the bowel with a new venous anastomosis apparatus. *Surgery* 1964; 55:796–802.

122. Grange TB, Quick CA. The use of revascularized ileocolic autografts for primary repair after pharyngolaryngoesophagectomy. *Am J Surg* 1978; 136:477–485.

123. Baudet J, Guinberteau JC, Traissac JL, et al. Reconstruction of the pharynx and cervical esophagus using free grafts from the intestine and stomach. *Chirurgie* 1978; 104(9):873–875.

124. Coleman J, Searles J, Hester T, et al. Ten years experience with the free jejunal autograft. *Am J Surg* 1987; 154:394–398.

125. Biel M, Maisel R. Free jejunal autograft reconstruction of the pharyngoesophagus: review of a 10-year experience. *Otolaryngol Head Neck Surg* 1987; 97:4:369–375.

126. Surkin M, Lawson W, Biller H. Analysis of the methods of pharyngoesophageal reconstruction. *Head Neck Surg* 1984; 6:953–970.

127. Petruzzelli G, Johnson J, Myers E, et al. The effect of postoperative radiation therapy on pharyngoesophageal reconstruction with free jejunal interposition. *Arch Otolaryngol Head Neck Surg* 1991; 117:1265–1268.

128. de Vries E, Myers E, Johnson J, et al. Jejunal interposition for repair of stricture or fistula after laryngectomy. *Ann Otol Rhinol Laryngol* 1990; 99:496–498.

129. Kato H, Watanabe H, Iizuka T, et al. Primary esophageal reconstruction after resection of the cancer in the hypopharynx or cervical esophagus: comparison of free forearm skin tube flap, free jejunal transplantation and pull-through esophagectomy. *Japan J Clin Oncol* 1987; 17:255–261.

130. Pukander J, Lahteenmaki T, Matikainen M, et al. Hypopharyngeal reconstruction with free microvascular jejunal transfer after total laryngopharyngectomy. *Acta Oncologica* 1990; 29:525–527.

131. Schusterman M, Shestak K, deVries E, et al. Reconstruction of the cervical esophagus: free jejunal transfer versus gastric pull-up. *Plast Reconstr Surg* 1990; 85:1:16–21.

132. Hester TR, McConnel FM, Nahal F, et al. Reconstruction of cervical esophagus, hypopharynx and oral cavity using free jejunal transfer. *Am J Surg* 1980; 140(4):487–491.

133. Katsaros J, Banis JC, Acland RD, et al. Monitoring free vascularized jejunal grafts. *Br J Plast Surg* 1985; 38:220–222.

134. Urken ML, Weinberg H, Vickery C, et al. Free flap design in head and neck reconstruction to achieve an external segment for monitoring. *Arch Otolaryngol Head Neck Surg* 1989; 115:1447–1453.

135. Harii K, Ebihara S, Ono I, et al. Pharyngoesophageal reconstruction using a fabricated forearm free flap. *Plast Reconstr Surg* 1985; 75:4:463–474.
136. Takato T, Harii K, Ebihara S, et al. Oral and pharyngeal reconstruction using the free forearm flap. *Arch Otolaryngol Head Neck Surg* 1987; 113:873–879.
137. Delaere P, Boeckx W, Ostyn F, et al. Hypopharyngeal stenosis and fistulas. *Arch Otolaryngol Head Neck Surg* 1988; 114:1326–1329.
138. Chen H, Tang Y, Noordhoff MS. Patch esophagoplasty with free forearm flap for focal stricture of the pharyngoesophageal junction and the cervical esophagus. *Plast Reconstr Surg* 1992; 90:1:45–52.
139. Hayden R. Lateral thigh flap. *Otol Clin N Amer* 1994; 27:1171–83.
140. Hayden RE, Fredrickson JM. The lateral cutaneous thigh flap. *Am J Otolargynol.* (in press).
141. Panje WR, Little AG, Moran WJ, et al. Immediate free gastro-omental flap reconstruction of the mouth and throat. *Ann Otol Rhinol Laryngol* 1987; 96:15–21.

Chapter 11

Neck Dissection

Alfio Ferlito and Carl E. Silver

The clinical significance of metastases to the cervical lymph nodes is of paramount importance in the treatment and prognosis of laryngeal and other upper aerodigestive tract carcinomas. Sooner or later, squamous cell carcinomas of the head and the neck usually metastasize to the cervical lymph nodes. Neck dissection in its various forms—radical, modified, and selective—is now the standard surgical treatment for malignant disease in the lymph nodes of the neck. Opinions vary, however, as to the indications for neck dissection and the type of dissection for particular conditions.

The nineteenth-century surgeons were aware that laryngeal and other upper aerodigestive tract carcinomas metastasized to the cervical lymph nodes. They often regarded the finding of metastatic lymphadenopathy as an indication of incurability, but occasionally they would include the resection of grossly involved lymph nodes with the excision of primary tumors of the larynx, the hypopharynx, and the oral cavity. These incomplete resections of lymph node disease were ineffective, justifying dismal prognostications.

In 1906, George Crile[1] published the results of treatment of 132 head and neck cancers. This landmark paper established the basis for effective treatment of such lesions by describing a block resection of the cervical lymph node–bearing tissue, to be removed either in continuity with the primary tumor or as a secondary operation for subsequent metastasis. Crile devised skin flaps for adequate exposure of the cervical field and indicated the planes of dissection that would encompass the entire lymphatic block. Although operative mortality was as high as 13%, Crile anticipated the great usefulness of this approach.

Further advances and clarifications in technique and indications for radical neck dissection during the pre–World War II period were described by Semken[2] and Ward and Hendrick,[3] although, as explained by Conley and Von Frankel,[4] the treatment of head and neck cancer during this period was generally dominated by the enthusiasm of many leading oncologists for radiation therapy. With the war came antibiotics, improvements in blood replacement and anesthesia, and a better understanding of the principles of preoperative and postoperative care. These factors combined to reduce surgical mortality to acceptable levels, whereas the results of radiation in the treatment of many head and neck tumors, particularly the advanced tumors, were found disappointing.

By 1944, Sylvestre-Benis,[5] in Argentina, had established the place of radical neck dissection in the treatment of laryngeal cancer. He recognized the possibility of "monoblock" extirpation of the primary lesion in the larynx together with its lymphatic shed and thus advocated simultaneous unilateral or bilateral neck dissection with total laryngectomy in patients with palpable nodes. Sylvestre-Benis performed "limited" neck dissections in cases in which he felt the disease was confined to the jugular nodes. For bilateral neck dissections, he preserved one of the jugular veins. Various other authors, particularly Del Sel and Agra,[6] Clerf et al.,[7] and Brown and McDowell,[8] published papers during the 1940s establishing the indications and techniques and reporting the results of radical neck dissection performed in association with total laryngectomy.

The greatest impetus for the development of radical surgery for treatment of head and neck cancer came from Martin, who compiled extensive experience in the treatment of these tumors by both radiation and surgery from the 1920s through the 1950s. In 1951, he and his colleagues published an analysis on 1450 cases of neck dissection.[9] This classic paper was most influential in defining the technique and gaining acceptance for radical neck dissection. The technical precepts described by Martin have been followed with almost religious consistency by many American surgeons until relatively recently, when some modifications in technique have begun to find acceptance. Martin advocated complete, rather than partial, neck dissection but did not favor "prophylactic" or elective neck dissection, except in cases in which he felt that dissection of the neck was really an integral part of the resection itself.

In 1952, Ogura and Bello[10] published an emphatic recommendation that one-stage total laryngectomy with radical neck dissection in continuity be the standard treatment for all advanced laryngeal carcinomas, with or without palpable nodes. They noted that metastatic carcinoma was the major cause of failure following laryngectomy and that postoperative cervical metastasis occurred in 30% of postlaryngectomy patients who had not had neck dissections but who, preoperatively, presented with clinically negative nodes. Results were significantly worse when the neck dissection was performed at a second stage.

Several important articles and monographs were published by Barbosa,[11, 12] which were influential in establishing the techniques and the standards for the treatment of laryngeal and other head and neck tumors with neck dissection in continuity with the primary site.

During the 1960s, Suarez[13] and Ballantyne[14] separately developed conservative neck dissections, maintaining the radical removal of the cancer. With these two similar techniques, the aponeurotic compartments of the neck were removed, preserving the accessory nerve, the sternomastoid and the omohyoid muscles, and the internal jugular and the common facial veins. Bocca and his staff popularized this surgical procedure by publishing several papers in the English-language literature.[15–18] Although Suarez did not write extensively on the fundamentals and surgical technique of functional neck dissection, he must be credited as the first surgeon to define the anatomic basis and surgical criteria for this procedure.[19]

Over the years, a number of changes to the standard radical neck dissection have been suggested to improve the functional and cosmetic results of the operation. A modified radical neck dissection was popularized at the M.D. Anderson Cancer Center in Houston, Texas,[20] based on Ballantyne's approach. Two different "functional" procedures were performed by this group. For tumors without palpable nodes, particularly tumors of the oral cavity and the oropharynx, the dissection involved bilateral removal of the jugular chains. If posterior triangle node involvement was suspected, all the nodal groups were removed, but the accessory nerve was preserved unless it was directly invaded. The sternomastoid muscle was preserved unless it was involved with tumor. Postoperative radiation was administered bilaterally if one side was found to be staged N2a (single positive ipsilateral node 3 to 6 cm in diameter) or higher on histologic examination. The M.D. Anderson group found the results after modified neck dissection to be at least as good as those after the conventional procedure.

At the present time, a number of different dissections are considered acceptable for the surgical treatment of the neck in patients with cancer of the larynx and hypopharynx, and these procedures are often proposed in order to improve the cosmetic and functional results without compromising cancer control.[21] Less radical procedures, employed with greater frequency and often bilaterally, usually combined with postoperative radiation therapy in patients found to have pathologically positive node disease, have significantly reduced the incidence of neck failure in the treatment of head and neck cancer.[22]

TOPOGRAPHY OF CERVICAL LYMPH NODES

It is worth emphasizing that there are approximately 300 lymph nodes in the head and neck region, about 30% of the total number occurring in the human body. The Memorial Sloan-Kettering group has defined six anatomic levels of cervical lymph nodes.[23] This classification is recommended

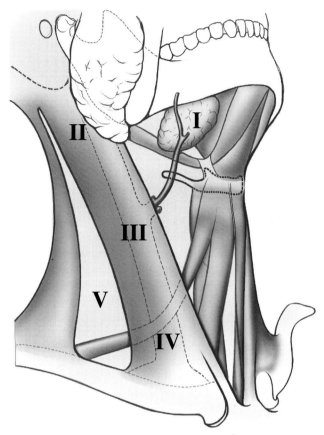

Figure 11–1. Schematic diagram of the neck showing levels of lymph node groups.

to standardize the terminology used to describe lymph node groups at risk for tumor metastases (Fig. 11–1).

Level I

Submental Group. This group consists of the lymph nodes within the triangular boundary of the anterior belly of the digastric muscles and the hyoid bone.

Submandibular Group. This group consists of the lymph nodes within the boundaries of the anterior and the posterior bellies of the digastric muscle and the body of the mandible. The submandibular gland is included in the specimen when the lymph nodes within this triangle are removed.

Level II

Upper Jugular Group. This group consists of the lymph nodes located around the upper third of the internal jugular vein and the adjacent spinal accessory nerve extending from the level of the carotid bifurcation (a surgical landmark) to the base of the skull. The posterior boundary is the posterior border of the sternocleidomastoid muscle, and the anterior boundary is the lateral border of the sternohyoid muscle.

Level III

Middle Jugular Group. This group consists of the lymph nodes located around the middle third of the internal jugular vein extending from the carotid bifurcation above to the omohyoid muscle (a surgical landmark) or the cricothyroid notch (a clinical landmark) below. The posterior boundary is the posterior border of the sternocleidomastoid muscle, and the anterior boundary is the lateral border of the sternohyoid muscle.

Level IV

Lower Jugular Group. This group consists of the lymph nodes located around the lower third of the internal jugular vein, extending from the omohyoid muscle above to the clavicle below. The posterior boundary is the posterior border of the sternocleidomastoid muscle, and the anterior boundary is the lateral border of the sternohyoid muscle.

Level V

Posterior Triangle Group. This group mainly comprises the lymph nodes located along the lower half of the spinal accessory nerve and the transverse cervical artery; the supraclavicular nodes are also included in this group. The posterior boundary is the anterior border of the trapezius muscle; the anterior boundary is the posterior border of the sternocleidomastoid muscle; and the inferior boundary is the clavicle.

Level VI

Anterior Compartment Group. This group comprises the lymph nodes surrounding the midline visceral structures of the neck extending from the level of the hyoid bone above to the suprasternal notch below. On each side, the lateral boundary is the medial border of the carotid sheath. Located within this compartment are the perithyroidal lymph nodes, the paratracheal lymph nodes, the lymph nodes along the recurrent laryngeal nerves, and the precricoid lymph nodes.

NECK DISSECTION TERMINOLOGY AND CLASSIFICATION

Several modifications to the classic neck dissection described by Crile[1] in 1906 have been pub-

lished. As each modification has prompted a new terminology, the "list" of operations has lengthened, with a diminishing uniformity in definitions and increasing confusion in terminology. In 1987, Suen and Goepfert[24] were the first to suggest a classification of neck dissections, which was simplified 2 years later by Medina.[25] The basic idea behind both proposed classifications was to identify three broad categories of neck dissections: (1) standard radical neck dissection, (2) comprehensive modified radical neck dissection, and (3) selective neck dissection, where one or more selected groups of nodes considered at risk are removed, depending on the site of the primary cancer and its expected lymphatic spread.

Subsequently, in order to eliminate potential misinterpretation, overlap, and lack of standardization, the Committee for Head and Neck Surgery and Oncology created by the American Academy of Otolaryngology-Head and Neck Surgery, in conjunction with the Education Committee of the American Society for Head and Neck Surgery, classified neck dissection procedures into four categories.[26] This classification has now been adopted by the American Academy of Otolaryngology-Head and Neck Surgery and should attain general acceptance (Table 11–1).

Radical Neck Dissection. Radical neck dissection refers to the removal of all ipsilateral cervical lymph node groups extending from the inferior border of the mandible above, to the clavicle below, and from the lateral border of the sternohyoid muscle, the hyoid bone, and the contralateral anterior belly of the digastric muscle anteriorly, to the anterior border of the trapezius muscle posteriorly. It includes all the lymph nodes from levels I through V (the submental group, the submandibular group, the upper jugular group, the middle jugular group, the lower jugular group, and the posterior triangle group). The spinal accessory nerve, the internal

---

Table 11–1. CLASSIFICATION OF NECK DISSECTIONS

Comprehensive Neck Dissection

Radical neck dissection
Modified radical neck dissection
  Type I
  Type II
  Type III

Selective Neck Dissection

Supraomohyoid neck dissection
Posterolateral neck dissection
Lateral neck dissection
Anterior neck dissection

Extended Neck Dissection

jugular vein, the sternocleidomastoid muscle, the submandibular gland, the tail of the parotid gland, the omohyoid muscle, and the cervical plexus nerves are also removed. The level VI lymph nodes are not included in radical neck dissection. Radical neck dissection is considered the standard basic procedure for cervical lymphadenectomy.

Modified Radical Neck Dissection. Modified radical neck dissection refers to the excision of all lymph nodes routinely removed in radical neck dissection with the preservation of one or more of the nonlymphatic structures routinely removed in radical neck dissection. This category includes three different types of neck dissection: type I, in which only one structure (the spinal accessory nerve) is preserved; type II, in which two structures (the spinal accessory nerve and the internal jugular vein) are preserved; and type III, in which all three structures (the spinal accessory nerve, the internal jugular vein, and the sternocleidomastoid muscle) are preserved. This last procedure corresponds to the Suarez functional neck dissection, and in the recent literature has often been termed "functional neck dissection" or "Bocca neck dissection."

Selective Neck Dissection. Selective neck dissection refers to any type of cervical lymphadenectomy preserving one or more lymph node groups removed by radical neck dissection. The four subtypes of selective neck dissection are the supraomohyoid neck dissection, the posterolateral neck dissection, the lateral neck dissection, and the anterior neck dissection.

Supraomohyoid neck dissection refers to the removal of lymph nodes contained in the submental and the submandibular triangle (level I), the upper jugular nodes (level II), and the midjugular lymph nodes (level III). This procedure is primarily indicated in the management of patients with stage T2 N0, T3 N0, or T4 N0, and selected patients with stage N1 squamous cell carcinomas of the oral cavity.[27] A study by Baredes et al.[28] revealed that supraomohyoid neck dissection at the time of supraglottic laryngectomy failed to benefit patients either by improving control of cervical metastasis or by improving survival. These findings correspond to the experience of many other surgeons. Supraomohyoid neck dissection is therefore not commonly employed for management of laryngeal carcinoma and will not be discussed further in this chapter.

Posterolateral neck dissection refers to the removal of the suboccipital lymph nodes, the upper, middle, and lower jugular lymph nodes (levels II, III, and IV), and the nodes of the posterior triangle (level V). This surgical procedure is primarily indicated to remove nodal disease from cutaneous melanoma of the posterior scalp and neck.[26] It may occa-

sionally be useful as an extension to radical or modified neck dissection in cancer of the larynx and the hypopharynx with involvement of the posterior triangle.

Lateral neck dissection includes the en bloc removal of the upper, middle, and lower jugular lymph nodes (levels II, III, and IV). These levels are the most commonly involved in cancer of the larynx and the hypopharynx.

Anterior compartment neck dissection consists of the removal of lymph nodes surrounding the visceral structures of the anterior aspect of the neck, that is, the pretracheal, the paratracheal, the perithyroid, and the precricoid (Delphian) nodes that form level VI, which can sometimes be involved in cancer of the larynx and hypopharynx.[29] The anterior compartment is dissected in total laryngectomy, particularly when it is performed for subglottic carcinoma, and is discussed in connection with those procedures (Chapter 7).

Extended Radical Neck Dissection. Extended radical neck dissection refers to the removal of one or more additional lymph node groups or nonlymphatic structures of the neck that are not routinely removed by radical neck dissection, such as the carotid artery, the hypoglossal nerve, the vagus nerve, and the paratracheal nodes.

Other Terminology

"Comprehensive" neck dissection includes radical neck dissection and the three types of modified radical neck dissection, where nodes from levels I to V are removed. The terms "classical neck dissection" and "functional neck dissection" were proposed by Conley to distinguish the radical (classical) procedure from the modified (functional procedure). The term "functional neck dissection" is less precise than "type III modified neck dissection" but has been used so extensively in the literature that it may be considered synonymous, and it is preferred by many authors. "Conservative" neck dissection usually refers to the same procedure, but the term should be avoided because of its lack of precision. "Therapeutic" neck dissection is performed for preoperatively diagnosed, usually palpable, cervical metastasis. Prophylactic or, preferably, "elective" neck dissection is employed for management of potential subclinical disease in the neck. The terms "therapeutic" and "elective" refer to the indication for neck dissection but do not specify the extent of dissection. In current surgical practice, however, "complete neck dissection," either modified or radical, is usually performed for a "therapeutic" indication, whereas selective neck dissection is often performed in "elective" situations (see below).

THE "CLINICALLY NEGATIVE" NECK

Elective Neck Dissection

The role of elective neck dissection has been recognized since the time of MacKenzie, who stated in 1900 that "early extirpation of the entire [larynx] with its tributary lymphatics and glands, whether the latter are apparently diseased or not, is the only possible safeguard against local recurrence or metastasis".[30] From the 1950s through the mid-1970s, radical neck dissection, or the Type I modified radical neck dissection, was employed by most surgeons for elective treatment of potential cervical metastasis in the clinically negative neck. Since that time the Type III modified radical neck dissection and, eventually, the selective "lateral" neck dissection, performed either unilaterally or bilaterally, have become favored for this purpose. Nevertheless, there are controversies among surgeons regarding the indication for and the extent of elective neck dissection, the role of preoperative diagnostic testing in the selection of patients for elective treatment of the neck, and the employment of elective radiation of the neck as an alternative to surgery.

Evaluation

Of course, no elective treatment of the neck would be necessary in the true absence of metastases. The problem is that it is almost impossible to diagnose the presence or absence of such disease with complete certainty. In the past, palpation of the neck was the only diagnostic method available for evaluation of the neck, which resulted in frequent failure to detect subclinical disease prior to treatment. The availability of modern imaging techniques of computed tomography (CT) and magnetic resonance imaging (MRI), abetted by needle aspiration cytology in some cases, has improved the ability to diagnose nonpalpable cervical disease, but even the most sophisticated of procedures may not be able to reveal micrometastases.[31, 32] Evidence of metastatic infiltrate in neck nodes may be minimal, showing no change in size, macroscopic morphology, or consistency. Metastases have been demonstrated in lymph nodes measuring only 4 to 6 mm in diameter. Although the issue is still debated, most clinicians feel that delay of treatment until such minimally involved nodes become radiographically or clinically positive may result in reduced survival.[33]

Even histologic examination may fail to reveal small nodes with micrometastases. Newer techniques employing monoclonal antibodies and immunohistochemical staining have enhanced the ability to detect metastases that had gone unnoticed in the original slides, while deep sections may detect metastases located at another level in the same lymph nodes.

The indication for and the extent of elective neck dissection may depend on the nature of the primary tumor. Friedmann and Mayer[30] divided patients with negative necks into low-risk and high-risk groups. The high-risk patients included those with T3 or T4 glottic lesions, T2 to T4 supraglottic lesions, or any subglottic lesion. These patients required further evaluation with CT, MRI, or ultrasound. Patients with radiographically positive necks were treated surgically, and the treatment of patients with radiographically negative necks was left to the discretion of the physician.

As there are currently no preoperative radiographic or clinical methods of documenting the presence or absence of occult metastatic disease before the operation, most practitioners suggest treating the clinically negative neck whenever there is a reasonably high likelihood of neck node metastases, even if they cannot be demonstrated preoperatively.

Elective Neck Irradiation as an Alternative to Surgery

Elective neck irradiation has been proposed as a valid alternative to modified radical neck dissection type III. Million and Cassisi[34] suggest that elective neck irradiation is not recommended when the risk of subclinical disease in the lymph nodes is small (less than 10%) because of the acute and late side-effects on the parotid glands and the normal mucosa. This treatment has been administered after excision of the primary tumor or together with radiation therapy for the primary tumor. Thus, a high-risk patient who would require total laryngectomy in order to control the primary tumor, but for whom adding a neck dissection to the procedure would present an unacceptable risk, should receive elective radiation to both sides of the neck after laryngectomy. Radiation is also useful to avoid the need for contralateral or bilateral neck dissection in patients with metastatic disease on the ipsilateral side. If positive nodes are found in the ipsilateral neck specimen, bilateral postoperative neck irradiation is recommended.

In certain situations, we prefer to rely on radiotherapy rather than on neck dissection for the control of subclinical lymph node metastases. A prime example would be an annular tumor of the postcricoid region or the cervical esophagus. Such tumors metastasize readily to both sides of the neck and the mediastinal lymph nodes and would require extraordinarily extensive surgery for control. It is simpler to remove the primary tumor and treat the areas of potential metastatic disease with radiotherapy.

In most instances, however, we do not feel it appropriate to abandon neck dissection and rely on postoperative irradiation for healthy patients who meet the criteria for elective treatment of the neck. In such patients, neck dissection does not significantly increase the operative risk, and the surgeon should not perform a procedure that is less than optimally curative once the patient is to undergo surgery. Postoperative complications, poor patient compliance, or other factors may interfere with timely or effective administration of radiotherapy.

Thus, irradiation is most useful to minimize the extent of surgery when appropriate or in cases in which the primary tumor is treated with irradiation. Neck irradiation, however, is not free of problems. Several disadvantages have been listed by Suen[35]:

1. Many patients may undergo unnecessary treatment if it is routinely administered.

2. Morbidity and mortality are increased if subsequent surgical therapy is needed.

3. A large field of irradiation increases problems during treatment, especially mucositis, pain, and weight loss; long-term side effects, such as dryness of the mouth and the pharynx, as well as fibrosis of the neck tissues, usually occur.

4. Irradiation fibrosis increases the difficulty of diagnosing recurrent disease, especially in patients with a thick neck.

SURGICAL TECHNIQUES FOR NECK DISSECTION

Neck Dissections for Advanced (Stage N2 or N3) Cervical Metastatic Disease: Standard Radical Neck Dissection and Type I Modified Radical Neck Dissection

The techniques of standard radical neck dissection and the type I modified radical neck dissection are discussed together because they are almost identical, with the exception of the preservation of the spinal accessory nerve in the type I modified dissection, and they are performed for similar indications. For many years we have preserved the spinal accessory nerve during otherwise radical neck dissection, if the nerve was not directly involved with tumor and could be safely dissected without violating the areas of gross tumor involvement. As the more conservative types of neck dissection have gained acceptance for elective as well as for therapeutic management of cervical disease, the more extensive procedures discussed here have been rele-

gated to the treatment of advanced neck involvement.

Indications

At the present time, radical neck dissection is indicated for multiple, clinically obvious, fixed lymph node metastases invading the neck structures. The diagnosis can be presumed or easily established when nodes are fixed or hard on palpation. Radical neck dissection is also indicated for persistent gross disease after previous irradiation of the neck, or when a fixed mass has become mobile after chemotherapy or irradiation.

Because less than 1% of cancers of the larynx and the hypopharynx metastasize to the submandibular triangle, it has been suggested that dissection of this region be omitted in the absence of clinical or radiographic evidence of metastatic spread.[36] Nevertheless, levels I and V may occasionally be involved, particularly if there is extensive involvement along the jugular chain.[37]

Whereas many surgeons feel that postoperative radiotherapy may improve regional control and prognosis and is indicated in every patient with histopathologically positive nodes,[38] others feel that a statistically significant effect can be demonstrated only in those patients with multiple pathologically positive nodes or extracapsular invasion. Extracapsular spread of carcinoma in cervical lymph nodes is universally recognized as an adverse prognostic factor, associated with a significant reduction in survival,[39–46] and is thus an indication for adjuvant therapy.

Contraindications to radical neck dissection include uncontrolled or uncontrollable primary cancer or documented distant metastases. Medical conditions that preclude general anesthesia or a patient's inability to provide informed consent are valid contraindications for neck dissection procedures. Cervical metastases may be unresectable because of invasion of the carotid artery, the spine, or the base of the skull.

Technique of Type I Modified Radical Neck Dissection

The procedure depicted here is identical to the "standard" radical neck dissection, with the exception that the accessory nerve is preserved. The specimen is mobilized from a lateral to a medial direction in order to enhance a broadly based "continuity" with the primary tumor. This dissection is commenced in the upper neck, affording a more controlled anatomic dissection of the upper carotid sheath region, easier identification of the

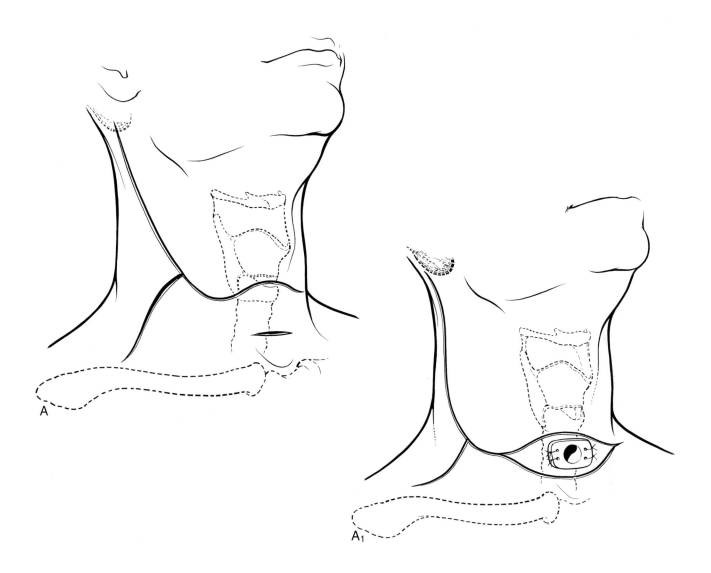

Figure 11–2. Type I modified radical neck dissection.

Illustration continued on page 309

structures, and higher ligation of the internal jugular vein than is achieved by the usual "below upward" procedure. In patients in whom resection is questionable, this approach allows evaluation of the operability of tumors early in the procedure, as inoperability often is manifest in the upper portion of the neck.

Figure 11–2A. Incisions. The single trifurcate incision with a large superior medial flap is preferred for total laryngectomy and neck dissection. The transverse limb of the incision is placed slightly higher for a supraglottic laryngectomy. If there is no previous tracheostomy, the tracheostoma is placed through a separate small incision in the inferior flap or through a midline vertical extension from the transverse skin incision.

Figure 11–2A_1. If a previous tracheostomy has been done, the entire tracheostomy site is excised elliptically. The tracheostoma is placed directly in the incision.

Figure 11–2*B.* Submental Triangle. Skin flaps are elevated in the subplatysmal plane as far as the mandible superiorly, the clavicle inferiorly, the trapezius muscle laterally, and, for laryngectomy, the opposite sternomastoid muscle. After the flaps are completely elevated, the submandibular branch of the facial nerve is identified as it crosses the anterior facial vessels (the anterior facial vein and the external maxillary artery). The vessels are transected and sutured to the superior skin flap, thereby retracting the nerve upward. The nerve is mobilized anteriorly and posteriorly before it is retracted.

Dissection of the submental triangle is commenced by incising along the border of the opposite (left) digastric muscle and dividing the deep cervical fascia along the anterior mandible. The specimen is reflected from the surface of the mylohyoid and the right digastric muscles as far as the hyoid bone, where it is left in continuity. After the right digastric muscle is exposed, the portion of mylohyoid muscle within the submandibular triangle is identified beneath the mandible, deep to the site of transection of the facial vessels. The attachments of the submandibular contents to the mandible and the mylohyoid vessels and nerve (not shown) are transected, uncovering the mylohyoid muscle.

Figure 11–2*C.* Submandibular (Digastric) Triangle. Dissection proceeds along the surface of the mylohyoid muscle, with reflection of the superficial portion of the submandibular gland laterally until the free posterior border of the mylohyoid muscle is reached. This is retracted anteriorly to reveal the deep portion of the submandibular gland, which lies on the hyoglossus muscle. Note the direction of the fibers of the mylohyoid, the digastric, and the hyoglossus muscles. The lingual nerve, Wharton's duct, and the hypoglossal nerve run across the hyoglossus muscle, deep to the submandibular gland.

The lingual nerve is identified by reflecting the submandibular gland downward. It is attached to the gland by the submandibular ganglion, as seen here. The ganglion is divided. Wharton's duct crosses deep to the lingual nerve and is divided. It is wise to identify the hypoglossal nerve with its accompanying vein by retracting the submandibular gland upward before transecting the remaining anterior attachments of the deep submandibular triangle. The specimen can now be reflected laterally after division of the attachments to the mandible.

The last structure encountered in the digastric triangle is the proximal end of the external maxillary artery, which crosses the medial aspect of the digastric muscle, entering the gland. This artery is carefully divided and ligated, permitting mobilization of the posterior belly of the digastric muscle.

Figure 11–2*D.* Upper Carotid Sheath. The posterior belly of the digastric muscle is a valuable landmark because it crosses superficial to and thus protects the vessels in the carotid sheath. The structures that cross superficial to the digastric muscle can be divided. These include the tail of the parotid gland and the sternomastoid muscle. The posterior belly of the digastric muscle (not the stylohyoid muscle) is identified and traced posteriorly as the overlying structures are transected. Further posteriorly the transverse process of C2 can be palpated deep to the digastric muscle. This marks the location of the internal jugular vein, which is immediately anterior. With a finger on the transverse process, the more posterior superficial structures can be divided, exposing the fibers of the splenius muscle. The hypoglossal nerve is identified posterior to the posterior belly of the digastric muscle. The nerve generally runs deep to a lingual vein, which is not divided until the nerve is identified.

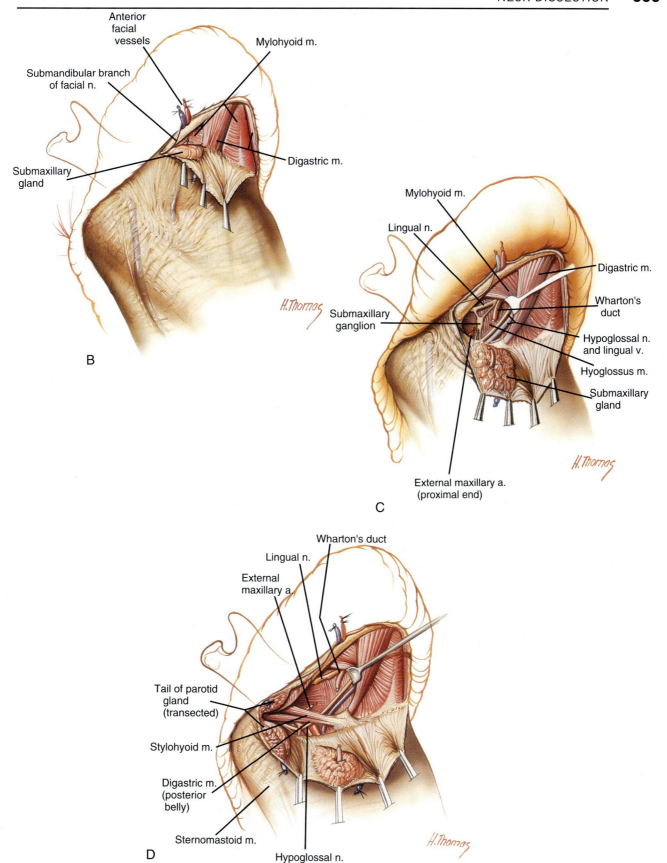

Anterior facial vessels

Submandibular branch of facial n.

Mylohyoid m.

Submaxillary gland

Digastric m.

H.Thomas

B

Mylohyoid m.

Lingual n.

Submaxillary ganglion

Digastric m.

Wharton's duct

Hypoglossal n. and lingual v.

Hyoglossus m.

Submaxillary gland

External maxillary a. (proximal end)

H.Thomas

C

Wharton's duct

Lingual n.

External maxillary a.

Tail of parotid gland (transected)

Stylohyoid m.

Digastric m. (posterior belly)

Sternomastoid m.

Hypoglossal n.

H.Thomas

D

Figure 11–2 *Continued* Type I modified radical neck dissection.

Illustration continued on following page

Figure 11–2E. Upper Carotid Sheath. The hypoglossal nerve is the key to identifying structures in the upper carotid sheath. The nerve crosses the carotid vessels and ascends in proximity to the jugular vein. As the nerve is traced posteriorly, the various structures that cross it (the lingual veins and the sternomastoid branch of the occipital artery) are divided. The carotid vessels can be palpated deep to the nerve. The descendens hypoglossal nerve (ansa hypoglossi) is eventually reached and divided. Further superiorly, the occipital vessels cross the nerve. If necessary, they are divided in order to free the jugular vein; if not necessary, they are left intact.

The internal jugular vein comes into view as the hypoglossal nerve is traced upward. The vein is mobilized, demonstrating the vagus nerve between the jugular vein and the internal carotid artery. The accessory nerve is identified on the superficial aspect of the jugular vein, coursing laterally. The

vein is mobilized, with care being taken to avoid injury to the carotid artery and the vagus, the hypoglossal, and the accessory nerves.

Figure 11–2E$_1$. The internal jugular vein is divided, ligated, and suture-ligated. It is wise to transfix the specimen side of the vessel also, as the tie is otherwise easily dislodged.

If the accessory nerve is to be preserved it is traced downward, whereas the overlying sternomastoid muscle is transected in a vertical direction. The sternomastoid branch of the accessory nerve is divided, leaving the trapezius branch intact.

Figure 11–2F. Omohyoid Region. With the upper half of the neck dissection completed, dissection is commenced below. The inferior end of the external jugular vein is divided, revealing the omohyoid muscle.

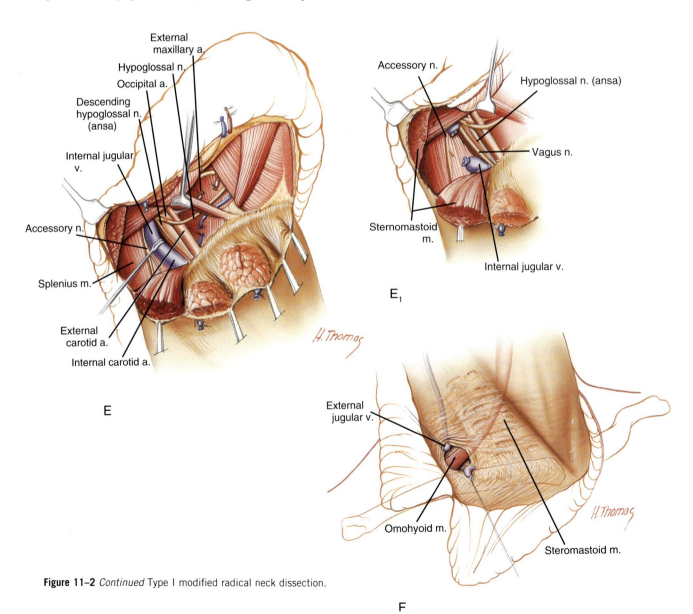

Figure 11–2 *Continued* Type I modified radical neck dissection.

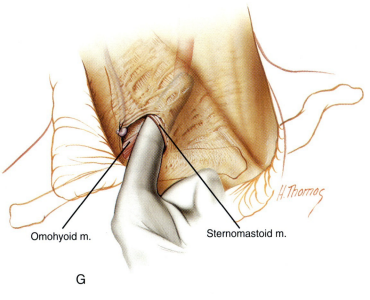

Omohyoid m.   Sternomastoid m.

G

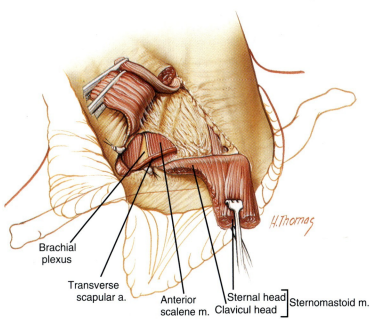

Brachial
plexus

Transverse
scapular a.   Anterior   Sternal head ⎤ Sternomastoid m.
                   scalene m.   Clavicul head ⎦

H

Figure 11–2 *Continued* Type I modified radical neck dissection.

Illustration continued on following page

Figure 11–2*G.* **Omohyoid Region** *(continued).* Like the digastric muscle, the omohyoid muscle crosses immediately superficial to the carotid sheath and can be used as a guide for the safe transection of the overlying sternomastoid muscle. Traced laterally, the superficial attachments to the clavicle can be divided without danger to the brachial plexus or the phrenic nerve, which are deep to the omohyoid muscle.

Figure 11–2*H.* **Lower Carotid Sheath.** Using the omohyoid muscle as a guide, the sternomastoid muscle is divided. The clavicular head is divided immediately above the clavicle. The sternal head is divided higher in the neck near where the omohyoid muscle crosses. Thus, the lower fourth of the sternomastoid muscle is preserved as a muscle flap for later coverage of the carotid artery. The muscle flap is temporarily retracted out of the field.

The omohyoid muscle is divided laterally and reflected medially. The transverse scapular artery is shown deep to the omohyoid muscle.

Figure 11–2*I*. Lower Carotid Sheath *(continued)*. The lower carotid end of the jugular vein is identified beneath the omohyoid fascia. Laterally, the transverse scapular artery is divided, revealing the scalene anterior muscle with the phrenic nerve on its anterior surface and the brachial plexus laterally. This step is often performed after division of the jugular vein.

Figure 11–2*I₁*. The jugular vein is mobilized, revealing the common carotid artery, which is situated medially and deep to the vein, and the vagus nerve, situated deeply between two vessels. The ansa hypoglossi, superficial and medial to the jugular vein, is divided.

Figure 11–2*J*. The lower end of the internal jugular vein is divided, ligated, and transfixed, and the specimen is reflected upward. The supraclavicular attachments are divided lateral to the brachial plexus, as far as the trapezius muscle, exposing the prevertebral muscles.

Figure 11–2*K*. Completion of Neck Dissection. The lateral attachments of the specimen are transected and the accessory nerve is identified and traced upward, dividing the overlying lymphoareolar tissues. It is impossible to preserve the accessory nerve without cutting through lymph node–bearing tissue, violating the theoretical "block" dissection—hence the objection to this procedure by some surgeons. As discussed, however, preservation of the nerve does not seem detrimental in elective dissection of the neck.

The specimen is reflected medially, toward the larynx, in the plane of the prevertebral fascia. This proceeds easily and can be done by sharp dissection. The branches of the cervical plexus are transected as they emerge through the prevertebral fascia and enter the specimen. The phrenic nerve, situated deep to the fascia, is preserved and traced upward until it joins the other cervical plexus branches that are transected.

For total laryngectomy, a broad base of continuity with the larynx is maintained, roughly from the hyoid bone to the sternohyoid muscle. For supraglottic laryngectomy, the necessity to preserve the intrahyoid muscles and to skeletonize the upper end of the thyroid cartilage makes it difficult to maintain continuity. The specimen must be reflected onto a narrow pedicle over the body of the hyoid bone. If preferred, the neck specimen may be removed for convenience, because the limited degree of continuity is probably of little benefit to the patient.

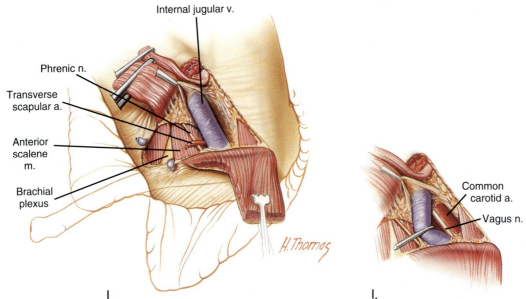

Figure 11–2 *Continued* Type I modified radical neck dissection.

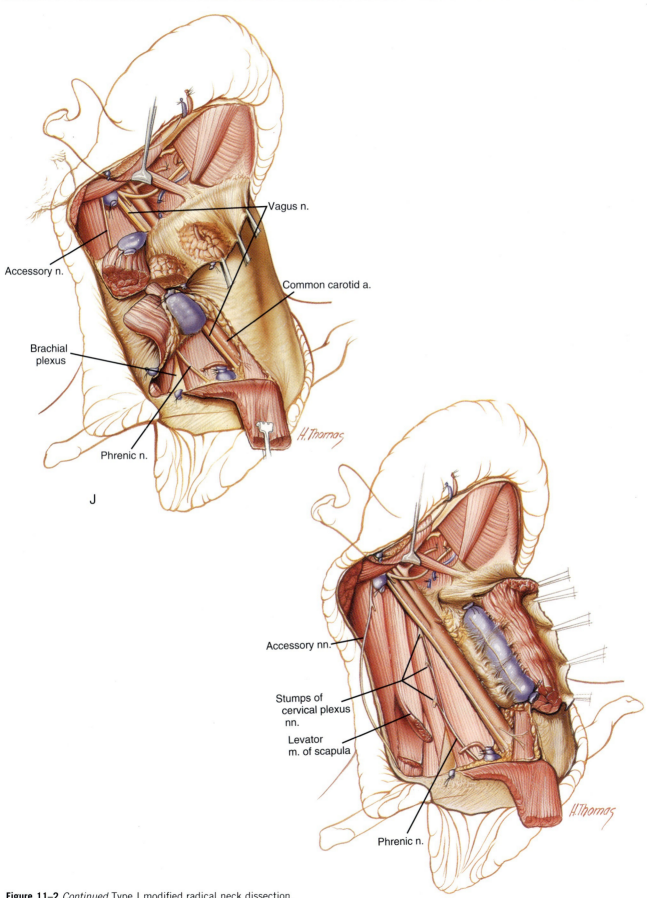

Vagus n.

Accessory n.

Common carotid a.

Brachial
plexus

Phrenic n.

J

H. Thomas

Accessory nn.

Stumps of
cervical plexus
nn.

Levator
m. of scapula

Phrenic n.

H. Thomas

Figure 11–2 *Continued* Type I modified radical neck dissection.

K

Illustration continued on following page

Figure 11–2L. Muscle Flap. We prefer to cover the carotid artery in all radical neck dissections. A combined flap from the levator muscle of the scapula and the sternomastoid muscle is used. The levator muscle is mobilized laterally and transected low in the neck. The scalene posterior muscle may be included in this flap. The muscle flap, when adequately mobilized, covers the upper two thirds to three fourths of the carotid artery. The preserved sternal head of the sternomastoid muscle envelops the lower portion of the vessel, thereby permitting complete coverage.

This technique of carotid coverage has proved quite successful. Over the years, we have encountered numerous instances of loss of skin coverage, usually in association with fistulae, in both irradiated and nonirradiated patients. In most instances, the muscle flap remained intact and prevented exposure of the carotid artery. The advent of the greater pectoral muscle and other myocutaneous flaps has made coverage of the carotid artery with a separate muscle flap unnecessary. The greater pectoral muscle provides adequate protection for the carotid artery.

An alternative method of covering the carotid artery is with a dermal graft. This deepithelialized skin graft "takes" on both superficial and deep aspects; thus, the skin flap heals over the skin graft, which heals over the artery.

To obtain the graft, a thin layer of skin is elevated from the donor site with a dermatome. A second layer, about 0.10 to 0.15 inch thick, is then removed as the graft. The superficial layer, which may remain attached at one end, is then placed over the graft bed. The dermal graft is sutured in place over the carotid artery.

Although many surgeons prefer the dermal graft for carotid artery coverage, it is employed on our service only in patients with extensive tumor or in cases of secondary surgery, in which there may not be sufficient muscle tissue available to cover the carotid artery. If muscles are available, however, their use is simpler and causes less postoperative discomfort than a dermal graft, particularly if the patient does not otherwise require a skin graft.

Neither the muscle flap nor the dermal graft compensates for poor surgical planning. In cases requiring massive mucosal resection, particularly if the site has been heavily irradiated, planned cutaneous or myocutaneous flaps, controlled stomas, or delayed closure must be employed. Neither muscle flaps nor dermal grafts can be expected to withstand massive early contamination and extensive tissue necrosis, such as may result from attempted closure under tension or from surgery performed on excessively irradiated tissue.

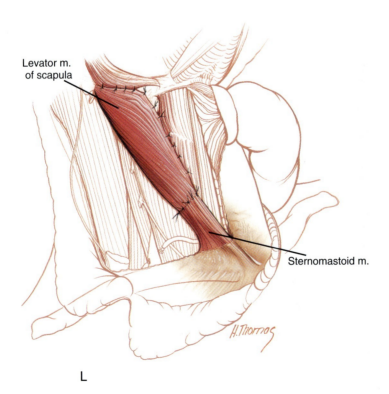

Levator m. of scapula

Sternomastoid m.

L

Figure 11–2 *Continued* Type I modified radical neck dissection.

Type III Modified Neck Dissection (Functional Neck Dissection)

Indications

The type III modified neck dissection may be used either as an elective or as a therapeutic procedure. The role of this operation for elective treatment of the neck has been discussed earlier. The current trend among many surgeons is to employ selective rather than modified radical neck dissection for staging or prophylaxis of cervical disease.

Modified radical neck dissection type III is indicated for many cases of significant metastatic disease. Molinari et al.[47] believe that this surgical procedure is indicated for the treatment of lymph node metastases when they are mobile and no larger than 2.5 cm. Gavilán et al.[19] feel that this surgical procedure is indicated for N0 or N1 tumors, whereas patients with N2 and N3 lesions should receive radical neck dissection. Bocca[48] extends the indications and believes that the only contraindication to the use of this procedure is the presence of node fixation.

Type III modified radical neck dissection has significant advantages over the more extensive procedures in cases in which equivalent cure rates can be demonstrated. The cosmetic and functional results are superior to those obtained by radical neck dissection, and simultaneous bilateral neck dissection can be performed with far less morbidity. This is particularly useful for the management of supraglottic carcinoma, which has a marked tendency to metastasize bilaterally and contralaterally.

Because different types of modified neck dissection techniques are available, surgical treatment of the clinically positive neck no longer means a rigid prescription of one operation. The procedure may be tailored according to the location of the primary tumor and the size, location, and extent of nodal metastases.[49]

Technique of Type III Modified Radical Neck Dissection

Figure 11–3A. The concept of this dissection is based on the fact that the lymph node–bearing tissues of the neck are contained within the fascial compartments. The lymphatics do not travel within the sternocleidomastoid (SCM) muscle, the jugular vein, or the other muscular, vascular, or neural structures. These structures may thus be preserved, provided they are not involved by direct extension from the tumor, and adequate exposure may be obtained without removing them. The illustration demonstrates the proposed fascial incisions (*dotted lines*) along the boundaries of the dissection (the midline, the mandible, the clavicle and the border of the trapezius muscle), as well as along the posterior border of the SCM muscle. The latter incision will divide the specimen into an anterior and a posterior portion. Most of the lymphatic tissue in the upper neck is located in the anterior portion and will be exposed by retracting the SCM muscle posteriorly. In the lower neck, most of the lymphoareolar tissue is situated in the posterior triangle and is exposed by retracting the SCM muscle anteriorly.

The procedure is commenced by incising the fascia along the mandible and reflecting it over the submandibular gland inferiorly. The salivary gland need not be resected, but any lymph nodes situated within the triangle should be included with the fascia.

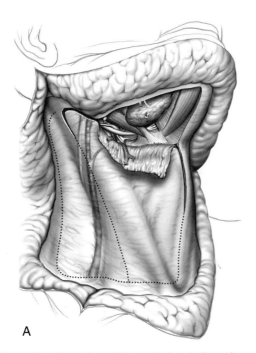

A

Figure 11–3. Type III modified radical neck dissection.
Illustration continued on following page

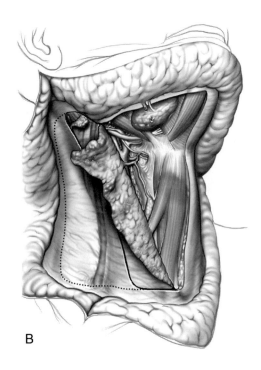

B

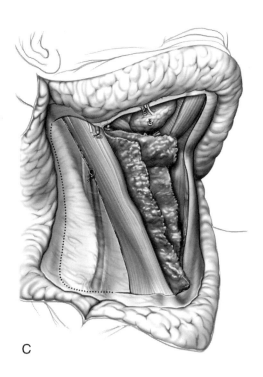

C

Figure 11–3 *Continued* Type III modified radical neck dissection.

Figure 11–3B. The fascial incision is continued downward in the anterior midline, and the fascia with the lymphoareolar tissue is reflected backward over the infrahyoid and the digastric muscles. The hypoglossal nerve and the common and the anterior facial vessels are exposed.

Figure 11–3C. The oblique fascial incision is made along the posterior border of the SCM muscle. The greater auricular nerve and the posterior facial vein are divided and the fascia is reflected anteriorly to expose the anterior border of the SCM muscle and to enter the carotid sheath.

Figure 11–3D. The mass of lymphoareolar tissue in the carotid sheath is now reflected downward from the surfaces of the carotid vessels and the internal jugular vein. The spinal accessory nerve is identified superiorly on the superficial lateral aspect of the internal jugular vein and is dissected free from the mass of tissue to be resected. Posterior retraction of the SCM muscle provides exposure of the structures within the carotid sheath and the anterior triangle.

Figure 11–3E. The posterior triangle is now dissected. The spinal accessory nerve is identified posterior to the SCM muscle, dissected free of surrounding structures, and retracted away from the lymphoareolar mass with an elastic tape. The fascia is incised along the clavicle and the anterior border of the SCM muscle. The SCM muscle is retracted anteriorly, exposing the posterior structures. The specimen is freed from the underlying prevertebral muscles. The brachial plexus and the phrenic nerve (not shown) are identified and preserved.

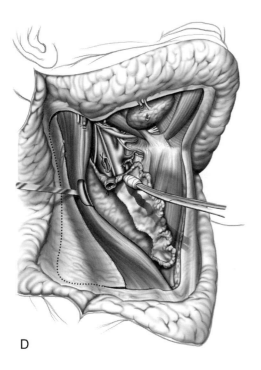

D

Figure 11–3 *Continued* Type III modified radical neck dissection.
Illustration continued on following page

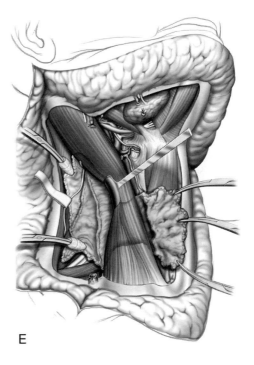

E

Figure 11–3*F.* The specimen is reflected from lateral to medial, beneath the SCM muscle, where it is continuous with the tissue mobilized from the anterior triangle. The specimen is now removed in the plane of the prevertebral muscles. The sensory branches of the cervical plexus nerves are sectioned, although they may be preserved by meticulous dissection if desired. The extent of sacrifice or preservation of such structures often depends on whether the dissection is being done for elective or for therapeutic purposes.

Figure 11–3*G.* The completed dissected neck is shown. The SCM and the omohyoid muscles, the internal jugular vein, the spinal accessory nerve, the brachial plexus, the phrenic nerve, the hypoglossal nerve, and the vagus nerve have been preserved. The common, the anterior, and the posterior facial veins; the greater auricular and the sensory cervical plexus nerves; and the lymphoareolar tissue of the anterior and the posterior triangles are preserved.

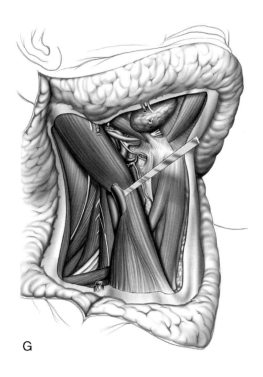

G

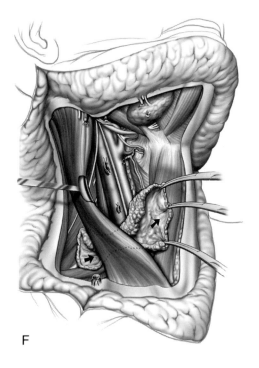

F

Figure 11–3 *Continued* Type III modified radical neck dissection.

Results of Type III Modified Neck Dissection

The test of success for modified neck dissection is a comparison of results obtained by this technique with those obtained by radical neck dissection for the same lesions. Chu and Strawitz[50] evaluated the results of "suprahyoid,"* modified radical, and standard radical neck dissections for metastatic squamous cell carcinoma. They demonstrated a high cervical recurrence rate after suprahyoid dissections in patients with histologically negative nodes. Modified radical neck dissections were done in some patients if nodal disease was confined above the jugulo-omohyoid group of nodes. Conventional radical neck dissection was done in some patients of this group and in all patients with histologic involvement at or below the level of the jugulo-omohyoid nodes. The modified radical neck dissection and the conventional neck dissection were comparable in terms of recurrence rates in the neck and 5-year-survival rates when the disease was confined above the jugulo-omohyoid nodes. The authors concluded that "suprahyoid" neck dissection should not be used at all as a procedure to control lymph node metastases and that modified neck dissection can be used instead of conventional neck dissection in selected patients.

Molinari et al.[47] reported the results of 175 patients treated with functional neck dissection at the Tumor Institute in Milan. This group of patients had palpable lymph node metastases smaller than 3 cm in size and not more than 3 in number. The results were compared with a historical group treated with radical neck dissection. The overall survival rate without recurrence in the neck was comparable in both groups even in the presence of positive lymph nodes.

Bocca et al.[16] reviewed the results of functional neck dissection in 843 cases treated at the Department of Otolaryngology of the University of Milan and compared them with results of "curative" (radical) neck dissection at the same institution during the same time period. The rate of tumor recurrence in the neck was 8.1% in the functional dissection group and 24.8% in the radical dissection group. When the results of 84 cases with N3 tumors treated by radical dissection were added to the results of the functional group, the overall recurrence rate was raised to 144 out of 927 cases (15.5%). Bocca concluded that the functional neck dissection had many advantages compared with radical neck dissection, including equal therapeutic effectiveness, avoidance of disfigurement, safety of simultaneous bilateral dissection, diminished incidence of large vessel necrosis, and widening of the indications for elective neck dissection.

Byers[51] reported the results of 967 patients treated at the M.D. Anderson Cancer Center by "modified neck dissection," which included "functional" (type III modified) and selective neck dissections either alone or in combination. The number of nodes removed by functional dissection was 31 compared to 44 removed by radical neck dissection, but this sampling difference was felt to be nonsignificant because the modified dissection removed the nodes predicted to be at highest risk. The functional neck dissection was usually reserved for necks with tumors staged N1 or higher and was often combined with selective dissection of the contralateral side. Byers concluded that functional neck dissection was effective treatment regardless of the stage of the disease. The incidence of neck recurrence was decreased with selective use of postoperative radiotherapy in patients with multiple positive nodes, a node more than 3 cm in diameter, or nodes with extracapsular invasion.

Selective Lateral Neck Dissection

Indications

Selective dissection of nodes in levels II, III, and IV is particularly applicable to carcinomas of the oropharynx, the hypopharynx, and the larynx. While this procedure is most often used for elective neck dissection, frequently bilateral, it has been successfully employed for therapeutic dissection, both with and without radiation therapy. Byers[51] termed this operation "anterior modified neck dissection" and employed the procedure bilaterally for tumors of the larynx staged clinically as N0 or N1. The procedure was considered adequate treatment, without completion neck dissection or postoperative irradiation, if multiple nodes were not involved, and if connective tissue involvement was not present. Postoperative irradiation was employed for the latter situations. Other authors have employed selective neck dissection for metastatic disease staged N1, N2a, or even N2b.[52]

---

*The "suprahyoid" dissection studied by Chu and Strawitz and found to be therapeutically ineffective should not be confused with the "supraomohyoid" dissection, discussed earlier, in which nodes in levels I, II, and III are thoroughly excised.

Technique of Selective Lateral Neck Dissection

Figure 11–4A. The lateral neck dissection may be performed through the same incision used for the total or partial laryngectomy. A transverse or oblique incision extending from the posterior to the ipsilateral SCM muscle to the contralateral SCM muscle will afford adequate exposure. These illustrations focus entirely on the neck dissection.

Figure 11–4B. The fascial incisions are the same as for the anterior half of a modified neck dissection type III. A triangular area is outlined inferior to the mandible, the midline of the neck, and diagonally along the SCM muscle.

Figure 11–4C. The fascia and the lymphoareolar attachments are reflected posteriorly from the midline toward the carotid sheath, exposing the infrahyoid muscles, the common facial vein, and the superior thyroid vessels.

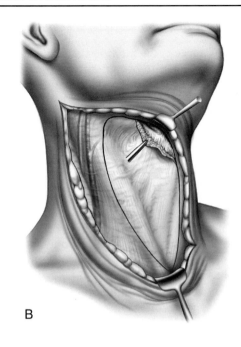

B

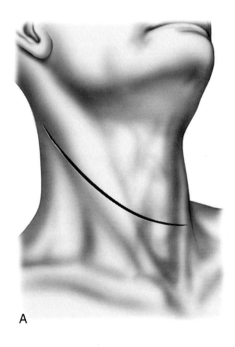

A

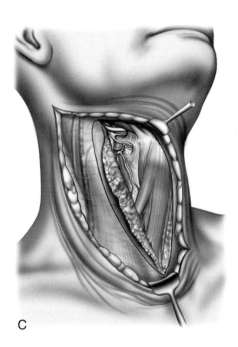

C

Figure 11–4. Selective lateral neck dissection.

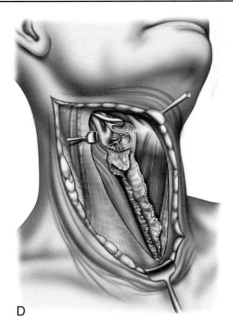

D

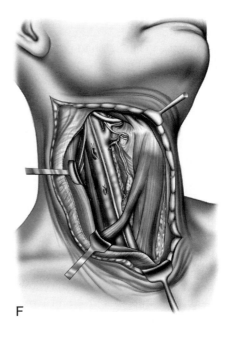

F

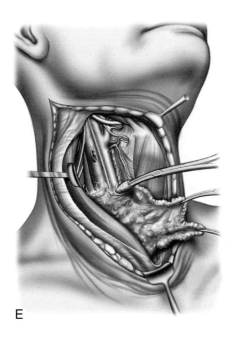

E

Figure 11–4 *Continued* Selective lateral neck dissection.

Figure 11–4*D.* Posteriorly, the fascia and the lymphoareolar tissue are reflected anteriorly from the SCM muscle to the carotid sheath. The great vessels, the digastric muscles, and the hypoglossal nerve are exposed, and the specimen is reflected downward from the level of the digastric muscle.

Figure 11–4*E.* At a further stage of dissection, the jugular vein and the spinal accessory nerve are exposed. It is important to remove the lymphoareolar tissue posterior to the jugular vein as far as the accessory nerve and the cervical nerve roots.

Figure 11–4*F.* The specimen has been completely removed, exposing the internal jugular vein inferior to the omohyoid muscle. Retraction of the SCM muscle permits adequate dissection and, in this illustration, exposes the entire operative field.

Results

Byers[51] reported 14 recurrences in 297 dissected necks (5%) in patients with primary laryngeal and hypopharyngeal cancer, at the 2-year follow-up (Table 11–2). Spiro et al.[53] reviewed the Memorial Hospital experience with 66 patients who had 85 "jugular node" (levels II, III, and IV) dissections between 1984 and 1991. Among 56 patients with clinically negative necks, 15 had pathologically positive nodes. Four patients with pathologically negative nodes developed neck recurrences; 2 had received postoperative radiation therapy. There were 2 instances of neck recurrences among 15 patients who had neck metastases within their neck dissection specimens. Both had received postoperative irradiation. The recurrent cancer was located outside of or at the limit of the operative field in all 6 patients with neck failure. Nearly all the recurrences involved the upper posterior or the mid posterior nodes, leading the authors to conclude that dissection of these areas should be carried lateral to the internal jugular vein. Nodal metastasis was confirmed in 8 out of 10 patients whose tumors were staged clinically as N1. Interestingly, there were no recurrences in this group of patients, all of whom received adjuvant radiation therapy.

CERVICAL LYMPHADENOPATHY UNRELATED TO PRIMARY CANCER OF THE LARYNX

Sometimes the presence of a palpable laterocervical lymph node in a patient with cancer of the larynx may be unrelated to the primary cancer itself. In addition to metastatic spread from a primary laryngeal tumor, the presence of lymphadenopathy may be associated with a variety of other pathologic situations, such as the following:

- reactive hyperplasia
- response to the infection and inflammation often associated with laryngeal cancer
- unrelated diseases, such as tuberculosis, anthracosis, or silicosis
- metastases unrelated to the primary laryngeal tumor (for example, metastases from cancer of the thyroid gland, the lungs, or the breast)
- metastases in the neck from a thyroid cancer with a clinically normal thyroid
- systemic neoplastic diseases, such as lymphoma or leukemia
- related dual lymph node pathology; for example, several lymph nodes may simultaneously contain laryngeal and thyroid metastases, or the same lymph node may contain neoplastic

Table 11–2. RECURRENCE RATES AFTER SELECTIVE LATERAL NECK DISSECTION: CANCER OF THE LARYNX AND THE HYPOPHARYNX*		
Pathologic Staging	Surgery Only	Surgery and Postoperative Radiotherapy
N0	10/130 (8%)	1/126 (1%)
N1	0/4 (0%)	0/17 (0%)
Multiple nodes or extracapsular invasion	. . .	3/20 (15%)

*Modified from Byers RM. Modified neck dissection: a study of 967 cases from 1970 to 1980. *Am J Surg* 1985; 150:414–421. Adapted with permission from American Journal of Surgery.

cells from a cancer of the larynx associated with chronic lymphocytic leukemia
- lymph nodes may be involved simultaneously by metastatic squamous cell carcinoma and tuberculosis
- metastases to cervical lymph nodes from an unknown primary site

The clinician should consider the possibility that cervical lymphadenopathy may be etiologically unrelated to the cancer of the larynx, because this will influence staging, management, and prognosis.[54]

NONSQUAMOUS MALIGNANT NEOPLASMS

Laryngeal tumors other than squamous cell carcinoma are uncommon, although these include several histologic varieties. The histologic types of neoplasms vary in their tendency to spread to the lymph nodes: some metastasize frequently, some do so only rarely, and some never do. Neck dissection is indicated in the following malignant neoplasms:

- spindle cell squamous carcinoma
- basaloid squamous carcinoma
- atypical carcinoid
- high-grade mucoepidermoid carcinoma
- malignant melanoma
- embryonal and alveolar rhabdomyosarcoma

Neck dissection is not indicated in the treatment of malignant lymphoma. It does not appear to be indicated in malignant fibrous histiocytoma or chondrosarcoma, unless clinical examination or imaging techniques suggest metastatic lymph node involvement. Neck dissection is not recommended in laryngeal melanoma because the incidence of regional lymph node metastases is considered low.[55] Therapeutic neck dissection is indicated only when there are cervical lymph node metastases in the absence of distant metastatic disease.[56] In addition, neck dissection is usually not indicated for the following tumors:

- verrucous squamous cell carcinoma
- adenoid cystic carcinoma
- typical carcinoid tumor
- small cell neuroendocrine carcinoma
- acinic cell carcinoma
- paraganglioma
- hemangiopericytoma
- synovial sarcoma
- liposarcoma

There may be various reasons for neck dissection not being indicated. For example, it is not indicated in verrucous squamous cell carcinoma because this tumor does not metastasize. Operative treatment should not include neck dissection, even when enlarged and tender lymph nodes may be palpated. In fact, histologic examination of these nodes has revealed only an inflammatory reaction. Cervical and distant metastases have not been reported in nonirradiated true verrucous carcinoma.[57] Prophylactic neck dissection is not indicated in laryngeal adenoid cystic carcinoma because this tumor does not usually metastasize to the cervical lymph nodes.[58, 59]

A cervical mass, even with a known primary tumor, is not always a metastatic lymph node. It may represent a recurrence or persistence of the primary tumor.[59, 60] A metastasis from a basaloid squamous cell carcinoma may be misdiagnosed as adenoid cystic carcinoma.[57] Neck dissection is not indicated in paraganglioma of the larynx because this tumor is benign. Essentially all reported cases of aggressive and metastasizing malignant paraganglioma of the larynx were actually atypical carcinoid tumors.[60] Neck dissection does not appear necessary in hemangiopericytoma because this neoplasm metastasizes hematogenously rather than via the lymphatic system.

In conclusion, it does not seem logical to perform a neck dissection for all malignant neoplasms of the larynx. It is important to understand the natural history of a particular neoplasm before it can be treated effectively.

REFERENCES

1. Crile G. Excision of cancer of the head and neck with special reference to the plan of dissection based upon one hundred thirty-two operations. *JAMA* 1906; 47:1780–1786.
2. Semken GH. Surgery of the neck. *In Nelson's Loose Leaf Surgery*, New York, Thomas Nelson & Son, 1932.
3. Ward GE, Hendrick JW. *Tumors of the Head and Neck.* Baltimore, Williams & Wilkins, 1950.
4. Conley JJ, Von Frankel PH. Historical aspects of head and neck surgery. *Ann Otol Rhinol Laryngol* 1956; 65:643–655.
5. Sylvestre-Benis C. Consideraciones sobre el problema del tratamiento quirurgico de los ganglios en los canceres de la laringe. *Actas II Congreso Sudamericano ORL*. Montevideo, Uruguay, 1944.
6. Del Sel J, Agra A. Cancer of the larynx: laryngectomy with systemic extirpation of the connective tissue and cervical lymph nodes as a routine procedure. *Trans Amer Acad Ophthalmol Otolaryngol* 1947; 51:653–655.
7. Clerf LH, Patney FJ, O'Keefe JJ. Carcinoma of the larynx. *Laryngoscope* 1948; 58:632.
8. Brown JH, McDowell F. Treatment of metastatic carcinoma in the neck. *Ann Surg* 1944; 119:543–555.
9. Martin HE, DeValle B, Ehrlich H, et al. Neck dissection. *Cancer* 1951; 4:441–491.
10. Ogura JH, Bello JA. Laryngectomy and radical neck dissection for carcinoma of the larynx. *Laryngoscope* 1952; 62:1–52.
11. Barbosa JF. Radical laryngectomy with bilateral neck dissection in continuity. *Arch Otolaryngol* 1965; 63:372–383.
12. Barbosa JF. *Surgical Treatment of Head and Neck Tumors.* New York, Grune & Stratton, 1974.
13. Suarez O. El problema de las metastasis linfaticas y alejadas del cancer de laringe y hipofaringe. *Rev Otorrinolaringol* 1963; 23:83–99.
14. Byers RM. Introduction at the Third International Conference on Cancer of the Neck. *In Johnson JT, Didolkar M (eds): Head and Neck Cancer*. Amsterdam, Excerpta Medica, 1993.
15. Bocca E. Supraglottic laryngectomy and functional neck dissection. *J Laryngol Otol* 1966; 80:831–838.
16. Bocca E, Pignataro O, Oldini C, et al. Functional neck dissection: an evaluation and review of 843 cases. *Laryngoscope* 1984; 94:942–945.
17. Bocca E, Pignataro O, Sasaki CT. Functional neck dissection: a description of operative technique. *Arch Otolaryngol* 1980; 106:524–527.
18. Calearo CV, Teatini G. Functional neck dissection: anatomical grounds, surgical technique, clinical observations. *Ann Otol Rhinol Laryngol* 1983; 92:215–222.
19. Gavilán J, Gavilán C, Herranz J. Functional neck dissection: three decades of controversy. *Ann Otol Rhinol Laryngol* 1992; 101:339–341.
20. Jesse RH, Ballantyne AJ, Larson D. Radical or modified neck dissection: a therapeutic dilemma. *Am J Surg* 1978; 136:516–519.
21. Khafif RA, Gelbfish GA, Asase DK, et al. Modified radical neck dissection in cancer of the mouth, pharynx, and larynx. *Head Neck* 1990; 12:476–482.
22. Spiro RH. Less can mean more. *Am J Surg* 1993; 166:322–325 (Hayes Martin Lecture to the Society of Head and Neck Surgeons).
23. Shah JP, Strong EW, Spiro RH, et al. Neck dissection: current status and future possibilities. *Clin Bull* 1981; 11:25–33.
24. Suen JY, Goepfert H. Standardization of neck dissection nomenclature. *Head Neck Surg* 1987; 10:75–77.
25. Medina JE. A rational classification of neck dissections. *Otolaryngol Head Neck Surg* 1989; 100:169–176.
26. Robbins KT, Medina JE, Wolfe GT, et al. Standardizing neck dissection terminology. Official report of the Academy's Committee for Head and Neck Surgery and Oncology. *Arch Otolaryngol Head Neck Surg* 1991; 117:601–605.
27. Medina JE, Byers RM. Supraomohyoid neck dissection: rationale, indications, and surgical technique. *Head Neck Surg* 1989; 11:111–122.
28. Baredes S, Nussbaum M, Som ML. The role of supraomohyoid dissection at the time of supraglottic laryngectomy. *Laryngoscope* 1985; 95:151–155.
29. Resta L, Micheau C, Cimmino A. Prognostic value of the prelaryngeal node in laryngeal and hypopharyngeal carcinoma. *Tumori* 1985; 71:361–365.
30. Friedman M, Mayer AD. Rationale for evaluation and treatment of the neck. *In Ferlito A (ed): Neoplasms of the Larynx*, pp 493–508. Edinburgh, Churchill, 1993.
31. Stern WBR, Silver CE, Zeifer BA, et al. Computed tomography of the clinically negative neck. *Head Neck* 1990; 12:109–113.
32. Mendelsohn MS, Shulman HS, Noyek AM. Diagnostic imaging. *In Ferlito A (ed): Neoplasms of the Larynx*, pp 401–423. Edinburgh, Churchill, 1993.

33. Feinmesser R, Freeman JL, Feinmesser M, et al. Role of modern imaging in decision-making for elective neck dissection. *Head Neck* 1992; 14:173–176.

34. Million RR, Cassisi NJ. General principles for treatment of cancers in the head and neck: selection of treatment for the primary site and for the neck. *In* Million RR, Cassisi NJ (eds): *Management of Head and Neck Cancer,* pp 58–59. Philadelphia, Lippincott, 1984.

35. Suen JY. Cancer of the neck. *In* Myers EN, Suen JY (eds): *Cancer of the Head and Neck,* 2nd ed, pp 221–254. New York, Churchill, 1989.

36. Wenig BL, Applebaum EL. The submandibular triangle in squamous cell carcinoma of the larynx and hypopharynx. *Laryngoscope* 1991; 101:516–518.

37. Candela FC, Shah J, Jaques DP, et al. Patterns of cervical node metastases from squamous carcinoma of the larynx. *Arch Otolaryngol Head Neck Surg* 1990; 116:432–435.

38. Leemans CR, Tiwari R, van der Waal I, et al. The efficacy of comprehensive neck dissection with or without postoperative radiotherapy in nodal metastases of squamous cell carcinoma of the upper respiratory and digestive tract. *Laryngoscope* 1990; 100:1194–1198.

39. Byers RM, Wolf PF, Ballantyne AJ. Rationale for elective modified neck dissection. *Head Neck Surg* 1988; 10:160–167.

40. Carter RL, Bliss JM, Soo KC, et al. Radical neck dissections for squamous carcinomas: pathological findings and clinical implications with particular reference to transcapsular spread. *Int J Radiat Oncol Biol Phys* 1987; 17:825–832.

41. Devineni VR, Simpson R, Sessions D, et al. Supraglottic carcinoma: impact of radiation therapy on outcome of patients with positive margins and extracapsular nodal disease. *Laryngoscope* 1991; 101:767–770.

42. Hirabayashi H, Koshii K, Uno K, et al. Extracapsular spread of squamous carcinoma in neck lymph nodes: prognostic factor in laryngeal cancer. *Laryngoscope* 1991; 101:502–506.

43. Johnson JT, Myers EN, Bedetti CD, et al. Cervical lymph node metastases: incidence and implications of extracapsular carcinoma. *Arch Otolaryngol* 1985; 111:534–537.

44. Kowalski LP, Franco EL, De Andrade Sobrinho J, et al. Prognostic factors in laryngeal cancer patients submitted to surgical treatment. *J Surg Oncol* 1991; 48:87–95.

45. Lefebvre JL, Castelain B, de la Torre JV, et al. Lymph node invasion in hypopharynx and lateral epilarynx carcinoma: a prognostic factor. *Head Neck Surg* 1987; 10:14–18.

46. Snyderman NL, Johnson JT, Schramm VL Jr, et al. Extracapsular spread of carcinoma in cervical lymph nodes: impact upon survival in patients with carcinoma of the supraglottic larynx. *Cancer* 1985; 56:1597–1599.

47. Molinari R, Cantù G, Chiesa F, et al. Retrospective comparison of conservative and radical neck dissection in laryngeal cancer. *Ann Otol Rhinol Laryngol* 1980; 89:578–581.

48. Bocca E. Surgical management of supraglottic cancer and its lymph node metastases in a conservative perspective. *Ann Otol Rhinol Laryngol* 1991; 100:261–267.

49. Medina JE. The role of surgery in the treatment of the neck. *In* Johnson JT, Didolkar M (eds): *Head and Neck Cancer,* pp 505–512. Amsterdam, Excerpta Medica, 1993.

50. Chu W, Strawitz JG. Results in suprahyoid, modified radical and standard radical neck dissections for metastatic squamous cell carcinoma: recurrence and survival. *Am J Surg* 1978; 136:512–515.

51. Byers RM. Modified neck dissection: a study of 967 cases from 1970 to 1980. *Am J Surg* 1985; 150:414–421.

52. Shah JP, Medina JE, Shaha AR, et al. Cervical lymph node metastasis. *Curr Prob Surg* 1993; 30:273–344.

53. Spiro RH, Gallo O, Shap JP. Selective jugular node dissection in patients with squamous carcinoma of the larynx or pharynx. *Am J Surg* 1993; 166:399–406.

54. Ratcliffe RJ, Soutar DS. Unexpected lymph node pathology in neck dissection for head and neck cancer. *Head Neck* 1990; 12:244–246.

55. Panje WR, Moran WJ. Melanoma of the upper aerodigestive tract: a review of 21 cases. *Head Neck Surg* 1986; 8:309–312.

56. Blatchford SJ, Koopmann CF, Coulthard SW. Mucosal melanoma of the head and neck. *Laryngoscope* 1986; 96:929–934.

57. Ferlito A. Atypical forms of squamous cell carcinoma. *In* Ferlito A (ed): *Neoplasms of the Larynx,* pp 135–167. Edinburgh, Churchill, 1993.

58. Ferlito A. Malignant laryngeal epithelial tumors and lymph node involvement: therapeutic and prognostic considerations. *Ann Otol Rhinol Laryngol* 1987; 96:542–548.

59. Ferlito A, Barnes L, Myers EN. Neck dissection for laryngeal adenoid cystic carcinoma: is it indicated? *Ann Otol Rhinol Laryngol* 1990; 99:277–280.

60. Ferlito A, Barnes L, Wenig BM. Identification, classification, treatment and prognosis of laryngeal paraganglioma. Review of the literature and eight new cases. *Ann Otol Rhinol Laryngol* 1994; 103:525–536.

Chapter 12

Laser Surgery for Cancer of the Larynx

Stanley M. Shapshay, Duncan R. Ingrams, and James Z. Cinberg

The birth of the laser, an acronym for *l*ight *a*mplification by *s*timulated *e*mission of *r*adiation, was announced in a three-paragraph article in the August 1960 issue of *Nature*.[1] The short statement reported Theodore Maiman's success at obtaining stimulated optical emission. The emission, which was within visible wavelengths, was of weak intensity. Since that time, laser technology has grown dramatically. In the past 30 years the surgical laser has evolved from a scientific curiosity into a fully accepted surgical instrument. A range of lasers is now available to the laryngeal surgeon, offering different characteristics for use in different tissues. However, the carbon dioxide (CO_2) laser remains the most widely used instrument, because its ability to excise tissue with precision and minimal damage to surrounding structures makes it suitable for almost all applications within the larynx.[2–4]

DEVELOPMENT OF THE LASER

The acronym "laser" describes the emission process in which an intense beam of electromagnetic radiation is generated. The broad idea of stimulated emission was contained in the theory of resonance developed by Lord Rayleigh in the late nineteenth century. Albert Einstein proposed the specific concepts of stimulated emissions, stimulated absorption, and spontaneous emission to explain the interaction between radiation and populations of atoms in the context of the quantum theory. His work provided the theoretical foundation for the laser and appeared in 1917 in his classic paper "Zur Quantum Theorie der Strahlung."[5]

Stimulated emission had been evaluated in studies of light absorption in the 1920s[6] and again in experiments with excited lithium nuclei in the early 1950s.[7] The potential application of these observations was not recognized at the time. In 1953, Weber[8] proved analytically that stimulated emission of amplified microwave radiation was possible. The following year, Gordon and coworkers[9] announced the successful generation of a coherent microwave beam resulting from stimulated emission and originated the acronym "maser" (microwave amplification by stimulated emission of radiation) to describe this phenomenon.

Schalow and Townes,[10] in 1958, published a now classic article, "Infrared and Optical Masers." They concluded that there were no theoretical obstacles to the development of stimulated emission in the visual spectrum. Soon thereafter, in 1960, Maiman, a research scientist for Hughes Aircraft, announced that he had succeeded in generating light amplification by stimulated emission, and lasers became a reality.

The first laser used a solid material, a ruby crystal, as the excitable medium and generated an ultrashort pulsed beam in the visible spectrum. Less than 6 months after Maiman's announcement, Javan and coworkers[11] at the Bell Telephone Laboratories were the first to use a gas as a "lasing medium." Their helium-neon laser provided the first continuous wave emission. In 1964, Patel[12] at the Bell Telephone Laboratories devised the first laser to permit conversion of electric power into a continuous laser wave at an efficiency and power intensity far greater than had been previously achieved. He used a CO_2 gas mixture as the active medium, and an emission in the infrared spectrum resulted. Current surgical lasers are direct descendants of this continuous wave CO_2 laser. Books by Goldman and Rockwell[13] and by Brotherton[14] are recommended to the reader interested in an in-depth review of the development of the laser.

PRODUCTION OF LASER RADIATION

Three components are basic to a laser: an energy source, a lasing medium, and a reflecting system. Energy may be supplied by high-voltage electric currents, chemical reactions, neutral atom discharge, optical pumping, or ionization. The wave length of a laser depends on the lasing medium. The lasing medium, which receives the energy, can be a solid, a liquid, a semiconductor diode, or a gas. Gas mixtures that can generate laser emission may be in the molecular, the atomic, or the ionic state.

The particles of a lasing medium do not all share the same energy level. The majority of the atomic population is at a "ground state," while a much smaller percentage is "excited" and occupies high energy levels. However, when the lasing medium is exposed to the energy source, the number of excited "high energy" particles increases greatly. These energized particles spontaneously discharge photons, or light quanta. They will also release photons in reaction to a stimulating radiation of appropriate wave length. A photon wave traveling through the lasing medium will collide with either excited or unexcited particles. If photons meet unexcited particles, they will be absorbed and their wave train will lose energy. When photons strike excited particles, additional photons are discharged, thus amplifying the wave. Photons traveling through the energized lasing medium will encounter more excited than unexcited particles, thus producing a net amplification of the original wave train.

The reflecting system, consisting of parallel mirrors aligned at opposite ends of the lasing medium container, keeps the wave train moving through the medium. Continuous amplification of stimulated emission in an axis perpendicular to the mirrors results. A "resonant cavity" occurs. However, the cavity is "leaky" because one of the mirrors is partially transparent. The leaked, or transmitted, emission is the laser output. The laser continues emitting in a stable equilibrium despite the leak, because the amplification process compensates for the loss. Duley[15] and Patel[16] provide a thorough review of laser physics.

PROPERTIES OF LASER RADIATION

Laser radiation has three basic properties: collimation, monochromaticity, and coherency. Collimation means that the emitted rays are parallel to each other. Monochromaticity refers to the fact that emitted rays are of the same wavelength. Coherency means that all the emitted rays are exactly in phase with each other in space and time. These three properties allow focused laser light to be concentrated on a single point with enormous energy density.

In reality, laser emission is not perfectly coherent. This is an important consideration for laser research. Slight variations in coherency do occur and result in different patterns of energy distribution at the focal point. Each pattern is called a mode. The transverse electromagnetic (TEM_{00}) mode is a pattern with maximum energy at its center and with a uniform decrease as the periphery extends. All current surgical lasers theoretically produce emissions in the TEM_{00} mode. Slight variations in the actual modes produced are clinically insignificant.

Laser strength is expressed in terms of power density. Power density is determined by dividing the average emission power by the average diameter of the beam cross-section and is expressed in watts per square centimeter. A 30-watt white light source will produce less than 1 watt per square centimeter at its focal point, whereas a 30-watt laser will produce more than 1000 watts per square centimeter.

BIOLOGY OF LASER-TISSUE INTERACTIONS

All matter selectively absorbs, scatters, and reflects incident electromagnetic radiation. The degree to which this occurs in a particular substance is dependent on the wavelength of the radiation. When laser light strikes biologic tissue, light energy is transformed into heat energy. The absorption

and intratissue scattering of the radiation and the resultant heat distribution determine the extent of the tissue changes that occur. The more laser energy that is absorbed by a mass of tissue, the less energy is transmitted to the surrounding tissue. The potential for incision is directly proportional to the degree of tissue absorption. On the other hand, the potential for hemostasis is proportional to the degree of transmission and scatter. However, if the tissue is completely transparent, with no absorption at all, no hemostasis will occur. Hemostasis is caused, in part, by moderate heating of the blood vessel. Increased hemostasis can be achieved by broadening the distribution zone of the heat source, which causes an increase in the width of the necrotic zone adjacent to the incision. Currently, lasers that have sufficient output to generate significant temperature gradients include the carbon-dioxide (CO_2), the neodymium:yttrium-aluminum-garnet (Nd:YAG), the ruby, the argon, and the potassium titanyl phosphate (KTP/532) lasers.

Of these, the CO_2 laser has the most precise soft tissue interaction. This is because its wavelength of 10.6 μm has a coefficient of absorption (AC) for water that is dramatically higher than for wavelengths produced by the other lasers. Almost all the applied energy is absorbed by the water-rich tissue, which is rapidly heated to 100°C. Cell water then evaporates. A high temperature gradient accompanies the "steaming" of the tissue and results in a localized necrotic zone formed by heat conduction. The temperature increase of the surrounding tissue during the ablation process, however, is minimal because of the rapidity of the process and the low thermal conductivity of tissue. The principal source of thermal energy is the steam produced by the tissue ablation process. This steam is dissipated almost instantaneously at the time of ablation, using an efficient suction device. The volume of tissue affected is directly related to the length of exposure. Longer laser pulses cause greater depths of ablation with only minimal increases in affected surface area. In addition, there is little forward or backward scattering of the energy, which enables the surgeon to see the effect of the radiation instantly.

The main disadvantage of the CO_2 laser is that its 10.6-μm wavelength cannot easily be transmitted by fiberoptic devices. Currently, our laboratory is evaluating new flexible fibers for delivering CO_2 laser energy, and it is to be hoped that eventually these fibers will increase the endoscopic uses of the CO_2 laser. At the moment, however, the CO_2 laser is most commonly used coupled with an operating microscope with an articulated series of mirrors. Micromanipulator devices have improved this method of delivery, allowing the surgeon to focus the energy onto a spot 250 μm in diameter, allowing very accurate incisions. This laser can also be used via a handpiece for less-precise excision of soft tissue. Hemostasis is largely restricted to capillaries and small vessels, but this is not normally a problem in poorly vascularized tissues such as the vocal cords.

The Nd:YAG laser has a wavelength of 1.06 μm and has a greater amount of scatter and a smaller AC than does the CO_2 laser. There is deeper penetration into tissue, depending on the amount of pigment far beyond the immediate area of the focal point. In addition, the maximal power density lies below the surface of the tissue, which makes it difficult for the surgeon to see the effect of the applied energy. This differs greatly from the CO_2 laser, with which the extent of tissue damage is clearly visible to the surgeon. The use of a contact tip with the Nd:YAG system allows a more predictable and precise destruction of soft tissue but is restricted by the manual dexterity of the surgeon and also eliminates the microprecision inherent in the micromanipulator operating microscope system. Hemostasis is comparable to that obtained with the CO_2 laser.

The argon laser, with a wavelength of either 488 or 515 nm, has the advantage of being suitable for delivery with either a fiberoptic or a micromanipulator system. The disadvantage of this laser (and the KTP/532 laser) is its selective absorption by pigmented tissue, such as hemoglobin, oxyhemoglobin, melanin, and carotene. The amount of forward and back scattering varies with the degree of pigmentation or vascularization of the tissue and is difficult to predict. It has limited usefulness for precise incision and ablation of nonpigmented soft tissue. Contact application can improve the cutting effect but is not as precise as a sharply focused CO_2 laser beam delivered by the micromanipulator.

It is for these reasons that although the Nd:YAG, the argon, and the KTP/532 lasers have specific applications in otolaryngology, the CO_2 laser remains the instrument of choice.

GENERAL CLINICAL CONSIDERATIONS

Our discussion of the laser as a treatment modality for cancer of the larynx will largely be confined to the CO_2 system for the reasons outlined above.

Equipment

The effect of the laser on the irradiated tissue is viewed through the surgical microscope. A micro-

manipulator system projects the beam to any direction of the visual field of the microscope. The micromanipulator consists of a mirror, seated in a double gimbal mount that is controlled by cams, which are linked to a lever. The mirror fully engages the laser beam. As the surgeon moves the lever, the mirror changes position and projects the laser beam to different quadrants of the microscope's field. An in-line lens made of zinc sulfide or a material with similar properties focuses the laser transmission to coincide with the focal length of the surgical microscope lens. A focal length of 400 mm is most suitable for endolaryngeal surgery. A 300-mm lens is used for surgery in the oral cavity.

The surgical laser has a visual aiming system to ensure precise control of the site of tissue destruction because the actual emission at the 10.6-μm wavelength is invisible. Different lasers use different strategies to align a controllable, visible light with the laser beam. In the earlier commercially available lasers, such as the Cavitron model AO-300, a minimal amount of the light from the microscope was diverted through a fiberoptic cable and passed through a green filter. The surgeon saw a green point ("virtual image") in the field of the microscope. Adjustments were then made so that the point of laser impact coincided with the virtual image. These preliminary adjustments were done by focusing and firing the laser onto a wooden tongue depressor or other material. In most of the more recent laser units, the aiming system is a visible light beam that is coaxial with the CO_2 laser emission, simultaneously transmitted through the microscope. The aiming light is often produced by a low-intensity visible laser, such as a helium-neon laser.

When the laser is fired through the laryngoscope, smoke and steam will obscure the field unless they are suctioned off. A microsuction cannula positioned in one of the light channels of the laryngoscope will permit uninterrupted smoke evacuation. The surgeon should also place a micro "whistle tip" suction close to the laser impact site to avoid damage to normal structures from the steam of vaporization.

Laser Safety

The CO_2 laser radiates light in the infrared spectrum. The emission is not radioactive or ionizing and, if unfocused, will cause only minimal skin damage. The main dangers of the CO_2 laser are those of ocular injury[17] and anesthesia fire hazard[18, 19] from the use of potentially flammable endotracheal tubes. The combustion of dry materials, such as surgical drapes, must also be avoided by constant moistening. The mid-infrared emission of the CO_2 laser produces deleterious effects primarily on the cornea, unlike the visible or the near-infrared emissions of other lasing media, which affect primarily the retina.

Although the danger of inadvertent direct contact is minimal, the focused laser beam can be reflected from shiny metal surfaces, thus representing a potential danger.[20] Ordinary glass or clear plastic lenses with side shields offer effective protection and should be worn by all operating room personnel. Because laser energy is well dissipated by water, the patient's eyes can be protected by being covered with wet cotton gauze or eye pads taped in position.

Pure oxygen or oxygen mixed with nonflammable gas will not be ignited by a laser beam. Biologic tissue cannot be made to support combustion even when it is destroyed by laser radiation in an atmosphere of oxygen. A flammable material must be present for combustion to occur. Thus, high-flow oxygen ventilation can be safely employed in laryngeal laser surgery, as discussed below. However, the impact of a laser beam of sufficient duration on a plastic or rubber endotracheal tube through which an oxygen-rich anesthesia gas mixture is passing can create an effect similar to that of an oxyacetylene torch, with disastrous consequences. This can be prevented by wrapping the endotracheal tube in aluminum foil or by using one of several commercially prepared laser-resistant tubes. A soaking-wet gauze or cottonoid inserted beneath the vocal cords will effectively prevent thermal injury to the trachea or to the balloon of the endotracheal tube. The tubes usually employed in current surgical practice contain two balloons that are inflated with water rather than with air. If one balloon is accidentally punctured by the laser beam, it will not ignite, and the closed-system airway can be maintained by inflating the second balloon.

Regardless of the choice of endotracheal tube, constant attention of the surgeon to proper technique is the most important safety factor. The lowest possible oxygen concentration consistent with adequate blood gases should be chosen by the anesthesiologist and supervised by the surgeon.

Anesthesia

Safety considerations with regard to anesthesia have been discussed in the preceding section. Of course, flammable or explosive inhalation anesthetics are not used. As with other microlaryngeal procedures, we prefer that the patient be paralyzed. Ventilation is accomplished either by a high-flow oxygen system coupled to the laryngoscope or through an endotracheal tube. In the high-flow technique, the oxygen is delivered through a 16-gauge needle or a pediatric bronchoscope suction tube placed in one of the light channels of the laryngoscope and insinuated at or just below the vocal cords. This cannula is connected to an adjustable pressure-reducing valve, which in turn is connected to pipeline oxygen. The technique, which was popularized by Carden and Ferguson,[21] allows unimpeded endolaryngeal visualization and manipulation. Alternatively, a clip-on proximal jet ventilating system can be constructed to fit onto the laryngoscope. Aspiration of blood or debris by the patient is a theoretical possibility with this system because of the absence of an endotracheal tube cuff. However, this complication is not known to be clinically significant, and this approach may be used routinely, except in patients with significantly diminished chest cage compliance because of excessive girth or skeletal disease. The high-flow system does not create a Venturi effect or air entrainment. Recently, special laryngoscopes have been designed for laser surgery, with multiple channels for positioning of the cannulae for high-flow oxygen, as well as for suction.

If an endotracheal tube is preferred, our preference is for a flexible metallic laser-resistant tube with balloons inflated with saline and methylene blue. This approach, however, affords significantly less access to the endolaryngeal structures than is possible with the high-flow system. Use of a tube also incurs the potential fire hazard associated with laser impact on the cuff or on an inadequately protected area. The tube does, however, protect the distal airway from blood and secretions, inhalation of which poses a particular hazard during major resections for laryngeal cancer. The surgical and anesthesia teams should be ready for a quick response in the event of ignition of a tube. The tube should be removed immediately and the airway restored. A bronchoscopy should be done to evaluate the extent of damage and to remove any foreign body. Antibiotics and steroids should be given to minimize the effects of the burn and to diminish the swelling.

APPLICATIONS FOR TREATMENT OF CANCER OF THE LARYNX

Lasers can be used in the initial evaluation of laryngeal lesions, including the sampling of tissue for histologic purposes or excisional biopsy, and in the treatment of frank carcinoma. Laser vaporization or excision may be the only therapy required in premalignant and early malignant lesions. In more invasive cancers, the laser can be used as part of a joint procedure to excise the affected area fully. Lasers can be used in the reconstruction of surgical defects through tissue welding or soldering of mucosal grafts. Lasers can be used to treat recurrences of tumors and can be used in palliation of non-resectable obstructing lesions. When used in conjunction with photosensitizing agents, laser photodynamic therapy may play a role in the treatment of superficial malignancies.

Excisional Biopsy with the Carbon Dioxide Laser

Endoscopic management of laryngeal neoplasia relies on adequate exposure of the larynx using a wide-bore laryngoscope that can be held in some form of suspension apparatus. Difficulty can be encountered owing to a narrow dental arch or scarring of the neck from previous surgery or radiotherapy. There may also be inadequate neck extension in patients with cervical arthritis. It is important to remember that traditional microsurgical techniques exist to treat early laryngeal neoplasia and that the CO_2 laser is not a magical tool. However, the laser has the advantage of providing noncontact microprecision in a relatively bloodless field. The laser may cause thermal damage to adjacent healthy tissue, causing inflammation and fibrosis. This can be minimized by using a small spot and intermittent exposure and by removing the specimen with constant tissue retraction. In general, tissue excision by thermal means, such as by laser, produces slower wound healing than with nonthermal surgical treatment; however, this delay in healing is not clinically significant.

Premalignant Lesions

Keratosis

After adequate exposure has been obtained, excess mucus is removed from the vocal cord. Using 25-fold magnification and a 400 mm-objective lens on the operating microscope, the vocal cords are carefully inspected. Fine microlaryngeal probes are used to palpate the vocal cords and retract the false cord on each side to inspect the ventricle. Mirrors or telescopes are used to examine the subglottic surface of the cord and the anterior commissure region. Toluidine blue (2%) is used to identify the surface areas of increased nucleic acid content.[22] These areas will stain deep purple and enable the surgeon to see multicentric areas of severe dysplasia and carcinoma in situ. It is important to remember that areas of inadvertent mechanical damage caused by surgical manipulation will also take up the stain, and that submucosal tumors will not (Fig. 12–1).

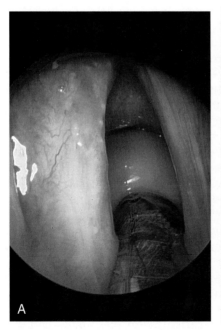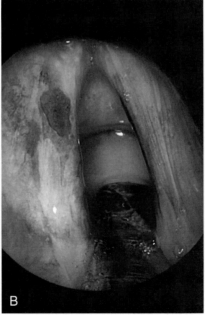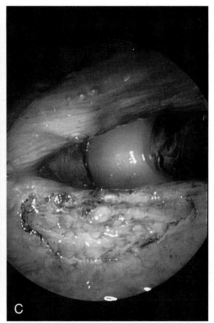

Figure 12–1. Excisional biopsy of vocal cord lesion. *(A)* Left vocal fold with superficial lesion. *(B)* Toluidine blue staining reveals early invasive carcinoma (dark stain) and adjacent areas of dysplasia. *(C)* Defect after excisional biopsy. (From Shapshay SM, Wang Z, Rebeizz EE, et al. "Window" laryngoplasty: a new combined laser endoscopic and open technique for conservation surgery. *Ann Otol Rhinol Laryngol* 1994; 103:679–685.)

Areas arousing suspicion should then be totally excised. The area is first outlined using the laser in a 0.1-second pulsed mode, using 2 watts of power and a spot size of 250 μm. Once this outline has been extended to the full depth of the lesion, the area can normally be "peeled off" the underlying tissue using microlaryngeal instruments. If the lesion is obviously restricted to the epithelium, such as with keratosis, the deep plane should be in the submucosal layer to preserve good vocal function. This cold technique is preferred because it reduces the thermal damage to the remaining vocal cord (the ligament and the underlying muscle), thereby minimizing the risk of subsequent scar formation. Some surgeons prefer to inject a saline-epinephrine solution into the submucosal space in order to raise the epithelial surface away from the underlying vocal ligament. The solution may also help provide hemostasis and may act as a heat sink for the laser.[23]

Dysplasia

A technique similar to the one described above is used in the treatment of dysplasia. The only differences for the removal of dysplastic lesions are the use of a slightly wider margin of excision of 1 to 2 mm and the excision of the full thickness of the epithelium, including Reinke's space. This thicker specimen is necessary because dysplasia may affect the full thickness of the epithelium, and it is also important to exclude invasion through the basement membrane. As in the case of keratosis, the specimen is first outlined with the laser and then dissected with microlaryngeal instruments. The laser incises the epithelium and provides a bloodless field for dissection. Frozen-section margins may be taken, and these often show incomplete clearance because dysplastic changes may occur across a wide field. It is important in these cases not to miss an area of carcinoma in situ or invasive carcinoma. Staining with toluidine blue helps to detect areas of severe dysplasia and carcinoma in situ.

Carcinoma in Situ

If the lesion is identified as carcinoma in situ, the excision should be deep enough to expose the vocal muscle. A 2- to 3-mm margin is necessary, and the specimen should be carefully orientated for the pathologist for examination. The full depth of the specimen is required to allow the pathologist to comment on any invasion of the basement epithelial membrane. This microprecise technique allows both cords to be treated simultaneously, provided that the dissection does not include the anterior commissure. The traditional "cord stripping" operation is no longer indicated because it results in an uneven plane of excision through Reinke's space, and some of the submucosal tissue may be missed.

Malignant Lesions

Early Invasive (Stage T1) Carcinoma

Strict criteria exist for the endoscopic management of invasive carcinoma with the laser.[24, 25] Exposure of the entire lesion must be possible. Vocal cord mobility must be unimpaired. The tumor must be limited to the membranous part of the vocal cord and must not involve the anterior commissure or the vocal process. Complete exposure of the anterior commissure is difficult endoscopically, and cartilage invasion is difficult to detect, thus rendering this region of the larynx less favorable for endoscopic treatment. It is important to note that attempts to extend laser resection of early vocal cord cancer to anterior commissure tumors have been associated with high rates of recurrence.[26, 27] Tumor involvement of 1 to 2 mm along the floor of the ventricle may be adequately resected by the endoscopic laser technique, but more extensive involvement makes lateral clearance very difficult.

After good exposure has been obtained, the lesion is held securely with microlaryngeal instruments. It is then outlined with a 2- to 3-mm margin, using a spot size of 300 μm for maximum precision. The CO_2 laser is efficient as a cutting tool, but hemostasis is limited to the microcirculation, and it is therefore important to have the electrocautery available for all cases, because blood vessels too large for coagulation with the CO_2 laser may be encountered. The laser is used in a pulsed or intermittent mode to minimize thermal effects at the tumor margins. The energy used is normally 4 watts in 0.1-second pulses. The pulse duration can be increased up to 1 second as required. The superpulsed mode is avoided because it leads to deeper tissue penetration and diminished hemostatic ability. The specimen is then dissected free as outlined earlier, after which it is placed on a strip of moist nonadhesive dressing on a wooden tongue depressor and stretched into position with 22-gauge needles. Holinger and Miller[28] have described the use of a slice of dehydrated cucumber for this purpose. As before, all specimens must be clearly labeled to allow accurate orientation. Longitudinal frozen sections are examined. If the margins show tumor involvement, or if the clearance is not sufficient, then further laser excision is carried out. Random biopsies are not helpful, as negative histologic results can encourage a false sense of security. It is important that the surgeon and pathologist cooperate closely in order to achieve the best chance of total excision (Fig. 12–2).

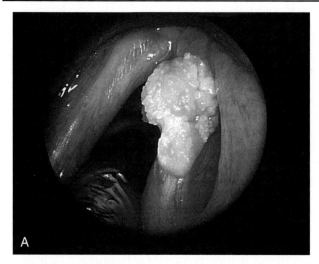
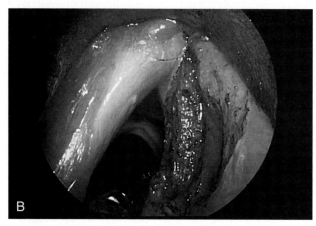

Figure 12–2. Excision of T1 glottic squamous cell carcinoma. *(A)* T1 lesion on anterior right vocal cord. *(B)* Defect after excision. (From Shapshay SM, Wang Z, Rebeizz EE, et al. "Window" laryngoplasty: a new combined laser endoscopic and open technique for conservation surgery. *Ann Otol Rhinol Laryngol* 1994; 103:679–685.)

Endoscopic treatment of appropriately selected T1 glottic carcinoma has proven as effective as radiotherapy in achieving a cure. In a retrospective study of 35 patients treated solely with laser excisional biopsy, 31 (89%) were disease free at 3 years.[29] When these patients were included in a literature review of 7 series totaling 142 patients, the local control rate was 87.3%, with an additional 4.2% of the patients undergoing successful salvage with further laser therapy alone. The overall rate of tumor control for patients successfully treated or salvaged by laser, more radical surgery, or radiotherapy was 98.6%. This compared with a local tumor control rate of 85.7% for 3,357 patients treated with radiotherapy and an ultimate control rate of 94.9% with all forms of salvage treatment[30] (Table 12–1). Although treatment with radiotherapy provides a better posttherapy voice than does treatment with laryngofissure techniques, endoscopic laser excision gives a posttreatment voice that is perceived as normal or near-normal by the patients themselves[31] and has been shown not to be significantly different to the postradiotherapy voice.[30] Ultimately, the quality of the voice after laser resection depends upon the extent of vocal muscle resection.

T2 Glottic Carcinoma

In more extensive glottic lesions the laser can be used with excisional biopsy techniques to define the extent of invasion accurately. This may result in restaging of the cancer from one that can be potentially cured by laser excision to a higher stage that cannot. Invasion of the cartilaginous skeleton of the larynx remains difficult to assess radiographically but can be seen directly with the operating microscope after initial blood-free dissection with the laser. Such tumors, restaged from T2 (radiographically) to T4 (after laser dissection), are then best managed with radiotherapy or more radical surgery.

Supraglottic Lesions

It is rare for patients with supraglottic carcinomas to be seen in the early stages of the disease, so the majority of the tumors are not suitable for simple laser therapy. T1 and T2 lesions are usually considered as being the same when the correct therapeutic approach is being determined. However, although the majority of these early lesions require

Table 12–1. LASER TREATMENT OF T1 GLOTTIC CARCINOMA*

Primary Therapy	Local Control Rate	Overall Control Rate After Further Excision, Surgery, or Radiotherapy
	Percentage of Patients Disease Free	*Percentage of Patients Disease Free*
Laser therapy	87.3%	98.6%
Radiotherapy	85.7%	94.9%

*Data from Cragle SP, Brandenburg JH. Laser cordectomy or radiotherapy: cure rates, communication, and cost. *Otolaryngol Head Neck Surg* 1993; 108:648–654.

supraglottic partial laryngectomy, there are cases of T1 lesions restricted to the suprahyoid epiglottis, the rim of the aryepiglottic folds, or both, which are suitable for excision with the laser. Some T2 lesions can be treated successfully by endoscopic laser partial laryngectomy, which is associated with better swallowing function and minimal aspiration when compared with conventional supraglottic partial laryngectomy. A major reason for the fewer side effects with the endoscopic approach is the preservation of the superior laryngeal nerve connection to the remaining larynx. This endoscopic approach can also be considered in those patients who are not medically fit or who decline other modalities of treatment.

Squamous cell carcinoma of the supraglottis behaves differently from that of glottic lesions. The rich lymphatic supply results in higher rates of metastasis to the local lymph nodes. If all T stages are considered, then 33% of supraglottic squamous cell carcinomas have cervical lymph node metastases.[32] A similar rate of metastasis of 37.6% was seen in a review of 731 male patients, and when tumor stages T1 and T2 only were considered, the rate was still 32.5%.[33] These nodes may not be clinically apparent at initial presentation, and therefore, treatment of one or both sides of the neck with either radiotherapy or modified neck dissection is advisable. Conventional supraglottic partial laryngectomy or total laryngectomy should always be considered when the pathology dictates this approach.

Recurrent Tumors

Endoscopic laser treatment of tumors that have recurred after initial treatment with the laser, open surgical excision, or radiotherapy must be employed selectively and with caution, as outlined earlier. However, the endoscopic approach is certainly useful in the treatment of recurrent premalignant or early invasive malignant lesions of the glottis. For superficial malignant recurrences, a subtotal cordectomy, with careful orientation and pathologic examination to determine clear resection margins, may be carried out. After radiotherapy, the recurrence is often multicentric, resulting in rates of tumor control as low as 50%,[29] and it is therefore difficult to recommend endoscopic excision unless no other option is available. If the tumor recurrence is clearly defined as a surface recurrence with discrete margins, then laser cordectomy should be attempted as a curative modality. If microscopic margins are free of cancer, close follow-up is indicated with no additional therapy.

It is possible that the use of oral *cis*-retinoic acid may reduce the rate of formation of second primary and recurrent tumors in the upper aerodigestive tract. Retinoids act directly on cells to suppress malignant transformation induced by drugs or radiation and, therefore, may be of use in stopping further malignant changes in the epithelium. The cessation of smoking tobacco and drinking alcohol would also have beneficial effects.[34]

Verrucous Carcinoma

This highly differentiated tumor does not metastasize systemically or to the lymph nodes but can be aggressively invasive locally. Verrucous carcinoma tends to be a "pushing type" of tumor rather than an invasive type at its borders, making endoscopic excision more feasible. Endoscopic laser excision is felt to be the correct initial treatment for T1 lesions, because low rates of recurrence can be obtained without exposing the patient to the sequelae of further radical surgery or radiotherapy. In our review of endoscopic treatment of T1 glottic cancer,[29] 12 cases of verrucous carcinoma had been treated by laser excision. All these patients were disease free at 3 years. T3 and T4 lesions, however, require hemilaryngectomy or total laryngectomy for treatment because of the extent of involvement.[35]

Other Uses of Lasers in Laryngeal Cancer

Avoidance of Tracheotomy Before Total Laryngectomy

Large exophytic lesions may cause airway obstruction. The traditional treatment for this problem has been to perform a tracheostomy before total laryngectomy. The tracheostomy itself, however, imposes the risks of local infection and, possibly, of stomal recurrence. These risks can be avoided if the patient can be intubated, usually while awake, with a small (5- to 5.5-mm) laser-resistant tube. The anterior portion of the tumor is then removed with the laser. Once a sufficiently large airway has been created, a Venturi jet ventilation needle can be fixed to the laryngoscope and the patient can be extubated, affording greater access to the posterior part of the glottis and, in particular, the subglottis for further tumor removal. This technique establishes a patent airway and provides tissue for histologic examination before carrying out definitive extirpative therapy. A similar technique can be used to preserve an airway in patients who decline or are not medically fit for curative surgery.

Cytoreduction or Tumor "Debulking"

As is the case with the preparation of patients with bulky tumors for surgery, "debulking" of the tumor before radiation provides tissue for diagnosis and usually improves the patient's airway and voice. In addition, there is a theoretical advantage in removing some of the bulk of large tumors before starting planned radiotherapy, although it has yet to be proven whether diminishing the tumor burden influences the outcome of subsequent radiotherapy.

Tissue Welding

Mucosal grafts can be used to cover deepithelialized areas of the larynx to reduce both the amount of scar formation and the risk of infection. Fibrin glue made from autologous blood products[36] can be used to maintain the position of these grafts. However, the length of time required for the glue to set can be a disadvantage. The addition of 1% indocyanin green to fibrin glue increases the coefficient of absorption of laser light at 810 nm, and the diode laser at this wavelength can then be used to set the glue within a few seconds.[37] We have developed a technique of combining CO_2 laser endoscopic excision with an open operation to excise bulky T1 glottic tumors. The technique minimizes the amount of tissue that needs to be excised without compromising oncologic clearance. The tissue is removed en bloc with the supporting portion of the

thyroid cartilage, making orientation of the specimen easier and helping the pathologist to determine the extent of the invasion. This approach also allows immediate reconstruction of the larynx with a pedicled sternohyoid muscle flap. If this flap is covered, before it is positioned, with a mucosal free graft welded in position with the 810-nm diode laser, there may be less chance of infection and scar formation. The technique is demonstrated in Figure 12–3. Early clinical results from our hospital indicate some benefit for this technique for laryngeal reconstruction after partial laryngectomy.[38]

Photodynamic Therapy

Photodynamic therapy (PDT) treatment of malignancies by selective destruction using light was first used in 1903.[39] The patient is first treated with a photosensitizing chemical that is selectively taken up by tumor cells. The agent is activated by light of an appropriate wavelength to produce selective damage either to the tumor cells or to the blood vessels that supply them. In areas where the tumors are readily accessible, such as in the skin and the bladder, PDT is felt to be an effective form of treatment in selected cases. However, the results of

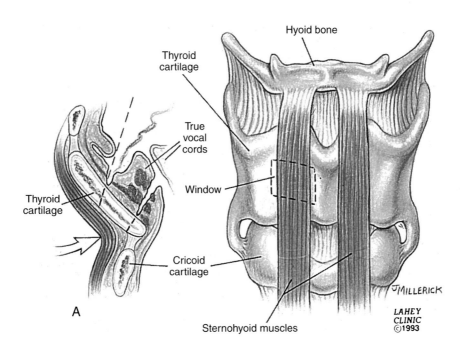

Figure 12–3. Window laryngoplasty. *(A)* Mucosal resection by laser. External view of larynx.

Illustration continued on following page

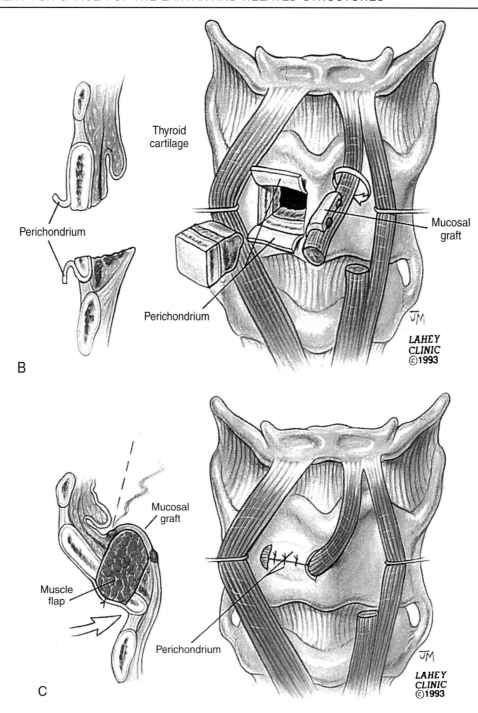

Fig. 12–3 *Continued (B)* Excision of "window" of thyroid cartilage by external approach. *(C)* Transfer of sternohyoid muscle flap with "welded" mucosal graft to resurface the defect. (From Shapshay SM, Wang Z, Rebeizz EE, et al. "Window" laryngoplasty: a new combined laser endoscopic and open technique for conservation surgery. *Ann Otol Rhinol Laryngol* 1994; 103:679–685.)

PDT for the treatment of laryngeal cancer have been generally disappointing, and its role must therefore be questioned.[40] At best, it should be used only as part of a well-constructed clinical trial, in cases where other treatment modalities are not indicated. The photosensitizers employed absorb light most strongly in the visible spectrum, so the CO_2 laser is not used. The energy required to produce cell damage can be delivered by a variety of lasers, including the argon pumped-dye laser or the gold laser.

REFERENCES

1. Maiman T. Stimulated optical emission in ruby masers. *Nature* 1960; 187:493–494.
2. Andrews AH, Goldenberg RA, Moss HW, et al. Carbon dioxide laser for laryngeal surgery. *Surg Ann* 1974; 6:459–476.
3. Lyons GD, Lousteau RJ, Mouney DF. CO_2 Laser laryngoscopy in a variety of lesions. *Laryngoscope* 1976; 86:1658–1662.
4. Vaughan CW, Strong MS, Jako GJ. Laryngeal carcinoma: transoral treatment utilizing the CO_2 laser. *Am J Surg* 1978; 136:490–493.
5. Einstein A. Zur Quanten Theorie der Strahlung. *Phys Z* 1917; 18:121.
6. Tolman RC. Duration of molecules in upper quantum states. *Phys Rev* 1924; 23:663.
7. Purcell EM, Pound PV. A nuclear spin system at negative temperature. *Phys Rev* 1951; 81:297.
8. Weber J. Amplification of microwave radiation by substances not in thermal equilibrium. *IRE Trans Elec Devices*, PGED 1953; 3:1.
9. Gordon JP, Zeiger HJ, Townes CH. Molecular microwave oscillator and new hyperfine structure in the microwave spectrum of NH. *Phys Rev* 1954; 95:282.
10. Schalow AL, Townes CH. Infrared and optical masers. *Phys Rev* 1958; 112:1940.
11. Javan A, Bennett Jr WB, Herriott TR. Population inversion and continuous optical maser oscillation in a gas discharge containing a He-Ne mixture. *Phys Rev* 1961; 6:106.
12. Patel CKN. Continuous wave laser action on vibrational rotational transitions of CO_2. *Phys Rev* 1964; 136:1187.
13. Goldman L and Rockwell Jr RJ. *Lasers in Medicine*. New York, Gordon and Breach Scientific Publishers, 1971.
14. Brotherton M. *Masers and Lasers*. New York, McGraw-Hill, 1964.
15. Duley WW. *CO_2 Lasers and Applications*. New York, Academic Press, 1976.
16. Patel CKN. High power carbon dioxide lasers. *Sci Am* 1968; 219:23–33.
17. Leibowitz HM, Peacock GR. Corneal injury produced by carbon dioxide laser radiation. *Arch Ophthalmol* 1969; 81:713–721.
18. Ketcham AS, Hoye RC, Riggle GC. A surgeon's appraisal of the laser. *Surg Clin North Am* 1967; 47:1249–1263.
19. Snow JC, Norton ML, Saluja TS, et al. Fire hazard during CO_2 laser microsurgery on the larynx and trachea. *Anaesth Analg* 1976; 55:146–147.
20. Strong MS, Jako GJ. Laser surgery in the larynx: early clinical experience with continuous CO_2 laser. *Ann Otol Rhinol Laryngol* 1972; 81:791–798.
21. Carden E, Ferguson GB. A new technique for microlaryngeal surgery in infants. *Laryngoscope* 1973; 83:691–699.
22. Strong MS, Vaughan CW, Incze J. Toluidine blue in diagnosis of cancer in the larynx. *Arch Otolaryngol Head Neck Surg* 1970; 91:515–519.
23. Zeitels SM, Vaughan CW. A submucosal true vocal fold infusion needle. *Otolaryngol Head Neck Surg* 1991; 105:478–479.
24. Strong MS. Laser excision of carcinoma of the larynx. *Laryngoscope* 1975; 85:1286–1289.
25. Wolfensberger M, Dort JC. Endoscopic laser surgery for early glottic carcinoma: a clinical and experimental study. *Laryngoscope* 1990; 100:1100–1105.
26. Krespi YP, Meltzer CJ. Laser surgery for vocal cord carcinoma involving the anterior commissure. *Ann Otol Rhinol Laryngol* 1989; 98:105–109.
27. Wetmore SJ, Key JM, Suen JY. Laser therapy for T1 glottic carcinoma of the larynx. *Arch Otolaryngol Head Neck Surg* 1986; 112:853–855.
28. Holinger LD, Miller AW III. A specimen mount for small laryngeal biopsies. *Laryngoscope* 1982; 92:524–526.
29. Blakeslee D, Vaughan CW, Shapshay SM, et al. Excisional biopsy in the selective management of T1 glottic cancer: a three year follow-up study. *Laryngoscope* 1984; 94:488–494.
30. Cragle SP, Brandenburg JH. Laser cordectomy or radiotherapy: cure rates, communication, and cost. *Otolaryngol Head Neck Surg* 1993; 108:648–654.
31. McGuirt WF, Blalock D, Koufman JA, et al. Voice analysis of patients with endoscopically treated early laryngeal carcinoma. *Ann Otol Rhinol Laryngol* 1992; 101:142–146.
32. McGavran MH, Bauer WC, Ogura JH. The incidence of cervical lymph node metastases from epidermoid carcinoma of the larynx and their relationship to certain characteristics of the primary tumor. *Cancer* 1961; 14:55–66.
33. Reid AP, Robin PE, Powell J, et al. Staging carcinoma: its value in cancer of the larynx. *J Laryngol Otol* 1991; 105:456–458.
34. Hong WK, Doos WG. Chemoprevention of head and neck cancer. Potential use of retinoids. *Otolaryngol Clin N Am* 1985; 8:543–549.
35. Hagen P, Lyons GD, Haindel C. Verrucous carcinoma of the larynx: role of human papillomavirus, radiation, and surgery. *Laryngoscope* 1993; 103:253–257.
36. Siedentop KH, Harris DM, Ham K, et al. Extended experimental and preliminary surgical findings with autologous fibrin tissue adhesive made from patient's own blood. *Laryngoscope* 1986; 96:1062–1064.
37. Pankratov MM, Wang Z, Rebeiz EE, et al. Endoscopic diode laser applications in airway surgery. *Proc* SPIE 1994; 2128:33–40.
38. Shapshay SM, Wang Z, Rebeiz EE, et al. "Window" laryngoplasty: a new combined laser endoscopic and open technique for conservation surgery. *Ann Otol Rhinol Laryngol* 1994; 103:679–685.
39. Tappenier H, Jesionek A. Theropeutische Reosuche met Fluoreszierenden Stoff. *Muench Med Wochsder*, 1903; 1:2042.
40. Gluckman JL. Haematoporphyrin photodynamic therapy: is there truly a future in head and neck oncology? Reflections on a 5-year experience. *Laryngoscope* 1991; 101:36–41.

Chapter 13

Tracheal Stomal Stenosis and Recurrence

Carl E. Silver and Hector Rodriguez

The postlaryngectomy tracheal stoma is essential to respiration and pulmonary toilet and may be the focus of a number of problems. The stoma itself is a source of embarrassment for the patient and requires constant care and attention. A well-functioning stoma is essential to currently employed methods of voice restoration. Numerous minor problems may be associated with the stoma, and patients often find support and advice in management of these daily vicissitudes in laryngectomy clubs and other sources of contact with laryngectomy patients. The major problems involving the tracheal stoma often require surgical attention. These problems are tracheal stomal stenosis and tracheal stomal recurrence of tumor.

TRACHEAL STOMAL STENOSIS

Definition

Under ideal circumstances, the tracheal stoma created after total laryngectomy should not require a cannula for stenting, should permit normal laminar flow of air with minimal turbulence during the ventilatory cycle, and should allow for normal clearing of tracheobronchial secretions. In current practice, the stoma should be wide enough to facilitate the insertion of a tracheoesophageal speech prosthesis, if one is to be considered. When the stoma is narrowed sufficiently to prevent these functions, tracheostomal stenosis, of some degree, may be considered to exist. Many surgeons consider it to be present in any patient who requires the use of a postoperative laryngeal cannula to maintain an adequate airway.[1, 2]

From a practical viewpoint, it is important to distinguish a stoma that may have less than optimal anatomic and functional characteristics from one that requires surgical correction. The need for the latter may vary according to the needs and expectations for the particular patient. For some patients, indefinite use of a laryngectomy tube or stoma button may be perfectly acceptable. Others may desire surgical revision in order to be relieved of the necessity for a laryngectomy tube, while other patients may require surgical enlargement (or narrowing) of the stoma to facilitate insertion of a voice prosthesis. In some cases, stenosis is so severe as to be life threatening and cannot be safely managed with a tube or a stent.

Incidence

The reported incidence of tracheal stomal stenosis varies according to the experience of the surgeon and the definition employed for stenosis (Table 13–1). Loewy and Larker[3] found only 6 occurrences in 138 patients (4%), all operated upon by a single surgeon, while Yonkers and Mercurio,[4] in a retrospective analysis of laryngectomies performed by various surgeons at 9 different hospitals, reported a much higher incidence of 46 out of 107 patients (42%).

Lam et al.[5] demonstrated the influence of the technique of stoma construction on the incidence of stenosis. In the initial phase of their series of 141 total laryngectomies, a 31% incidence of stenosis occurred. After modifying the technique of stoma construction, the incidence was reduced to 4%.

Classification

Montgomery[6, 7] categorized stenosis into three different types according to the possible etiology and the external stomal configuration. The most common was "concentric stenosis," caused by circumferential scar contracture or keloid formation, which represented more than 60% of the instances of stenosis in his series. The next most frequent form of stenosis was "vertical shelf stenosis," caused by lateral encroachment from the sternomastoid muscle or the remaining thyroid lobe. "Inferior shelf stenosis," caused by redundant skin folds, accounted for fewer than 10% of Montgomery's cases

		No. of Patients with	
Author	No. of Patients with Laryngectomy	Tracheal Stomal Stenosis	Percentage of Patients with Stenosis
Yonkers and Mercurio[4]	107	46	43%
Langebrunner and Chandler[2]	124	43	36%
Lam et al.[5]	116*	36	31%
	25†	1	4%
Griffith and Luce[8]	89	19	21%
Loewy and Larker[3]	138	6	4%

Table 13–1. INCIDENCE OF TRACHEAL STOMAL STENOSIS

*Early experience.
†Later experience.

of stenosis. This classification serves as a practical guide for formulation of a strategy for effective correction of stenosis.

Risk Factors for Stomal Stenosis

There are inherent risk factors for the development of tracheal stomal stenosis, as well as intraoperative and postoperative events that may produce this problem.

Inherent Risk Factors

Race, sex, and body habitus all may influence the development of stenosis. It has been well established that blacks have a higher incidence of keloid and hypertrophic scar formation than does the general population. Hence, this racial group is more susceptible to concentric stenosis from exuberant scar or keloid formation. Women have a smaller tracheal circumference (up to 30% smaller) and thinner, less rigid tracheal cartilages than do men. The smaller, softer trachea is more easily affected by extrinsic pressure, leading to stenosis. Individuals with short, thick cervical habitus are at a higher risk because of excess skin laxity and thick subcutaneous tissue that tends to bulge into the stoma, often resulting in a "pseudostenosis," in which the stoma is obstructed by the extrinsic tissue, although the mucocutaneous junction itself may be of adequate diameter. Prominent thyroid glands and hypertrophic muscles may cause encroachment upon the tracheal walls. A rare occurrence is the congenital absence of tracheal rings.

There is debate as to the effect of radiation therapy on the incidence of stomal stenosis. Griffith and Luce[8] noted a 14% incidence of stomal stenosis in patients receiving postoperative radiation therapy, but other authors have not found this to be the case.[1, 2, 5]

Intraoperative Risk Factors

Technical factors during surgery may contribute to the development of tracheal stomal stenosis. Stenosis is encouraged by the failure to displace tissues that encroach upon the stoma, to obliterate dead space, or to approximate the mucocutaneous junction precisely. A common cause of stenosis is mucocutaneous separation produced by excessive tension at the tracheocutaneous junction. The gap created by the separation will heal by secondary intention, with deposition of scar tissue and reduction in luminal size. This problem is inherent when a short tracheal stump results after laryngectomy following a previous tracheostomy or after resection of subglottic tumors. Tracheocutaneous separation may also occur in patients who are hypoproteinemic or who are receiving corticosteroid therapy.

Postoperative Risk Factors

Salivary fistulae are frequently associated with subsequent tracheal stomal stenosis. Balle and Bretlau[9] reported a 61% incidence of stomal stenosis in association with postoperative fistula formation. Other authors[4, 5] feel that only pharyngostomal fistulae, rather than all pharyngocutaneous fistulae, play a contributory role, because of the ultimate scarring adjacent to the stoma. Tracheitis at the mucocutaneous junction caused by irritation from the prolonged use of postoperative respirators, vigorous suctioning with rigid catheters, and ill-fitting cannulas are also considered to be contributory factors.

Most authors[1, 3, 9–12] agree that benign scar contracture, in the absence of other factors, plays a major role in the etiology of tracheal stomal stenosis. The basic problem is the natural tendency of cutaneous wounds to contract and shorten. Contraction of circular scars will reduce the luminal diameter. The area most vulnerable to contraction is the posterior membranous tracheal wall, because of the absence of cartilaginous support in this area.

Recurrent tumor is responsible for fewer than 5% of the cases of stomal stenosis but constitutes an important cause of late stenosis (see section on tracheal stomal recurrence).

Pathophysiology

Because the need for surgical revisions varies according to the needs and expectations of the patient, the ability to tolerate various degrees of stenosis differs from patient to patient depending on the size of the opening relative to the respiratory reserve. Bain[13] determined that a 50% stenosis in all diameters produces a 75% reduction in surface luminal area. Individuals with normal lung function can tolerate this extent of stenosis, but the same deficit may produce considerable respiratory disability in patients with pulmonary disease. Spirometric analysis of patients with stomal stenosis demonstrates a reduction in the forced expiratory volume (FEV) at 1 second and in maximal voluntary ventilation (MVV) at 1 minute.

Another problem generated by a stenotic tracheal stoma is the increase in air turbulence at the cutaneous opening, which causes desiccation and crusting. This, in turn, impedes the proper clearing of tracheal secretions, which may contribute to pulmonary infections. The problem may be temporarily solved by use of a tracheal cannula to bypass the stenotic area, but in some patients, persistent irritation and crusting from the compression of the tracheal wall will begin a cycle of progressive deterioration if the problem is left untreated.

Principles of Tracheal Stoma Construction

The principles of tracheal stoma construction apply both in primary stoma construction at the time of laryngectomy and in procedures to correct established tracheal stomal stenosis. While there are various accepted methods of stoma construction, most authors agree on three major steps to prevent tracheal stomal stenosis. These include tension-free anastomosis, displacement of encroaching tissues, and elongation and interruption of the tracheal stomal perimeter.

Tension-Free Anastomosis

The trachea must be exteriorized at the proper level of the neck to avoid anastomotic tension. This is easily accomplished in patients with adequate tracheal stump length. The surgeon can either incorporate the tracheal stump into the transverse incision joining the superior and the inferior skin flaps or place it in the inferior flap, either through a separate incision or through a vertical extension from the junction of the flaps. Clairmont[14] suggested the use of tension-releasing sutures of heavy suture material (1–0 or 2–0 silk or nylon) placed through at least two cartilaginous rings and skin, in cases where the tracheal stump is too short for simple tension-free anastomosis.

In extreme cases in which the remaining trachea cannot reach the level of the suprasternal notch without excessive tension, a manubriectomy with creation of a mediastinal tracheostomy may be necessary.[15] Alternatives to this approach may include funneling skin to the trachea by cutaneous advancement or by pedicled or mycocutaneous flaps.[10, 16]

Displacement of Encroaching Tissues

Lateral displacement or partial resection of bulky thyroid lobes and transection of the sternal attachments of the sternomastoid muscle, particularly in those patients with stomas located at the level of the suprasternal notch, will prevent the formation of vertical shelf stenosis. The identification and resection of excessive cutaneous laxity and subcutaneous fat-laden tissue, particularly in obese individuals, will avoid the formation of inferior shelf stenosis or pseudostenosis. Proper trimming of protruding tracheal cartilaginous rings, in order to obtain exact mucocutaneous approximation, will facilitate primary healing and help avoid concentric stomal stenosis.

Elongation and Interruption of the Tracheal Stomal Perimeter

These maneuvers are aimed at avoiding circumferential stomal stenosis secondary to benign scar contracture. A simple means of increasing tracheal stomal circumference at the time of laryngectomy is by tracheal beveling, as demonstrated in Chapter 6. A 45-degree angle cut in an anteroposterior direction by transecting across at least two cartilaginous rings will change the configuration of the opening from circular to elliptical and create a satisfactorily large stoma.[1, 14, 17, 18] Interruption of the tracheal stomal perimeter is in keeping with the time-honored principle of avoiding a linear scar with its natural tendency to contract. Numerous techniques have been employed for interruption of the perimeter, which include single and multiple Z-plasties,[1, 5, 17] single and double tracheal relaxing incisions with V-Y advancement,[19–21] and complex combinations of Z-plasty with V-Y advancement.[11, 22]

Repair of Stomal Stenosis

Nonsurgical Methods

A variety of nonsurgical techniques are often used initially or in mild cases. These include the placement of progressively larger tracheostomy tubes or "stomal" buttons. Such measures may provide only a temporary solution, because removal of the stent will often result in recurrent stenosis.

Multiple Radial Incisions

A simple method for correction of circumferential stenosis was described by Montgomery[6, 7] and later by Callins and Applebaum.[23] Multiple radial incisions are made with an electrocautery and carried through the mucous membrane, the skin, the soft tissues, and the fibrous bands of the stenotic area. Care is taken not to extend the incisions more than 6 to 8 mm laterally to avoid injury to the major vessels. This is followed by the insertion of a No. 10 laryngeal cannula, which is left in place for 1 month. The results and long-term follow-up have not been reported. The procedure can be performed under local anesthesia, and it represents a relatively noninvasive attempt to correct stenosis in patients who may not be candidates for more extensive procedures.

Excision of the Concentric Scar with Mobilization of the Trachea and the Skin

This is the basic initial procedure used with all techniques for formal correction of tracheal stomal stenosis. The "donut" excision of the scar associated with the mobilization of the trachea and the surrounding skin may be followed by tension-free reapproximation of the skin to the trachea or may be combined with one of the procedures (described later) to enlarge and interrupt the perimeter (Figs. 13–2, 13–3, and 13–4).

Figure 13–1A. A concentric tracheal stenosis is shown. The narrowing may exist just at the tracheocutaneous junction as a result of simple scar contraction, but often there is heaped-up scar tissue surrounding the stomal orifice.

Figure 13–1B. The length of the stenotic segment can be appreciated in this sagittal view. If stenosis has been caused by tracheal cutaneous separation, there may be an appreciable stenotic fibrous segment between the skin and the normal distal trachea. The cutaneous ring and the fibrous stenotic segment are dilated until a tube adequate for administration of anesthesia can be inserted.

Figure 13–1C. After induction of anesthesia, a circumferential incision is created around the stenotic stoma and extended horizontally on each side sufficiently to obtain adequate exposure, as well as to permit generous mobilization of the surrounding skin.

Figure 13–1D. Dissection is commenced, with the normal skin being elevated in all directions around the stoma.

Figure 13–1E. The circular scar and the stenotic fibrous segment are dissected from the surrounding tissues, with care being taken to not tear the fibrous tube, if possible. Normal tracheal cartilage is eventually encountered. Dissection continues on the surface of the trachea. With the help of traction sutures and with the continued liberation of the cartilaginous walls, the normal portion of the trachea is brought to the level of the skin. This phase of the operation is the most difficult and is essential to the success of any subsequent technique employed to reconstruct the mucocutaneous junction.

Figure 13–1F. The scar and fibrotic portion of the stenotic tube are excised, leaving normal trachea circumferentially at skin level. At this point, the skin may be simply approximated to the tracheal edge, but most surgeons would prefer to employ one of several methods of elongating and interrupting the stomal perimeter, as described below.

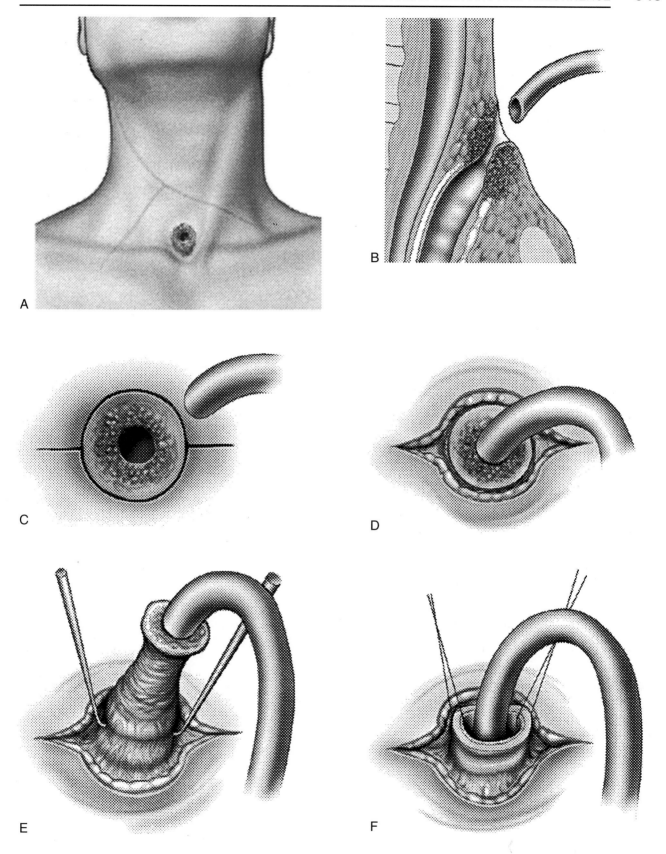

Figure 13–1. Concentric tracheal stomal stenosis. Excision of stenotic area and mobilization of normal trachea.

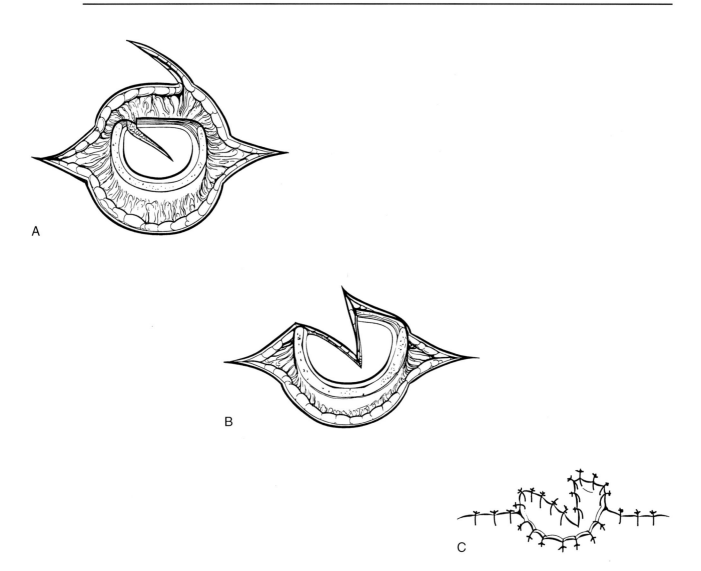

Figure 13–2. Creation of stomal perimeter by Z-plasty.

Creation of Stomal Perimeter by Z-Plasty

Relaxing incisions in the trachea in combination with Z-plasties or cutaneous flaps will alter the configuration of the stoma, creating an irregular perimeter and redistributing the forces of scar contraction, thus avoiding concentric stenosis. Both single and multiple Z-plasties have been described.[1, 5] The single Z-plasties are usually placed in the posterior membranous tracheal wall, allowing for transposition of both the skin and the mucosal triangles. Trail et al.[17] reported effective reduction of stenosis in 50 patients with single posteriorly located Z-plasties.

Figure 13–2A. A single posterior Z-plasty is demonstrated. Parallel diagonal incisions are made in the skin and posterior tracheal wall, creating skin and mucosal flaps. Chandler[1, 2] stressed the importance

of making the posterior Z-plasties sufficiently large by incising 2 to 3 cm of posterior tracheal wall.

Figure 13–2B. The skin and mucosal flaps are transposed, interposing a triangle of skin into the posterior tracheal wall and a triangle of mucosa into the posterior stomal skin.

Figure 13–2C. The flaps are sutured. The procedure results in interruption and elongation of the stomal perimeter.

A second Z-plasty may be constructed on the anterior tracheal wall. Dual Z-plasties, when employed, are usually created in the anterior and posterior portions of the stoma. Flaps created by incising through the cartilaginous rings may be deficient in a blood supply if angulated too sharply and may be cumbersome to transpose because of the rigidity of the cartilage if the angulation is excessively broad.

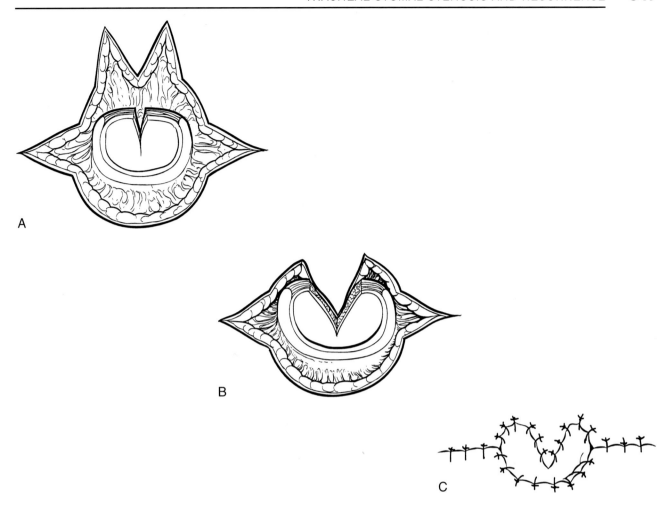

Figure 13–3. Single posterior relaxing incision.

Single Posterior Relaxing Incision

Relaxing incisions in the trachea are created by simple perpendicular transection of the trachea or by wedge excisions. They usually extend through two cartilaginous rings or 1.5 to 2.5 cm of the tracheal wall. The incisions may be placed at the 12, 3, 6, and 9 o'clock positions of the tracheal perimeter and are reported as being single (usually posterior), double (either anteroposterior or lateral), or multiple (all four quadrants). Skin may be interposed into the gaps created by the relaxing incisions by reapproximation of the preserved skin wedges or by advancement or rotation advancement flaps.

Figure 13–3A. Hartwell and Dykes,[19] in 1967, and Carlton,[20] in 1968, reported success with the use of a posterior tracheal relaxing incision, followed by the advancement of a superiorly based triangular flap. They employed this technique both for primary construction and for secondary revision. The tracheal incision extends 2.5 cm in length, and two lateral cutaneous triangles are excised before the advancement of the flap.

Figure 13–3B. The triangular cutaneous flap is advanced into the posterior tracheal defect, enlarging and disrupting the perimeter.

Figure 13–3C. The mucocutaneous junction is sutured. Myers and Gallia[21] reported a similar technique but utilized a posterior tracheal wedge excision and a transposition cutaneous flap to fill the space.

The final result is similar to that achieved with a single posterior Z-plasty. Both techniques have the disadvantage of rendering subsequent placement of a tracheoesophageal voice prosthesis difficult. The thickness of the newly interposed skin may not accept even the longest of the voice prosthetic devices, and creation of the puncture at the posterior mucocutaneous junction may lead to undue widening of the tracheoesophageal fistula.

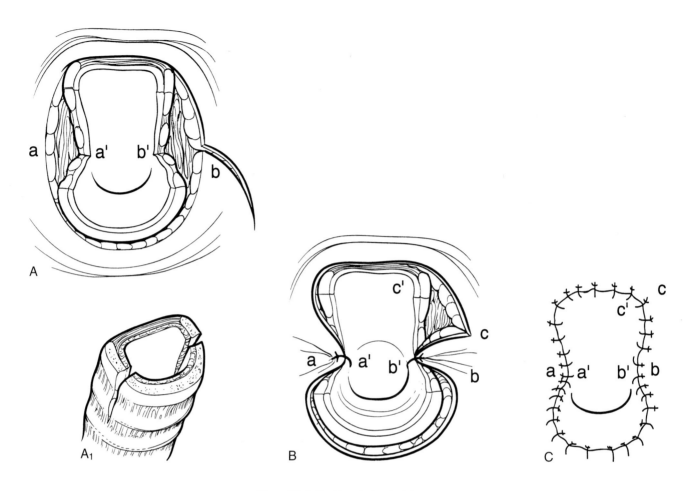

Figure 13–4. Double relaxing incisions.

Double Relaxing Incisions

Double relaxing incisions have been employed by numerous authors.[8, 14, 19] When performed at the anterior and posterior tracheal walls, followed by the interdigitation of triangular cutaneous advancement flaps, they create an external stomal configuration of a "bow tie" or a "butterfly."

The anterior and posterior relaxing incisions have the same disadvantage as the posterior Z-plasty and the single relaxing incision with regard to interfering with the subsequent placement of a tracheoesophageal prosthetic device. Double relaxing incisions placed on the lateral tracheal walls with interdigitation of lateral cervical skin triangles avoid this problem and are favored if a voice prosthesis is contemplated.[6, 12]

Figures 13–4A and 13–4A₁. Relaxing incisions from 2.0 to 2.5 cm in length are made through both lateral walls of the trachea. After excision of all cutaneous scar tissue, the surrounding skin is mobilized sufficiently to permit the creation of the necessary flaps for reconstruction. A diagonal incision from point b to point c is made on the (patient's) left side, as shown, creating a triangular skin flap.

Figure 13–4B. On the (patient's) right side, as shown, point a is advanced into the tracheal defect and sutured to point a'. Traction on the skin produced by advancing point a on the right side will cause the triangular flap created by the incision between points b and c to rotate into the left-sided defect, where point b is sutured to point b'. The remaining skin will rotate, opening the linear space produced by the incision between points b and c, thus bringing point c in proximity with point c' on the tracheal wall.

Figure 13–4C. The skin is now sutured around the entire perimeter to the tracheal edge, creating a butterfly shaped stoma. The perimeter has been elongated and interrupted, and a tracheoesophageal puncture can be performed in the superior medial portion of the tracheostoma without interference by a skin flap.

Other Procedures

Lam et al.[5] have employed a procedure involving the creation of multiple relaxing incisions at the 12, 3, 6, and 9 o'clock positions around the circumference of the tracheostoma, followed by interdigitation of triangular flaps from the surrounding skin to create a serrated stomal configuration. This has been employed predominately for initial tracheostoma construction, with a 96% success rate. Other local alternatives include the five-flap procedure described by Murayama et al.,[22] which consists of a combination of two Z-plasties and a V-Y advancement flap interposed in the posterior suture line. More extensive procedures include transposition of lateral cervical skin flaps sutured to the lateral tracheal walls and the use of fenestrated deltopectoral flaps. These have been advocated mostly for patients with severe skin compromise secondary to radiation therapy.[10, 16]

The technique of anterior mediastinal tracheostomy, created by resecting the manubrium of the sternum and transposing the trachea inferiorly into the chest skin as described by Sisson et al.,[24] Grillo,[15] and Orringer and Sloan,[25] is utilized for patients who require excision of larger segments of the tracheal stump for stomal recurrence (see below).

Tracheal stomal stenosis after laryngectomy can be caused by underlying anatomic, genetic, or medical predisposition; excessive anastomotic tension caused by the extent of resection or faulty operative technique; or by postoperative events, such as infection. Surgical techniques employed to prevent stenosis by maximizing the tracheostomal perimeter or by minimizing anastomotic tension range from the simple beveling of the tracheal end to complex procedures involving the transfer of local or distant skin flaps. Anterior mediastinal tracheostomy may be necessary in cases of extensive tracheal resection.

The question of whether to correct tracheal stenosis surgically depends on the amount of functional impairment present and the requirements of the particular patient. Procedures employed to correct stenosis include the excision of the circumferential scar, the advancement of sufficient skin to permit tension-free anastomosis, and the use of techniques in primary construction that interrupt and lengthen the tracheostomal perimeter in order to prevent stenosis.

The decision as to which measures should be taken during initial laryngectomy in order to prevent postoperative stenosis may depend on circumstances related to individual patients and may vary among surgeons. Some employ special techniques for interrupting and lengthening the perimeter in all laryngectomy cases; others, including ourselves, are satisfied with the results obtained by simple construction, provided the basic mechanical requirements, such as avoiding tension and tissue redundancy, have been met.

TRACHEAL STOMAL RECURRENCE OF CANCER

Recurrence of tumor at the tracheostoma is a devastating sequel to total laryngectomy. The combination of airway obstruction, bleeding, and invasion of the deep mediastinal structures combine to make the mortality high and the treatment of the problem challenging. In the past, death would often result from complications of attempted surgical treatment, particularly from rupture of the great vessels. The development of newer surgical techniques combined with a better understanding of the nature and the different types of tracheal stomal recurrences has created a more optimistic outlook in some cases.

Incidence, Predisposing Factors, and Prevention

In a literature review, Batsakis et al.[26] reported 48 cases of stomal tumor recurrence out of 827 laryngectomies (5.8%), with the incidence ranging from 1.7% to 14.7%. Josephson and Krespi,[27] reported the incidence to range from 5% to 15% in most series. Predisposing factors include inadequate resection margins, residual disease in paratracheal lymph nodes, and residual disease in unresected thyroid tissue; all these factors are more likely to exist in association with subglottic carcinoma than with other laryngeal tumors. Numerous authors agree that previous tracheostomy is a predisposing factor in stomal recurrence because of implantation of tumor cells in the wound.[26, 28–30]

It is easier to prevent stomal recurrences than to treat them. Avoidance of preliminary tracheostomy, if possible, meticulous paratracheal dissection, and microscopic control of the resection margins are the most effective surgical measures.[28, 31] Preliminary tracheostomy may be avoided in some cases by reducing the bulk of the neoplasm with the CO_2 laser or by "emergency laryngectomy," in which the patient, admitted with airway obstruction, is rapidly evaluated, prepared, and treated with total laryngectomy as the primary procedure.[32] Postoperative radiation is also effective in preventing tracheal stomal recurrence. Tong et al.[33] gave elective post-operative radiation to 26 patients felt to be at high risk for stomal recurrence. In 22 patients the stomas were included in the field of radiation and no stomal recurrences developed. In 4 patients the stomas were shielded, and stomal recurrence developed in 2 of the 4 patients. Similar results were reported by Schneider et al.[34]

Classification of Tracheal Stomal Recurrence

Tracheal stomal recurrence has been classified into four types, related to the location and the extent of involvement, by Sisson et al.[35] Type I recurrence is localized to the superior aspect of the stoma and has no esophageal involvement. Type II recurrence is localized to the superior aspect of the stoma and involves the esophagus. Type III recurrence

originates from the inferior aspect of the stoma and involves the superior mediastinum. Type IV recurrence extends laterally beneath the clavicles and into the superior mediastinum (Fig. 13–5).

Treatment of Tracheal Stomal Recurrence

Despite an occasional report of successful treatment with radiation therapy[36] or chemoradiation,[37] most authors feel that salvage can be accomplished only by an aggressive surgical approach, with wide excision of the skin, the manubrium, the trachea, and the mediastinal lymphatics.[28, 30, 38] In the past, the major problems involved in this surgery were related to coverage of the often irradiated great vessels in the mediastinum and to the low tracheal resection. Any necrosis of the overlying skin or separation of the tracheostoma would usually result in exposure and rupture of the innominate artery, which was a frequent complication of this surgery. Progress was made with a two-stage approach devised by Sisson et al.[39, 40] Sisson and coworkers' approach stressed wide excision of the skin with manubrial resection, mediastinal dissection, low transection of the trachea, and a staged reconstruction with pectoral muscle to cover the mediastinal vessels and a delayed bipedicled thoracic cutaneous flap that was rotated over the defect. This approach began to improve survival, although considerable morbidity and lengthy hospitalization were still associated with the staged operations. The prognosis remained poor, however. In 1977, Sisson et al.[35] reported a 5-year survival of 11.3%.

Biller et al.'s[41] introduction of the greater pectoral muscle myocutaneous flap for one-stage reconstruction after transsternal resection of tracheal stomal recurrence produced a major improvement in postoperative morbidity and mortality. The pectoral muscle served to cover the great vessels and to obliterate mediastinal dead space. The well-vascularized skin island could be transferred in one stage and provided excellent replacement for the irradiated, tumor-involved skin resected with the stomal recurrence. Josephson and Krespi[27] combined the use of the greater pectoral myocutaneous flap with blunt total pharyngoesophagectomy and gastric transposition for treatment of type II tracheal stomal recurrence with esophageal involvement. In the current surgical environment, the use of free revascularized flaps provides the surgeon with many options for safe reconstruction of the formidable defects resulting after adequate resection of tracheal stomal recurrences of various types.

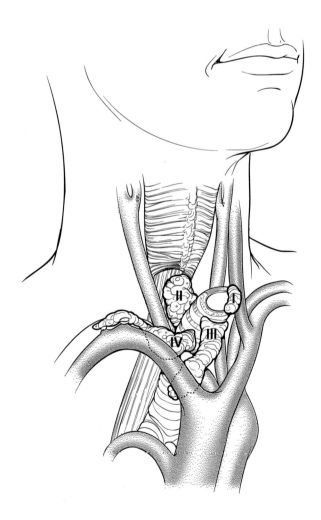

Figure 13–5. Types of tracheal stomal recurrence of cancer.

Results of Treatment

A significant contribution to the management of tracheal stomal recurrence was made by Gluckman et al.[42] in 1987. These authors reported the results of surgery in 41 patients operated upon for stomal recurrence. Overall 2-year survival was only 16% for all patients, but further analysis revealed a 5-year survival of 45% with type I and type II lesions and a survival of 9% for type III and type IV lesions. This work demonstrated that acceptable cure rates can be expected in the treatment of the less advanced stomal recurrences, while surgical treatment for type III and type IV stomal recurrence, even when feasible, must be considered palliative. The risk should be evaluated in relation to the possible benefit. In many cases, supervoltage radiation therapy or aggressive chemotherapy may produce symptomatic relief and survival comparable to that obtainable by extensive surgery.

Surgical Procedures for Tracheal Stomal Recurrence

In accordance with the discussion above, only procedures for the treatment of type I and type II stomal recurrence will be demonstrated. Type III and type IV recurrences are considered nonresectable.

Technique of Transsternal Neck Dissection with Thoracotracheostomy for Stomal Recurrence Type I and Repair by Greater Pectoral Myocutaneous Flap

Figure 13–6A. The site of the lesion, the outline of the skin incisions, and the anatomic relations of the surrounding structures are shown. A generous margin of skin around the stoma is included in the resection. The paddle of the pectoral muscle myocutaneous flap is outlined.

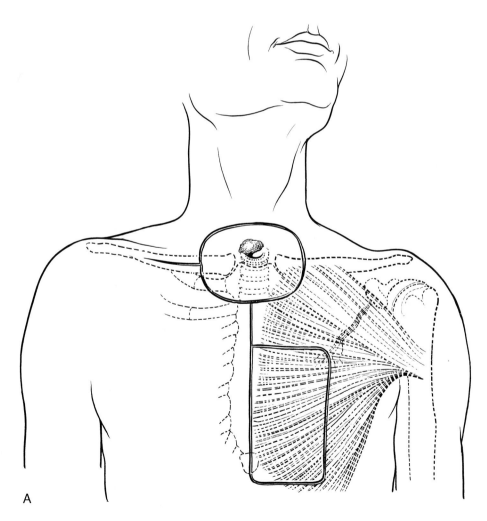

A

Figure 13–6. Transsternal neck dissection with thoracotracheostomy for stomal recurrence type I. Repair by greater pectoral muscle myocutaneous flap.

Illustration continued on following page

Figures 13–6*B*, **13–6***B₁*, **and 13–6***B₂.* The upper half of the manubrium is resected. The internal mammary vessels are ligated and divided within the first intercostal space. The sternum is transected with a Gigli saw (Fig. 13–6*B₁*). An oscillating saw may be used if desired. The first costal cartilages and the medial ends of the clavicles are transected with a Gigli saw, an oscillating saw, or bone cutters. A simpler approach may be used for the elective resection of subglottic carcinoma, in which the low resection of the trachea and the elective removal of the paratracheal lymph nodes are desired. Adequate exposure of the superior mediastinum is obtained by resecting a "V" from the manubrium, as shown (Fig. 13–6*B₂*).

Figure 13–6*C.* The mediastinal structures are dissected. It is best to identify the major vascular structures and dissect the lymphoareolar tissue from the surface of the innominate and the left common carotid arteries. The left innominate vein may be retracted downward or may be divided. Cervical skin flaps are raised appropriately to permit dissection of the vessels in the neck as far as necessary. The lymphoareolar tissue is mobilized toward the trachea, which is visualized and finally divided low enough to allow an adequate resection margin. Division of the trachea releases the specimen.

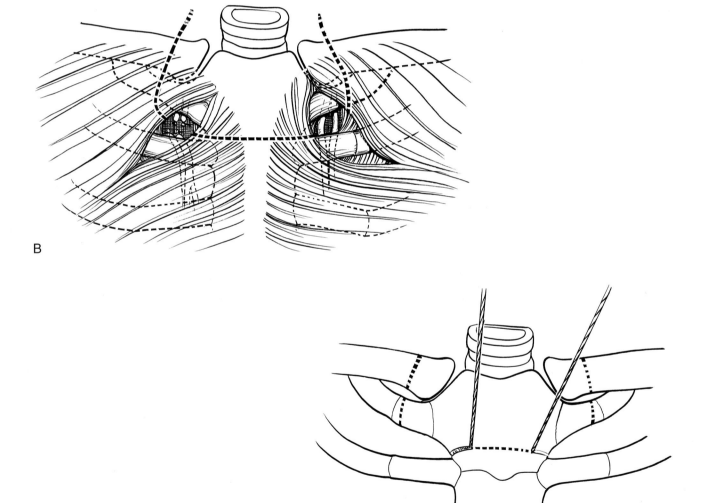

B

B₁

Figure 13–6 *Continued* Transsternal neck dissection with thoracotracheostomy for stomal recurrence type I.

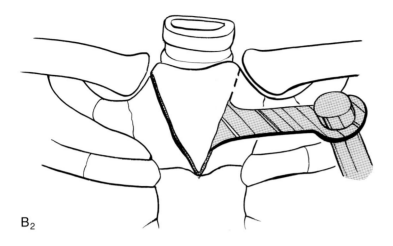

B₂

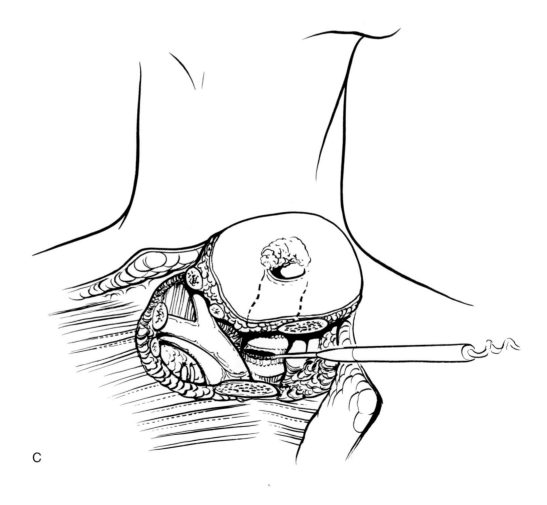

C

Figure 13–6 *Continued* Transsternal neck dissection with thoracotracheostomy for stomal recurrence type I.

Illustration continued on following page

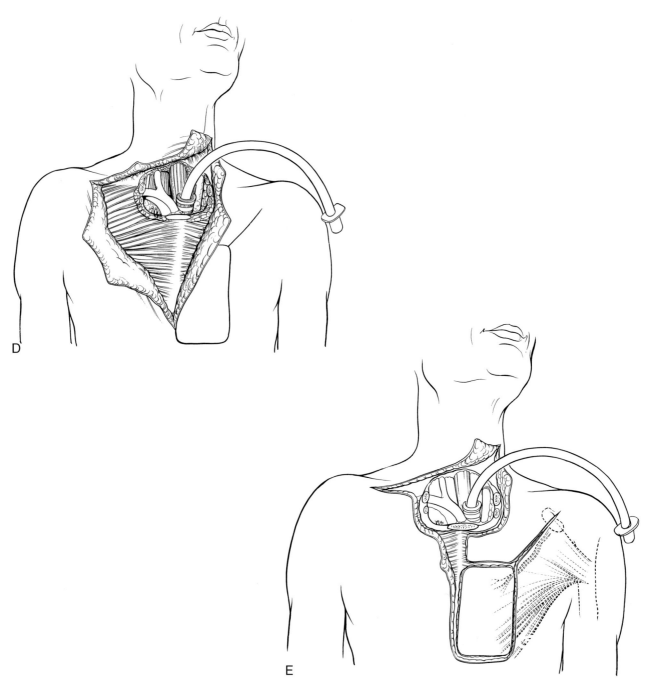

Figure 13–6 *Continued* Transsternal neck dissection with thoracotracheostomy for stomal recurrence type I.

Figure 13–6D. The surgical field is shown after completion of the resection. The specimen includes the manubrium, the overlying skin with the stoma and the tumor, several centimeters of the trachea, and the contiguous lymphoareolar tissue. The innominate and the left common carotid vessels have been dissected. In this case, the left innominate vein has been divided.

Figure 13–6E. The skin incisions for the pectoral myocutaneous flap are shown. The flap extends to the midline over the sternum and overlies the lower medial portion of the greater pectoral muscle. An oblique incision extends toward the clavicle for exposure of the muscle. Note the location of the thoracoacromial vessels.

Figure 13–6*F.* The greater pectoral muscle is incised without separating the overlying skin paddle. The insertion onto the humerus is severed. The muscle is left attached to the clavicle in the region of the thoracoacromial vessels. The vessels are readily seen on the deep surface of the greater pectoral muscle. The muscle may be detached from the clavicle as much as necessary to permit unhampered rotation of the flap, as long as the thoracoacromial vessels are not compromised.

Figure 13–6*G.* The myocutaneous flap is rotated into the superior mediastinal defect. The stoma is implanted into a small incision in the center of the flap and sutured in place. The blood supply of the myocutaneous flap is sufficient to withstand this disruption of its integrity.

Figure 13–6*H.* The donor site usually can be closed primarily without a skin graft, even in male patients. The female breast must not be permitted to exert tension on the paddle of the myocutaneous flap by its weight. It should be fixed to the chest wall with heavy sutures and should not be sutured directly to the paddle.

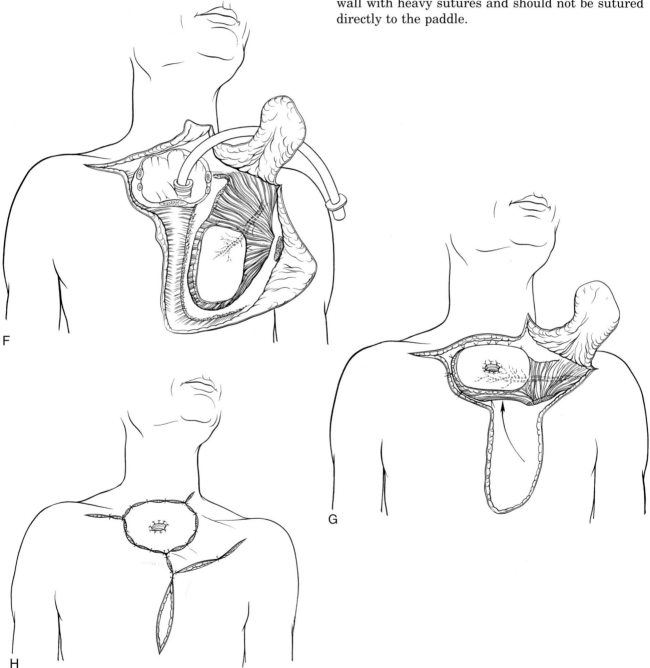

Figure 13–6 *Continued* Transsternal neck dissection with thoracotracheostomy for stomal recurrence type I.

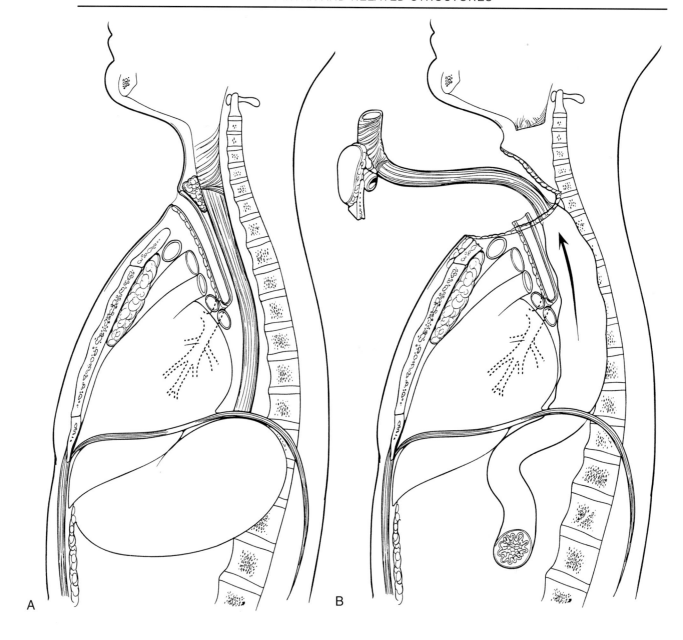

Figure 13–7. Transsternal neck dissection with thoracotracheostomy and esophagectomy for stomal recurrence type II. Repair by greater pectoral muscle myocutaneous flap and gastric transposition.

Technique of Transsternal Neck Dissection with Thoracotracheostomy and Esophagectomy for Stomal Recurrence Type II and Repair by Greater Pectoral Muscle Myocutaneous Flap and Gastric Transposition

Figure 13–7A. A sagittal section through the neck and the thorax demonstrates a type II tracheal stomal recurrence situated on the posterior superior stomal wall and extending into the cervical esophagus.

Figure 13–7B. The initial resection is similar to the procedures shown in Figures 13–6A through 13–6D, mobilizing the skin, the trachea, and a portion of manubrium if necessary. The trachea is not separated from the esophagus in the region of the tumor but is left in continuity, while the cervical pharyngoesophagus is liberated, and a blunt closed chest total esophagectomy is performed as shown in Figures 10–4A through 10–4G. The esophagus is extracted while the liberated stomach is transposed into the posterior mediastinum.

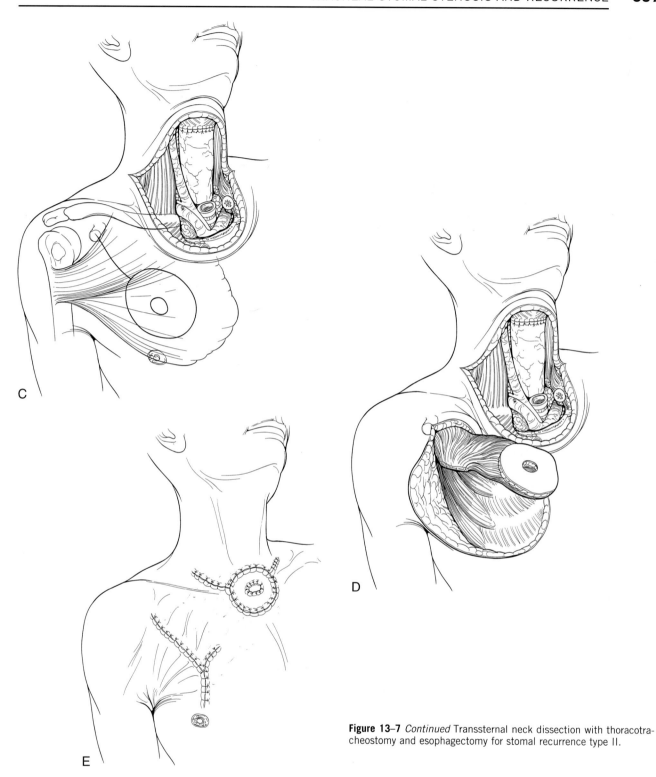

C

D

E

Figure 13–7 *Continued* Transsternal neck dissection with thoracotracheostomy and esophagectomy for stomal recurrence type II.

Figure 13–7*C.* After transection of the cardioesophageal junction, an incision is made in the gastric fundus and a pharyngogastrostomy is created. The surgical defect is now similar to that shown in Figure 13–6*D.* A greater pectoral myocutaneous flap is created on the chest wall (in this example, shown on the right side).

Figure 13–7*D.* The pectoral muscle myocutaneous flap is elevated and will be rotated into the defect in order to resurface the area.

Figure 13–7*E.* The flap has been rotated, the defect resurfaced, and a thoracotracheostomy created in the center of the cutaneous "paddle." The thoracic donor site can usually be closed primarily.

Complications

Josephson and Krespi[27] have classified complications as intraoperative, immediate postoperative, or late postoperative. The most common intraoperative complication is an injury to the great mediastinal vessels that causes massive hemorrhage. The hemorrhage may be difficult to control, and if vascular repair is required, subsequent infection in the mediastinum may lead to "blowout" of the repair. Ligation of the innominate artery may lead to cerebral vascular complications. Air embolism may result from venous injury, and pneumothorax is always a danger, either from mediastinal dissection or from blunt esophagectomy. Chyle leaks may occur, particularly in cases requiring esophagectomy. The leak should be detected and sutured immediately with nonabsorbable material to avoid formation of a postoperative chyle fistula or chyloma.

The first 5 to 7 days after surgery comprise the immediate postoperative period. During this time airway obstruction, pneumothorax, and mediastinitis are the most frequent complications. Mediastinitis is most likely in cases with esophagectomy and usually results from disruption of a suture line. Such a problem must be identified and treated immediately by surgery, with adequate drainage and closure or diversion, if possible, of the leak.

The most dangerous problem in the late postoperative period is the possibility of a late disruption of a major vessel, in particular, the fistulization of the innominate or the left common carotid artery into the trachea. This problem may result from tracheocutaneous separation or from tracheal necrosis caused by pressure from an overinflated cuff. Flap necrosis may lead to exposure and rupture of a great vessel, although this problem has been minimized by the well-vascularized myocutaneous flaps now in use. Nevertheless, while major flap loss is rare, minor flap necrosis occurs in approximately 10% of the patients.[43]

Many of the problems that may occur after resection for stomal recurrence are the same as those after extended total laryngectomy or pharyngolaryngoesophagectomy. These include loss of thyroid and parathyroid function and nutritional and respiratory difficulties. Aspiration pneumonia, particularly if a salivary fistula is present, is a significant cause of both morbidity and mortality in all major head and neck procedures of this nature.

Conclusions

While tracheal stomal recurrence of tumor is still a formidable problem, much progress has been made in its management. The employment of well-vascularized myocutaneous flaps for one-stage reconstruction has resulted in a significant decline in the operative and postoperative morbidity and mortality. The availability of reliable methods for esophageal replacement has facilitated the safe resection of tumors involving the esophagus. A better understanding of the nature of stomal recurrence has permitted the selection of those patients for surgical treatment who have a reasonable chance for cure. Patients with lesions too advanced for surgery are treated palliatively with nonsurgical methods.

REFERENCES

1. Chandler JR. Construction and reconstruction of the laryngeal stoma. *Int Surg* 1967; 48:233–239.
2. Langebrunner DJ, Chandler JR. Tracheal stomal stenosis: causes and correction. *South Med J* 1968; 61:838–842.
3. Loewy A, Larker HI. Tracheal stoma problems. *Arch Otolaryngol* 1968; 87:477–481.
4. Yonkers AJ, Mercurio GA Jr. Tracheostomal stenosis following total laryngectomy. *Otolaryngol Clin North Am* 1983; 16:391–405.
5. Lam KH, Wei WI, Wong J, et al. Tracheostoma construction during laryngectomy: a method to prevent stenosis. *Laryngoscope* 1983; 93:212–215.
6. Montgomery W. Stenosis of tracheostoma. *Arch Otolaryngol* 1962; 75:76–79.
7. Montgomery W. *Surgery of the Upper Respiratory System*, 2nd ed, Vol 2. Philadelphia, Lea and Febiger, 1979.
8. Griffith GR, Luce EA. Tracheal stomal stenosis after laryngectomy. *Plast Reconstr Surg* 1982; 70:694–698.
9. Balle VH, Bretlau P. Tracheostomal stenosis following total laryngectomy. *J Laryngol Otol* 1985; 99:577–580.
10. Doyle PJ, Dubeta KR. Post laryngectomy tracheostoma stenosis: etiology and treatment. *J Otolaryngol* 1977; 6:284–289.
11. Ishiki N, Tanabe M. A simple technique to prevent stenosis of the tracheostoma after total laryngectomy. *J Laryngol Otol* 1980; 94:637–642.
12. Panje WR, Kitt VV. Tracheal stoma reconstruction. *Arch Otolaryngol* 1985; 111:190–192.
13. Bain J. Late complication of tracheostomy and prolonged endotracheal intubation. *Int Anesth Clin* 1972; 10:255–264.
14. Clairmont AA. Tracheostoma construction during laryngectomy: techniques to prevent stenosis. *J Laryngol Otol* 1978; 92:75–78.
15. Grillo HC. Terminal or mural tracheostomy in the anterior mediastinum. *J Thorac Cardiovasc Surg* 1966; 51:422–427.
16. East CA, Flemming AF, Brough MD. Tracheostomal reconstruction using a fenestrated deltopectoral skin flap. *J Laryngol Otol* 1988; 102:282–283.
17. Trail ML, Chambers R, Leonard JR. Z-Plasty of tracheal stoma at laryngectomy. *Arch Otolaryngol* 1968; 88:84–86.
18. Catlin D. Making a large tracheal stoma during laryngectomy. *Ear Nose Throat J* 1966; 45:87–90.
19. Hartwell SW, Dykes ER. Construction and care of the end tracheostomy. *Am J Surg* 1967; 113:498–500.
20. Carleton JS. Revision of the tracheal stoma. *Laryngoscope* 1970; 80:260–266.
21. Myers EN, Gallia LJ. Tracheostomal stenosis following total laryngectomy. *Ann Otol Rhinol Laryngol* 1982; 91:450–453.
22. Murayama Y, Kubota J, Nakasima H. A 5 flap procedure for repair of stenosed tracheostoma. *Acta Chir Plast* (Prague) 1980; 22:107–110.
23. Callins WP, Applebaum EL. Correction of laryngectomy stomal stenosis. *Laryngoscope* 1980; 90:159–161.

24. Sisson GA, Straechley CJ Jr, Johnson NE. Mediastinal dissection for recurrent cancer after laryngectomy. *Laryngoscope* 1962; 72:1064–1077.
25. Orringer MB, Sloan H. Anterior mediastinal tracheostomy. *J Thorac Cardiovasc Surg* 1979; 78:850–859.
26. Batsakis JG, Hybels R, Rice DH. Laryngeal carcinoma: stomal recurrences and distant metastasis. *In* Alberti PE, Bryce DP (eds), *Workshops from the Centennial Conference on Laryngeal Cancer*, pp 868–876. New York, Appleton Century-Crofts, 1976.
27. Josephson JS, Krespi YP. Management of stomal recurrence. *In* Silver CE (ed), *Laryngeal Cancer*, pp 240–245. Thieme, New York, 1991.
28. Bonneau, RA, Lehman RH. Stomal recurrence following laryngectomy. *Arch Otolaryngol* 1975; 101:408–412.
29. Keim WF, Shapiro MJ, Rosen HO. Study of postlaryngectomy stomal recurrences. *Arch Otolaryngol* 1965; 81:183–186.
30. Stell PM, van den Broek P. Stomal recurrence after laryngectomy: aetiology and management. *J Laryngol Otol* 1971; 85:131–140.
31. Harris HH, Butler E. Surgical limits in cancer. *Arch Otolaryngol* 1968; 87:490–493.
32. Hoover WB, King BD. Emergency laryngectomy. *Arch Otolaryngol* 1954; 59:431–433.
33. Tong D, Moss WT, Stevens KR. Elective irradiation of the lower cervical region in patients at high risk for recurrent cancer at the tracheal stoma. *Radiology* 1977; 124:809–811.
34. Schneider JJ, Lindberg RD, Jesse RH. Prevention of tracheal stoma recurrences after total laryngectomy by postoperative irradiation. *J Surg Oncol* 1975; 7:187–190.
35. Sisson GA, Bytell DE, Becker SP. Mediastinal dissection 1976: indications and newer techniques. *Laryngoscope* 1977; 87:751–759.
36. Gunn WG. Treatment of cancer recurrent at the tracheostoma. *Cancer* 1965; 18:1261.
37. Balm AJ, Snow GB, Karim AB, et al. Long-term results of concurrent polychemotherapy and radiotherapy in patients with stomal recurrence after total laryngectomy. *Ann Otol Rhinol Laryngol* 1986; 95:572–575.
38. Sisson GA, Bytell DE, Edison BD, Yeh S. Transsternal radical neck dissection for control of stomal recurrences—end results. *Laryngoscope* 1975; 85:1504–1510.
39. Sisson GA, Strachley CJ, Johnson NE. Mediastinal dissection for recurrent cancer after laryngectomy. *Laryngoscope* 1962; 72:1064–1077.
40. Sisson GA, Edison BP, Bytell DE. Transsternal radical neck dissection: postoperative complications and management. *Arch Otolaryngol* 1975; 101:46–49.
41. Biller HF, Krespi YP, Lawson W, et al. A one-stage flap reconstruction following resection for stomal recurrence. *Otolaryngol Head Neck Surg* 1980; 88:357–360.
42. Gluckman L, Hamaker RC, Schuller DE, et al. Surgical salvage for stomal recurrence: a multi institutional experience. *Laryngoscope* 1987; 97:1025–1029.
43. Withers EH, Davis L, Lynch JB. Anterior mediastinal tracheostomy with a pectoralis major musculocutaneous flap. *Plast Reconst Surg* 1981; 67:381–383.

Chapter 14

Prosthetic Voice Rehabilitation

Gianfranco Recher and Alfio Ferlito*

---

*Deceased

Despite progress in therapeutic modalities, total laryngectomy remains one of the most effective treatments at certain stages of laryngeal disease, and subsequent voice restoration is still one of the major problems facing laryngeal surgeons and speech pathologists. A number of patients prove incapable of learning esophageal speech,[1] and the electrolarynx produces a monotonous, mechanical voice that is often unacceptable to patients. New prosthetic techniques have been developed, however, especially over the last few decades, to restore a link between the airway and the digestive tract, and acoustic measurements have demonstrated that a prosthetic voice is greatly superior to the esophageal voice, both in vocal quality and in success rate.[2, 3]

HISTORICAL BACKGROUND

The problem of voice restoration has existed ever since Billroth's first total laryngectomy in 1873, when his coworker Gussenbauer[4] used a special cannula consisting of tracheal and pharyngeal tubes to introduce expired air into the pharynx. The pharyngeal extremity was covered with a lid, or "pseudoglottis," that closed with swallowing and opened for speech, while a vibrating metal membrane, or "tongue," was placed in the airstream for sound production. Three weeks after surgery, the patient was able to speak with an intelligible but monotonous voice. He died a few months later from recurrent carcinoma.

In 1894, Gluck was the first to perform a primary closure of the pharyngeal defect after total laryngectomy.[5] This overcame the need for a pharyngostoma but prevented voice production with a prosthesis communicating between the trachea and the esophagus. Primary pharyngeal closure thus forced the introduction of esophageal speech in voice rehabilitation.

During the 1950s, a renewed interest developed in surgical techniques for restoring a connection between the airway and the digestive tract. In 1952, Briani[6] introduced a method for creating a pharyngocutaneous fistula connected to the tracheostoma by means of a variety of acrylic and polyethylene prostheses.

In 1958, Conley et al.[7] created a shunt using a reversed esophageal mucosal tube and later employed a free reversed vein graft for this purpose.[8]

In 1965, Asai[9] developed a three-stage skin tube construction forming a long vertical internal shunt. Other surgical procedures were developed[10–13] but were rarely used because of their high failure rates and postoperative complications. In 1973, Staffieri[13]

reported satisfactory functional results with a tracheal hypopharyngeal shunt called the "phonatory neoglottis," but the technique encountered serious problems with aspiration and fistula closure. Amatsu,[14] in 1978, suggested a new one-stage laryngectomy procedure involving speech preservation with an internal tracheoesophageal shunt. All of these techniques relied on the principle of shunting pulmonary air into the pharyngoesophageal tract, and all shared the risk of aspiration of food and liquids if the shunt diameter was too wide, and the risk of closure if the diameter was too narrow. Creation of the various shunts also requires fairly elaborate surgical techniques.

The field of prosthetic voice restoration after total laryngectomy was revolutionized in 1978 when Singer and Blom[15] described an uncomplicated endoscopic method for phonatory shunt construction. A simple silicone prosthesis was inserted into a small direct tracheoesophageal fistula and worked as a one-way valve. The device reduced inhalation problems and prevented fistula closure. Despite initial skepticism, the method has since been widely used.[16] The work of Singer and Blom stimulated a renewed interest in prosthetic voice rehabilitation, and other prostheses based on the same principle were introduced around the world.[15] Various other methods for secondary tracheoesophageal puncture for voice rehabilitation were also advocated.[3, 17–19]

Singer and Blom[15] initially reported the use of their endoscopic technique on patients who had undergone an earlier total laryngectomy. Panje,[20] Maves and Lingeman,[21] and Hamaker et al.[22] subsequently demonstrated that the prosthesis could be applied immediately, during the course of the total laryngectomy. Some debate followed as to whether the primary or the secondary application produced the best results,[23–30] but with consequent improvements in surgical procedure and in the prosthetic devices, the trend has increasingly been to prefer primary tracheoesophageal puncture during total laryngectomy because a second operation is avoided, and speech is rapidly restored.

PATIENT SELECTION

Patient selection criteria have varied somewhat according to whether rehabilitation is to be a primary or a secondary procedure. For primary voice restoration, the surgical procedure can be tailored to the needs of prosthetic rehabilitation, and the patient can be suitably prepared psychologically (the failure of prosthetic voice restoration is often attributable to psychologic factors[31]). The option of associating the laryngectomy with pharyngeal constrictor myotomy or neurectomy to overcome the risk of pharyngoesophageal hypertonicity can be considered, and adequate stoma construction will help prevent peritracheostomal surface inadequacy, thus facilitating the application of the prosthesis and the tracheostoma valve.

Patients who fail to achieve useful esophageal or electrolaryngeal speech, or who are dissatisfied with either, are candidates for secondary prosthetic voice rehabilitation. For secondary endoscopic voice restoration after laryngectomy, patients must have normal visual acuity, reasonable manual dexterity, and satisfactory lung capacity. A barium swallow is indicated before the puncture to evaluate the size and mobility of the pharyngoesophageal tract. The patient's motivation to learn a new verbal communication method deserves careful attention. Uncontrolled alcoholism is often a severe limitation to the use of a prosthesis. Patients being rehabilitated many years after total laryngectomy often have trouble using the prosthesis because they have already adapted to communicating by nonverbal methods.

The esophageal insufflation test described by Blom et al.[32] is an important procedure that precedes secondary prosthetic voice rehabilitation. The test enables the evaluation of muscular resistance in the pharyngoesophageal tract in relation to the patient's lung capacity. Hypertonicity of this segment may force pulmonary air from the prosthesis downward into the esophagus, rather than upward into the pharyngobuccal region, thus precluding voice production. If a voice cannot be produced by insufflated air introduced accurately into the pharyngoesophagus (a "negative" test result), then simultaneous performance of pharyngeal constrictor myotomy at the time of tracheoesophageal puncture may be indicated. If the test is positive, the patient can undergo tracheoesophageal puncture without additional procedures. If test results are equivocal, application of the prosthesis and rehabilitation may proceed without myotomy. If phonatory results prove inadequate, secondary pharyngeal constrictor myotomy may be suggested on the basis of the outcome of a percutaneous pharyngeal plexus nerve block. The esophageal air insufflation test is generally reliable, although false-positive and false-negative results are known to occur.

Radiotherapy may be implemented before or after installing the prosthesis,[5, 33, 34] although there is still a question as to whether this entails a higher risk of complications.[30, 35] Radical neck dissection and even extensive operations involving reconstruction of the hypopharynx and cervical esophagus with a deltopectoral skin flap, myocutaneous flaps, a cutaneous revascularized graft, or transposition of the viscera do not preclude this type of rehabilitation, and favorable results have been reported.[36–40]

VOICE PROSTHESES AND TRACHEOSTOMA VALVES

Singer and Blom[41] made various structural and material changes to their original prosthesis, while different models were also developed by others. Table 14–1 illustrates the different types of prostheses introduced since the end of the 1970s.[20, 41–50] The most commonly applied prostheses are produced by Inhealth and Bivona. The Gronigen, Herrman, and Provox prostheses are also widely used, particularly in Europe.

The original Blom-Singer prosthesis had a valve mechanism (called a "duckbill") in the distal section, which came into contact with the esophageal walls and caused an increase in resistance to air flow.[41] A low-pressure prosthesis was developed,

Table 14–1. TYPES OF VOICE PROSTHESIS

Voice Prosthesis	Reference	Manufacturer
Duckbill	Singer and Blom[41]	Bivona
Duckbill with retention collar	Singer and Blom[41]	Bivona
Duckbill	Singer and Blom[41]	Inhealth
Low-pressure	Singer and Blom[41]	Inhealth
Herrmann	Herrmann and Koss[42]	Eska
Panje button	Panje[20]	Xomed
Bonelli valve	Bonelli et al.[43]	
Groningen	Nijdam et al.[44]	Entermed
Periscope	Shapiro and Ramanathan[45]	Bivona
Henley-Cohn	Henley-Cohn et al.[46]	Dow Corning
Colorado		Bivona
Ultra-low resistance		Bivona
Pull-out	Staffieri and Staffieri[47]	
Algaba	Algaba et al.[48]	
Traissac	Traissac et al.[49]	Atos Medical
Provox	Hilgers and Schouwenburg[50]	Entermed

employing a flap rather than a duckbill-type valve, with shifting of the valve mechanism inside the prosthesis. This type of prosthesis is more complex and somewhat more difficult for the patient to insert than the original duckbill type, but it is more satisfactory for certain patients who have difficulty generating sufficient stomal pressure for good vocal function with the original prosthesis. Other improvements have been made, which include changing from two retention flanges to one, eliminating the air flow port in the proximal inferior section of the prosthesis, and using more-flexible silicone.

During the 1980s, two main types of prosthesis were developed: one type is not self-retaining and requires regular maintenance and periodical removal by the patient; the other type (developed mainly by Dutch researchers[44, 50, 51]) is self-retaining and requires limited maintenance and no actual removal. To produce a sound, the patient either manually occludes the tracheostoma or uses a "hands-free" valve, which consists of a housing fixed around the tracheostoma by means of an adhesive and a curved latex diaphragm that remains open during breathing and closes with increased expiratory flow, for speech.

The original model of the hands-free tracheostoma valve made by Bivona is fitted with a choice of four curved diaphragms (ultralight, light, medium, or firm) according to the patient's lung capacity and resistance to air flow in the pharyngoesophageal tract. A more complex Bivona tracheostoma valve is based on a single diaphragm, with a set of interchangeable springs to suit the needs of various patients. Inhealth produces a model similar to the first Bivona type but has also recently introduced a new self-regulating valve: this has a single diaphragm with an airflow resistance adjustable by the patient.

The problem with all these hands-free devices is one of making the housings adhere to the tracheostoma skin. This may be hindered by an irregular peritracheostomal surface, bronchial secretions, or continuous movements produced by the airflow. Progress has recently been made with new adhesive disks, often made of foam material.

An alternative is the tracheostoma valve used by Herrmann et al.,[42] which is inserted directly in the trachea and does not need to adhere to the skin. The distal tract of the trachea has to be specially reconstructed during total laryngectomy in order to accommodate the valve. Nevertheless, problems have been reported with the application and use of this type of valve, particularly in relation to coughing and sneezing.[52]

SURGICAL TECHNIQUES

Primary, or Immediate, Tracheoesophageal Puncture

The tracheoesophageal puncture (TEP) for voice prosthesis is demonstrated using a modification of the technique described by Hamaker et al.[22] In most cases we perform cricopharyngeal myotomy in patients in whom primary TEP is to be performed, because this maneuver is easily accomplished at the same time and presents no significant risk.

Figure 14–1*A*. A right-angle hemostat is placed through the pharyngotomy against the back wall of the trachea, where a horizontal incision about 4 mm long is made approximately 8 mm from the cut edge of the trachea.

Figures 14–1*B* and 14–1*C*. If necessary, the trachea and the esophagus are tacked together with fine sutures in order to create a broad "party wall." A No. 14 silicone catheter is passed through the incision from the trachea into the esophagus.

Figures 14–1*D* and 14–1*D₁*. The catheter is pushed from the pharyngeal gap into the midesophagus, and the distal end is passed into the stomach. This catheter is used to keep the fistula patent, and it also functions as a feeding tube until the patient is able to feed orally. The catheter is fixed to the skin with a suture and tape and is cut short when it is no longer needed for feeding. The catheter is kept in situ for approximately 3 weeks, when it is exchanged for a prosthesis. There is considerable variation in the time that various surgeons wait before exchanging the catheter for a prosthesis. On our service, the 3-week interval has been chosen in order to permit good epithelialization of the tracheoesophageal puncture and minimize the possibility of "false passage" formation during prosthesis insertion.

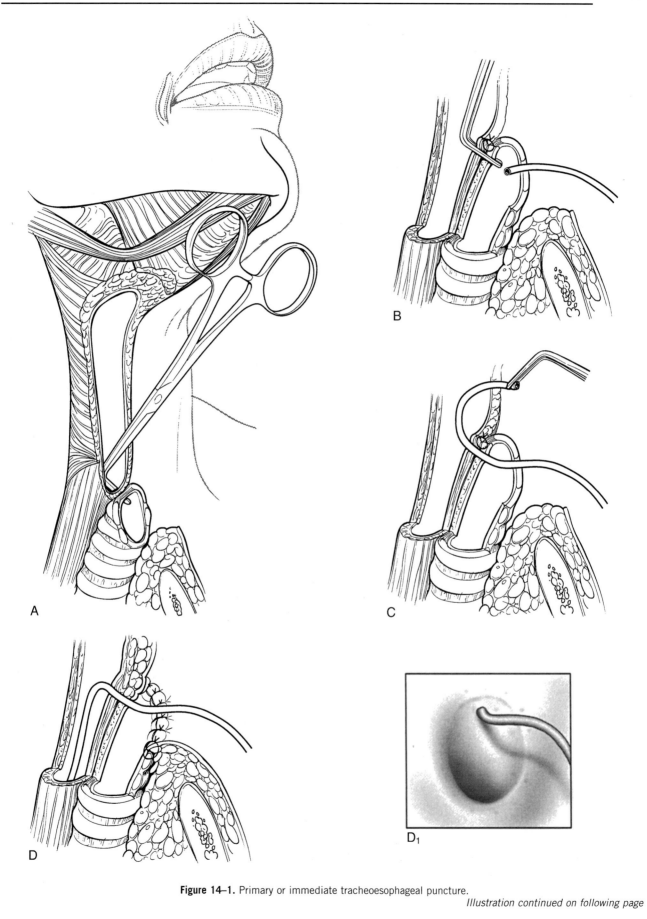

Figure 14–1. Primary or immediate tracheoesophageal puncture.

Illustration continued on following page

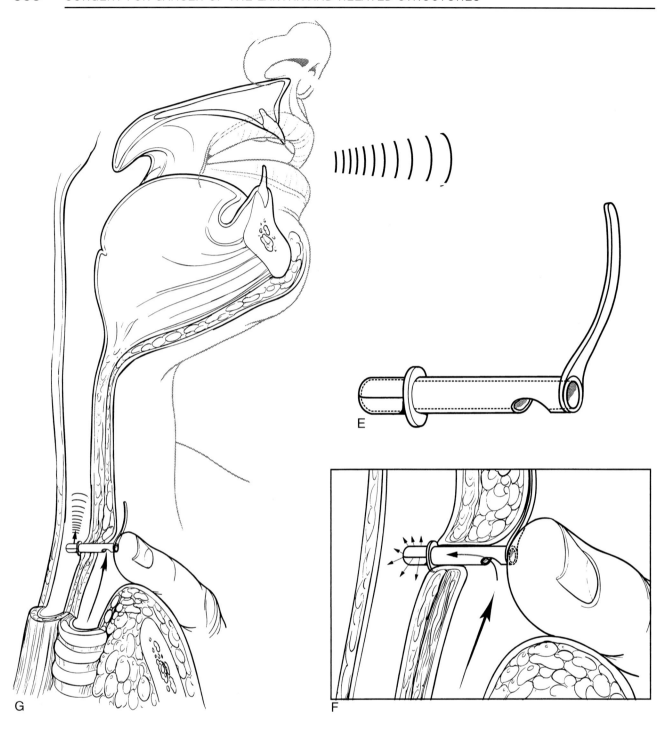

Figure 14–1 *Continued* Primary or immediate tracheoesophageal puncture.

Figures 14–1*E*, 14–1*F*, and 14–1*G*. The catheter is removed and a suitably sized prosthesis is inserted in the fistula. The prosthesis demonstrated here is the Blom-Singer duckbill type of prosthesis (Fig. 14–1*E*). The depth of the tract is measured, and a prosthesis of suitable length is inserted. When properly seated, the mucosal surface of the anterior esophageal wall is engaged by the flange on the prosthesis, preventing extrusion (Fig. 14–1*F*). The Blom-Singer prosthesis is further secured by taping the vertical tab to the skin above the tracheostoma (not shown). This tape must be changed daily, and the skin and peristomal area must be kept clean and free of crusts and other debris. The patient phonates by occluding the stoma with a finger, causing exhaled air to pass through the duckbill valve into the pharyngoesophageal segment (Figs. 14–1*F* and 14–1*G*).

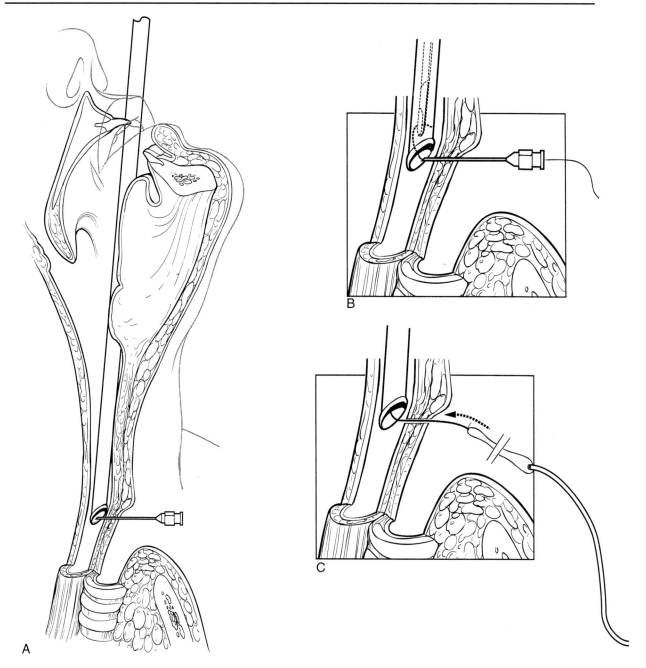

Figure 14–2. Secondary or delayed tracheoesophageal puncture.

Illustration continued on following page

Secondary, or Delayed, Tracheoesophageal Puncture

The procedure requires rigid esophagoscopy and thus often is best performed under general anesthesia with relaxation,[3, 15, 17, 19, 34] although some surgeons prefer local and topical anesthesia.[18, 53, 54] If general anesthesia is employed, ventilation is maintained with a small endotracheal tube.

Figure 14–2A. The patient lies supine with the chin on the median line and the neck fully extended. The first surgeon performs esophagoscopy with a rigid esophagoscope. On reaching the posterior wall of the tracheostoma, the esophagoscope is rotated 180 degrees. A second surgeon performs the tracheoesophageal puncture with a trocar on the rear wall of the trachea, 2 to 4 mm from the junction between the skin and the mucosa (or 0.5 to 1 cm for the Provox prosthesis), while the endoscopist checks the position.

Figures 14–2B and 14–2C. A nylon thread carrying a suitably modified No. 14 urethral catheter is inserted in the esophagus through the trocar.

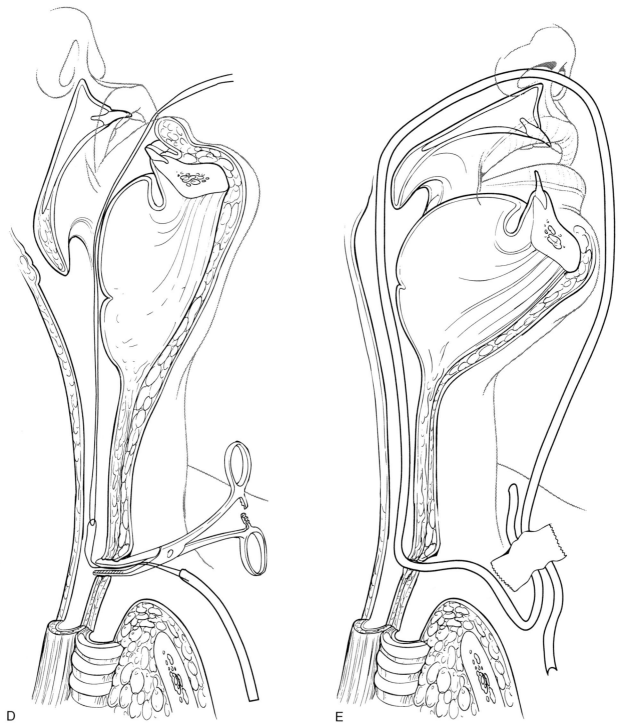

D   E

Figure 14–2 *Continued* Secondary or delayed tracheoesophageal puncture.

Figures 14–2D and 14–2E. The endoscopist pulls the catheter into the esophagus, removes the esophagoscope, and passes the catheter through the nose. The puncture site is dilated with a hemostat or another instrument, if necessary, to accommodate the passage of the catheter. If the anesthesia tube interferes with the creation of the tracheoesophageal puncture, it can be removed, leaving the patient in apnea for up to 1 minute. The nasotracheal catheter is secured in place as shown (Fig. 14–2E). Again, there is considerable variation among surgeons in the time interval before the catheter is exchanged for a prosthesis. This interval may vary from 48 hours to 3 weeks. The placement and function of the prosthesis is exactly the same as shown in Figs. 14–1E, 14–1F, and 14–1G.

Choice of Prosthesis and Patient Instruction

Prostheses that patients can replace themselves (for example, the Inhealth, the Bivona, and the Herrmann prostheses) are usually preferable, although considerable training in the application and maintenance of the prosthesis is required. Patients with poor manual dexterity or with insufficient family support may have difficulty in applying these devices on their own, which may lead to fistula closure if the prosthesis is not properly seated. In these patients, a self-retaining prosthesis, such as the Provox prosthesis, may be a better choice.

Once the prosthesis has been inserted, the patient is instructed by a speech therapist in maintenance of the prosthesis and correct pneumophonic mechanism. Whenever possible, a tracheostoma valve is preferable to manual occlusion, but this requires even further training of the patient in achieving consistent adherence of the retaining ring to the peritracheostomal skin. Much of the rehabilitative process is accomplished on an outpatient basis or in a convalescent facility.

Modifications of the Laryngectomy Technique for Tracheoesophageal Puncture

As the use of primary and secondary TEP has become widespread, certain modifications of the total laryngectomy procedure can facilitate the performance of the procedure and have been found to improve results both quantitatively and qualitatively. Yoshida et al.[55] consider certain steps crucial: incision of the skin, stoma construction, pharyngeal constrictor myotomy or pharyngeal plexus neurectomy, use of buttress sutures, and hypopharyngeal closure.

Pharyngeal Constrictor Myotomy

As discussed earlier, pharyngoesophageal muscle spasm can prevent sound production. Extramucosal myotomy of the pharyngeal constrictor muscle fibers and the tunica muscularis of the first section of the cervical esophagus, with the pharyngeal gap open, is used to prevent this risk.

A limited lateral myotomy on the posterolateral side, in line with the tracheostoma, reaching only 4 to 5 mm upward and involving only the fibers of the inferior pharyngeal constrictor muscle and the tunica muscularis of the first segment of the cervical esophagus, has the advantage of producing a vibratory segment capable of giving intensity and sonority to the nonlaryngeal voice without offering excessive resistance to the injection of air. Myotomy

during laryngectomy is easy to perform and adds no more than 10 minutes to the length of the procedure.[56]

Pharyngeal constrictor myotomy for secondary voice rehabilitation in patients who cannot develop a useful prosthetic voice because of excessive hypertonicity of the pharyngoesophageal tract has been described by Singer and Blom.[57] The air insufflation test for identification of such patients before TEP has been discussed earlier.

Clevens et al.[58] believe that the need for pharyngeal constrictor myotomy or pharyngeal plexus neurectomy may be obviated by employing a nonmuscle closure of the pharyngeal defect after laryngectomy.

Primary Neurectomy of the Pharyngeal Plexus

The pharyngeal plexus neurectomy described by Singer et al.[59] in 1986 is an effective treatment for muscular hypertonicity of the pharyngeal-esophageal segment, either as an alternative to posterior myotomy or as an adjuvant procedure.[55]

The pharyngeal plexus can be identified before or after removal of the larynx. The plexus fibers emanate from the vagus nerve on each side, at the level of the middle pharyngeal constrictors, often associated with the superior thyroid artery. Separation of the pharynx from the carotid artery at the prevertebral level renders the area accessible. The identity of the delicate fibers is confirmed with an electrostimulator, which produces fasciculation of the ipsilateral pharynx. The identified fibers are divided by electrocautery. This technique produces minimal delay in performing the total laryngectomy.

Tracheostoma Construction

The construction of an adequate tracheostoma, in terms of site and size, is crucial to facilitate prosthesis and tracheostoma valve application and maintenance. For easy prosthesis replacement and maintenance, it is essential to construct an adequately wide tracheostoma, well clear of the sternum. It is often advisable to incorporate the stoma in the laryngectomy incision.[60] The peritracheostomal surface must also be sufficiently smooth for firm adhesion of the tracheostoma valve. In cases where the tracheal stump can be easily brought to skin level without tension, this can be accomplished without difficulty. The posterolateral edges of the cartilage rings are simply pushed aside and sutured to the inferior skin flaps. The problem of a small trachea can be dealt with by one of the methods discussed in detail in Chapter 13. A simple, effective procedure has been described by Yoshida et al.[55] The upper two tracheal rings are incised laterally at the 3 o'clock and 9 o'clock positions. Triangular skin flaps created from the inferior skin flap are inserted in the lateral tracheal defects. This adaptation, proposed by Yoshida et al.,[55] enables the tracheostoma to be widened and is useful in preventing stenosis.

A short retrosternal tracheal stump can be anchored with two sutures of heavy, slowly absorbed material, such as polyglactin, to the anterior margin of the sternal ends of the sternocleidomastoid muscles before the cut tracheal edge is sutured to the inferior skin flap. This will bring the tracheostoma superficial to the sternocleidomastoid muscles and the thyroid lobes, rendering it more accessible for prosthesis insertion and creating a better surface for application of a valve housing.

OUTCOME OF PROSTHETIC VOICE RESTORATION METHODS

Results

The results obtained with TEP vary considerably but are nonetheless favorable in comparison with other surgical and nonsurgical voice restoration methods.[2] The variability in the results may stem from the patient selection criteria, the type of prosthesis used, and the length of follow-up. Bailey[61] feels that 1 year is a suitable interval for final evaluation of the results.

Table 14–2 summarizes the results reported in the literature by various authors.[2, 15, 24, 30, 50, 62–73] Extensive resection and reconstruction of the pharynx and cervical esophagus with subsequent skin or myocutaneous flap reconstruction or visceral transposition does not prevent this type of rehabilitation, although results are qualitatively inferior to those achieved with uncomplicated total laryngectomy. Favorable results have been reported by various authors.[37–39, 74, 75]

Complications

Voice rehabilitation by means of TEP is relatively simple and has a high success rate, but it is not without complications. The incidence of severe clinical complications has been significantly reduced by improvements in surgical technique for the tracheoesophageal puncture, in the prostheses themselves, and in the instruments used for their insertion or replacement.

The incidence of complications reported in the literature varies from 15% to 55% of the cases.[28, 33, 69, 76]

Study	Year	No. of Cases	Restoration of Voice	
			Immediate	*Long-Term*
Singer and Blom[15]	1980	60	90%	
Wetmore et al.[62]	1981	63	89%	71%
Annyas et al.[63]	1984	36	86%	
Hall et al.[64]	1985	30	57%	
Wetmore et al.[65]	1985	66		64%
Perry et al.[66]	1987	50	94%	73%
Stienberg et al.[67]	1987	20		65%
Lavertu et al.[68]	1989	117		85%
Maniglia et al.[69]	1989	33*	94%	85%
		62†	77%	69%
Singer et al.[24]	1989	128		80%
Hilgers and Schouwenburg[50]	1990	79	NR	80%
Recher et al.[70]	1991	70‡	86%	64%
		32§		91%
Camilleri and MacKenzie[71]	1992	30	83%	
Hilgers and Balm[72]	1993	132		92%
Kerr et al.[73]	1993	25*		54%
		29†		37%
Izdebski et al.[2]	1994	95		92%
Kao et al.[30]	1994	106*		93%
		30†		83%

Table 14–2. RESULTS REPORTED IN THE LITERATURE WITH PRIMARY OR SECONDARY TRACHEOESOPHAGEAL PUNCTURE

*Patients proving unable to learn esophageal speech.
†Patients selecting prosthesis as treatment of choice.
‡Primary (immediate) tracheoesophageal prosthesis application.
§Secondary (delayed) tracheoesophageal prosthesis application.

Such a wide range probably stems from the fact that some authors report only severe problems, while others take into account even basic handling difficulties.

Local Complications

The most frequent complications are of a local character. The formation of granulation tissue in the tracheoesophageal shunt[70, 76, 77] and biodegradation of the prosthesis by microflora, especially *Candida albicans*, settling on its surface are probably the most important complications.[78–80] Granulation tissue at the tracheal orifice can be removed under local anesthesia by electrocautery, and the prosthesis can be reapplied immediately (after reducing its length in some cases).

Most prostheses made from Silastic or polyurethane remain useful for about 6 months, but this interval varies from one individual to another. As the prosthesis ages and loses its resiliency, its valve function is lost, producing aspiration of saliva or food. Increasing rigidity of the material requires greater opening pressure for phonation. As these problems become sufficiently severe, the prosthesis must be replaced.

Other, relatively rare, complications have been reported, which include fistula closure after unwanted dislocation of the prosthesis from the shunt, persistence of a fistula after final removal of a prosthesis from the shunt,[50] fistula dilatation,[78] false tract formation,[76] fistula migration,[33, 70] allergy to the material used for the prosthesis,[33] acute inflammation in the tracheoesophageal shunt, and fistula wall necrosis.[70, 81]

Patients can undergo repuncture for fistula closure, false tract formation, and fistula migration. Fistula incontinence with salivary leakage around the prosthesis is treated by silver nitrate cauterization, by replacing the prosthesis with a more suitable model, or by injecting sclerosing substances in the fistula wall (this can be repeated several times). Necrosis of the fistula walls is generally observed in patients who have had prior radiotherapy. It sometimes requires a prolonged hospital stay, treatment with antibiotics and frequent medication to achieve spontaneous fistula closure, or shrinkage of the fistula and subsequent reapplication of the prosthesis. A persistent fistula after the definitive removal of a prosthesis, or uncontrolled dilatation, requires surgical treatment by direct suture, or by use of a local flap in severe instances. Allergy to the prosthetic material requires removal of the prosthesis; after recovery, a new prosthesis made of another material can be tried.

Regional Complications

The most frequent regional complications are hypertonicity or spasticity of the pharyngoesophageal tract and dysphagia. Odynophagia and cephalalgia have been reported.[48] More severe, although less common, complications are progression of chronic obstructive lung disease, pneumothorax,[82, 83] aspiration pneumonia,[33] peristomal or cervical cellulitis,[33, 76] subcutaneous emphysema,[70, 84] stomal stenosis,[33, 85, 86] esophageal stenosis,[33] esophageal perforation,[33] paraesophageal abscess,[69, 87] cervical spine fracture,[76] osteomyelitis of the vertebra,[87, 88] hematoma,[59] tracheostoma diverticula,[85] and mediastinitis.[76]

Treatment for hypertonicity or spasticity of the pharyngoesophageal segment by myotomy or pharyngeal plexus neurectomy has been discussed in an earlier section. Should the prosthesis evoke pain or pressure, the reason should be sought and the prosthesis should be replaced with another of a more convenient shape and size. To prevent any progression of chronic obstructive lung diseases, the low-pressure type of prosthesis is preferable.

Inflammatory complications caused by bacteria or fungi require temporary removal of the prosthesis and treatment of the patient with antibiotics or antimycotics. Soft-tissue cellulitis of the neck and tracheobronchial inflammation can occur in the immediate postoperative period and will respond to antibiotic and corticosteroid treatment. Subcutaneous emphysema may be overcome by suspending the use of the prosthesis for a few days. Tracheostoma stenosis can be treated using the Colorado prosthesis or a Blom-Singer prosthesis with a fenestrated tracheostoma vent.

Esophageal perforation is a rare, but severe, consequence of esophagoscopy that must be identified without delay. Treatment involves applying a nasoesophageal tube and administering massive doses of antibiotics. If the problem becomes complicated by mediastinitis, surgical drainage may be indicated.

Aspiration of certain types of prosthesis has occurred very rarely,[33] usually while coughing or changing the prosthesis. The prosthesis can be retrieved by flexible fiberoptic bronchoscopy under local anesthesia.

The onset of complications does not necessarily mean abandoning the prosthesis, and sufficiently motivated patients prove able to overcome most of these problems, which are usually relatively mild. It is important to stress that the outcome depends on a multidisciplinary team effort, involving the surgeon, the speech therapist, and the oncologic nurse, but the motivation of the patient remains the key element for success.

REFERENCES

1. Singer MI. Voice rehabilitation after total laryngectomy. *In* Ferlito A (ed): *Neoplasms of the Larynx*, pp 541–544. Edinburgh, Churchill Livingstone, 1993.
2. Izdebeski K, Reed CG, Ross JC, et al. Problems with tracheo-esophageal fistula voice restoration in totally laryngectomized patients: a review of 95 cases. *Arch Otolaryngol Head Neck Surg* 1994; 120:840–845.
3. Brown DH, Rhys Evans PH. A simplified method of tracheo-esophageal puncture for speech restoration. *Laryngoscope* 1992; 102:579–580.
4. Gussenbauer C. Über die erste durch Th. Billroth am Menschen ausgeführte Kehlkopf-Extirpation und die Anwendung eines künstlichen Kehlkopfes. *Arch Klin Chir* 1874; 17:343–356.
5. Singer MI. Tracheoesophageal speech: vocal rehabilitation after total laryngectomy. *Laryngoscope* 1983; 93:1454–1465.
6. Briani A. Riabilitazione fonetica di laringectomizzati a mezzo della corrente aerea espiratoria. *Arch Ital Otol Rinol Laringol* 1952; 63:469–475.
7. Conley JJ, DeAmesti F, Pierce MK. A new surgical technique for the vocal rehabilitation of the laryngectomized patient. *Ann Otol Rhinol Laryngol* 1958; 67:655–664.
8. Conley JJ. Vocal rehabilitation by autogenous vein graft. *Ann Otol Rhinol Laryngol* 1959; 68:990–995.
9. Asai R. Laryngoplasty after total laryngectomy. *Arch Otolaryngol* 1965; 95:114–119.
10. Arslan M. Reconstructive laryngectomy: report on the first 35 cases. *Ann Otol Rhinol Laryngol* 1972; 81:479–487.
11. Arslan M, Serafini I. Restoration of laryngeal functions after total laryngectomy: report on the first 25 cases. *Laryngoscope* 1972; 82:1349–1360.
12. Iwai H, Koike Y. Primary laryngoplasty. *Laryngoscope* 1975; 85:929–934.
13. Staffieri M. Laringectomia totale con ricostruzione di "glottide fonatoria". *Nuovo Arch Ital Otol Rinol Laringol* 1973; 1:181–198.
14. Amatsu M. A new one-stage surgical technique for postlaryngectomy speech. *Arch Otorhinolaryngol* 1978; 220:149–152.
15. Singer MI, Blom ED. An endoscopic technique for restoration of voice after laryngectomy. *Ann Otol Rhinol Laryngol* 1980; 89:529–533.
16. Lopez MJ, Kraybill W, McElroy TH, et al. Voice rehabilitation practices among head and neck surgeons. *Ann Otol Rhinol Laryngol* 1987; 96:261–263.
17. Deeb ZE, Arenstein MH, Lerner DN. A new simple technique for tracheoesophageal puncture. *Laryngoscope* 1992; 102:837–838.
18. Gross M, Hess M. A new method for tracheoesophageal puncture under topical anesthesia. *Laryngoscope* 1994; 104:233–234.
19. Heatley DG, Anderson AG. Tracheoesophageal puncture for speech rehabilitation after laryngectomy. *Laryngoscope* 1992; 102:581–582.
20. Panje WR. Prosthetic vocal rehabilitation following laryngectomy: the voice button. *Ann Otol Rhinol Laryngol* 1981; 90:116–120.
21. Maves MD, Lingemann RE. Primary vocal rehabilitation using the Blom-Singer and Panje voice prostheses. *Ann Otol Rhinol Laryngol* 1982; 91:458–460.
22. Hamaker RC, Singer MI, Blom ED, et al. Primary voice restoration at laryngectomy. *Arch Otolaryngol* 1985; 111:182–186.
23. Cantrell RW. The case against immediate neoglottic reconstruction. *Head Neck Surg* 1988; 10:135–138.
24. Singer MI, Hamaker RC, Blom ED, et al. Applications of the voice prosthesis during laryngectomy. *Ann Otol Rhinol Laryngol* 1989; 98:921–925.
25. Trudeau MD, Schuller DE, Hall DA. Timing of tracheoesophageal puncture for voice restoration: primary vs secondary. *Head Neck Surg* 1988; 10:130–140.
26. Trudeau MD, Hirsch SM, Schuller DE. Vocal restorative surgery: why wait? *Laryngoscope* 1986; 96:975–977.
27. van Weissenbruch R, Albers FWJ. Voice rehabilitation after total laryngectomy. *Acta Otorhinolaryngol Belg* 1992; 46:221–246.
28. Ward PH, Andrews JC, Mickel RA, et al. Complications of medical and surgical approaches to voice restoration after total laryngectomy. *Head Neck Surg* 1988; 10:124–128.
29. Wenig BL, Mullooly V, Levy J, et al. Voice restoration following laryngectomy: the role of primary versus secondary tracheoesophageal puncture. *Ann Rhinol Laryngol* 1989; 98:70–73.
30. Kao WW, Mohr RM, Kimmel CA, et al. The outcome and techniques of primary and secondary tracheoesophageal puncture. *Arch Otolaryngol Head Neck Surg* 1994; 120:301–307.
31. Cheesman AD, Knight J, McIvor P, et al. Tracheo-oesophageal "puncture speech": an assessment technique for failed oesophageal speakers. *J Laryngol Otol* 1986; 100:191–199.
32. Blom ED, Singer MI, Hamaker RC. An improved esophageal insufflation test. *Arch Otolaryngol* 1985; 111:211–212.
33. Andrews JC, Mickel RA, Hanson DG, et al. Major complications following tracheoesophageal puncture for voice rehabilitation. *Laryngoscope* 1987; 97:562–567.
34. Recher G. Riabilitazione fonatoria dopo laringectomia totale con protesi tracheo-esofagee. *In* Veronese U, Molinari R, Bonfi A, Santoro A (eds): *I Tumori della Testa e del Collo*, pp 243–249. Milano, Casa Editrice Ambrosiana, 1990.
35. Silverman AH, Black MJ. Efficacy of primary tracheoesophageal puncture in laryngectomy rehabilitation. *J Otolaryngol* 1994; 23:370–377.
36. Cumberworth VL, O'Flynn P, Perry A, et al. Surgical voice restoration after laryngopharyngectomy with free radial forearm flap repair using a Blom-Singer prosthesis. *J R Soc Med* 1992; 85:760–761.
37. Izdebeski K, Ross JC, Hetzler D, et al. Speech restoration post-pharyngolaryngoesophagectomy using tracheogastric fistula. *J Rehabil Res Dev* 1988; 25:33–40.
38. Juarbe C, Shemen L, Wang R, et al. Tracheoesophageal puncture for voice restoration after extended laryngopharyngectomy. *Arch Otolaryngol Head Neck Surg* 1989; 115:356–359.
39. Medina JE, Nance A, Burns L, et al. Voice restoration after total laryngopharyngectomy and cervical esophagectomy using duckbill prosthesis. *Am J Surg* 1987; 154:407–410.
40. Wilson PS, Bruce-Lockhart FJ, Johnson AP, et al. Speech restoration following total laryngo-pharyngectomy with free jejunal repair. *Clin Otolaryngol* 1994; 19:145–148.
41. Singer MI, Blom ED. Vocal rehabilitation after laryngectomy. *Otolaryngol Clin N Am* 1985; 18:605–611.
42. Herrmann IF, Koss W. Experience with the ESKA-Herrmann tracheostoma valve. *In* Herrmann IF (ed): *Speech Restoration via Voice Prosthesis*, pp 184–186. Berlin, Springer Verlag, 1986.
43. Bonelli L, Aluffi E, Aversa AS, et al. Shunt phonatoire avec deglutition normal. *Riv ORL Aud Fon* 1982; 1:96–100.
44. Nijdam HF, Annyas AA, Schutte HK, et al. A new prosthesis for voice rehabilitation after laryngectomy. *Arch Otorhinolaryngol* 1982; 237:27–33.
45. Shapiro MJ, Ramanathan VR. Trachea stoma vent voice prosthesis. *Laryngoscope* 1982; 92:1126–1129.
46. Henley-Cohn JL, Hausfeld JN, Jakubczak G. Artificial larynx prosthesis: comparative clinical evaluation. *Laryngoscope* 1984; 94:43–45.
47. Staffieri M, Staffieri A. La "pull-out prosthesis": un nuovo voice button per la riabilitazione della voce dopo laringectomia totale. *Acta Otorhinolaryngol Ital* 1986; 6:19–26.
48. Algaba J. Recuperation de la voix pour les patients laryngectomises. *Revue Laryngol Otol Rhinol* 1987; 108:139–142.
49. Traissac L, Devars F, Gioux M, et al. La rèhabilitation vocale du laryngectomisé total par implant phonatoire: résultats actuels. *Rev Laryngol Otol Rhinol* 1987; 108:157–159.
50. Hilgers FJM, Schouwenburg. A new low-resistance, self-retaining prosthesis (Provox/tm) for voice rehabilitation after total laryngectomy. *Laryngoscope* 1990; 100:1202–1207.

51. Manni JJ, van de Broek P, de Groot MAH, et al. Voice rehabilitation after laryngectomy with the Groningen prosthesis. *J Otolaryngol* 1984; 13:333–336.
52. Mahieu HF. Voice and speech rehabilitation following laryngectomy. Doctoral thesis. Groningen, The Netherlands, Groningen University, 1988.
53. Motta G, Galli V, Tedesco S, et al. La riabilitazione vocale dei laringectomizzati mediante protesi tracheoesofagee. Tecnica chirurgica originale in anestesia locale. *Acta Otorhinolaryngol Ital* 1986; 6:27–38.
54. Spofford B, Jafek B, Barcz D. An improved method for creating tracheoesophageal fistulas for Blom-Singer or Panje voice prostheses. *Laryngoscope* 1984; 94:257–258.
55. Yoshida GY, Hamaker RC, Singer MI, et al. Primary voice restoration at laryngectomy: 1989 update. *Laryngoscope* 1989; 99:1093–1095.
56. Mahieu HF, Annyas AA, Schutte HK, et al. Pharyngoesophageal myotomy for vocal rehabilitation of laryngectomies. *Laryngoscope* 1987; 97:451–457.
57. Singer MI, Blom ED. Selective myotomy for voice restoration after total laryngectomy. *Arch Otolaryngol* 1981; 107:670–673.
58. Clevens RA, Esclamado RM, Hartshorn DO, et al. Voice rehabilitation after total laryngectomy and tracheoesophageal puncture using nonmuscle closure. *Ann Otol Rhinol Laryngol* 1993; 102:793–796.
59. Singer MI, Blom ED, Hamaker RC. Pharyngeal plexus neurectomy for a laryngeal speech rehabilitation. *Laryngoscope* 1986; 96:50–54.
60. Nigam A, Campbell JB, Dasgupta AR. Does the location of the laryngectomy stoma influence its ultimate size. *Clin Otolaryngol* 1993; 18:193–195.
61. Bailey BJ. Editorial footnote. *Arch Otolaryngol Head Neck Surg* 1988; 114:1421.
62. Wetmore SJ, Johns ME, Baker SR. The Singer-Blom voice restoration procedure. *Arch Otolaryngol* 1981; 107:674–676.
63. Annyas AA, Nijdam HF, Escajadillo JR, et al. Groningen prosthesis for voice rehabilitation after laryngectomy. *Clin Otolaryngol* 1984; 9:51–54.
64. Hall JG, Dahl T, Arnesen AR. Speech prostheses: failures, problems and successes. *In* Myers EN (ed): *New Dimensions in Otorhinolaryngology - Head and Neck Surgery*, Vol 1, pp 418–421. Proceeding of the 13th World Congress, Miami Beach, FL, 26–31 May 1985. Amsterdam, Excerpta Medica, 1985.
65. Wetmore SJ, Krueger K, Wesson K, et al. Long-term results of the Blom-Singer speech rehabilitation procedure. *Arch Otolaryngol* 1985; 111:106–109.
66. Perry A, Cheesman AD, McIvor J, et al. A British experience of surgical voice restoration techniques as a secondary procedure following total laryngectomy. *J Laryngol Otol* 1987; 101:155–163.
67. Stiernberg CM, Bailey BJ, Calhoun KH, et al. Primary tracheoesophageal fistula procedure for voice restoration: the University of Texas Medical Branch experience. *Laryngoscope* 1987; 97:820–824.
68. Lavertu P, Scott SE, Finnegan EM, et al. Secondary tracheoesophageal puncture for voice rehabilitation after laryngectomy. *Arch Otolaryngol Head Neck Surg* 1989; 115:350–355.
69. Maniglia AJ, Lundy DS, Casiano RC, et al. Speech restoration and complications of primary versus secondary tracheoesophageal puncture following total laryngectomy. *Laryngoscope* 1989; 99:489–491.
70. Recher G, Pesavento G, Cristoferi V, et al. Italian experience of voice restoration after laryngectomy with tracheoesophageal puncture. *Ann Otol Rhinol Laryngol* 1991; 100:206–210.
71. Camilleri AE, MacKenzie K. The acceptability of secondary tracheo-oesophageal fistula creation in long standing laryngectomees. *J Laryngol Otol* 1992; 106:231–233.
72. Hilgers FJM, Balm AJM. Long-term results of vocal rehabilitation after total laryngectomy with the low-resistance, indwelling Provox voice prosthesis system. *Clin Otolaryngol* 1993; 18:517–523.
73. Kerr AIG, Denholm S, Sanderson RJ, et al. Blom-Singer prosthesis: an 11 year experience of primary and secondary procedures. *Clin Otolaryngol* 1993; 18:184–187.
74. Bleach N, Perry A, Cheesman A. Surgical voice restoration with the Blom-Singer prosthesis following laryngopharyngoesophagectomy and pharyngogastric anastomosis. *Ann Otol Rhinol Laryngol* 1991; 100:142–147.
75. Cristoferi V, Pighi GP, Narne S, et al. Voice restoration with tracheo-gastric puncture after hypopharyngolaryngoesophagectomy. *In* Motta G (ed): *The New Frontiers of Oto-Rhino-Laryngology in Europe*, Vol 4, pp 113–116. Second European Congress of Otorhinolaryngology Cervico-Facial Surgery, Monduzzi, Bologna, 1992.
76. Silver FM, Gluckman JL, Donegan JO. Operative complications of tracheosophageal puncture. *Laryngoscope* 1985; 95:1360–1362.
77. Lobe L. Problems and failures of a long-term application of Wurzburg type voice prostheses. *Rev Laryngol Otol Rhinol* (Bord) 1987; 108:123–124.
78. Mahieu HF, van Saene HKF, Jeroen Rosingh H, et al. *Candida* vegetations on silicone voice prostheses. *Arch Otolaryngol Head Neck Surg* 1986; 112:321–325.
79. Palmer MD, Johnson AP, Elliott TSJ. Microbial colonization of Blom-Singer prostheses in postlaryngectomy patients. *Laryngoscope* 1993; 103:910–914.
80. Šebová I, Lobe LP, Sandow D, et al. Biodegradation and biocompatibility of voice prostheses and laryngectomees. *In* Motta G (ed): *The New Frontiers of Oto-Rhino-Laryngology in Europe*, vol 4, pp 103–107. Second European Congress of Otorhinolaryngology and Cervico-Facial Surgery, Monduzzi, Bologna, 1992.
81. McConnel FMS, Duck SW. Indications for tracheoesophageal puncture speech rehabilitation. *Laryngoscope* 1986; 96:1065–1068.
82. Lacau St Guily J, Baril P, Cadranel J, et al. Une nouvelle cause de pneumothorax: les fistules phonatoires aprés laryngectomie total. *Presse Med* 1990; 19:1505–1506.
83. Odland R, Adams G. Pneumothorax as a complication of tracheoesophageal voice prosthesis use. *Ann Otol Rhinol Laryngol* 1988; 97:537–541.
84. Singer MI, Blom ED, Hamaker RC. Further experience with voice restoration after total laryngectomy. *Ann Otol Rhinol Laryngol* 1981; 90:498–502.
85. Ho CM, Wei WI, Lau WF, et al. Tracheostomal stenosis after immediate tracheoesophageal puncture. *Arch Otolaryngol Head Neck Surg* 1991; 117:662–665.
86. Wang RC, Bui T, Sauris E, et al. Long-term problems in patients with tracheoesophageal puncture. *Arch Otolaryngol Head Neck Surg* 1991; 117:1273–1276.
87. Ruth H, Davis WE, Renner G. Deep neck abscess after tracheoesophageal puncture and insertion of a voice button prosthesis. *Otolaryngol Head Neck Surg* 1985; 93:809–811.
88. Cullen JR, Primrose WJ, Vaughn CW. Osteomyelitis as a complication of a tracheo-oesophageal puncture. *J Laryngol Otol* 1993; 107:242–244.

Index

Note: Page numbers in *italics* refer to illustrations; page numbers followed by t refer to tables.

377

ISBN 0-7216-5266-2

90038

9 780721 652665